Advances in Wearables and Nearables for Healthcare Applications

Wearable and nearable technologies are revolutionizing modern healthcare by enabling continuous, noninvasive, and real-time monitoring of physiological, behavioral, and environmental factors. Advancements in sensing technologies, embedded electronics, signal processing, and artificial intelligence (AI) have greatly enhanced the capabilities of wearables and nearables, making them integral to preventive healthcare, personalized medicine, remote patient monitoring, and digital therapeutics. From smartwatches and rings to ambient, nearable sensors installed in homes and healthcare settings, these technologies are revolutionizing how health data is collected, processed, and interpreted.

This edited book covers original research, implementations, and comprehensive reviews to discuss recent achievements and emerging trends in wearable and nearable technology for health-related applications. The book covers aspects of signal acquisition, preprocessing, feature extraction, machine learning (ML), and deep learning (DL) methodologies specific to data from wearable and nearable technologies. It also covers practical issues related to data reliability, clinical validation, regulatory issues, and ethical issues, as well as cloud computing, Internet of Things (IoT), and Internet of Medical Things (IoMT) infrastructures.

Features:

- Explores advanced sensing and signal processing techniques for wearable and nearable health technologies.
- Discusses real-time monitoring, cloud-based analytics, and IoT/IoMT integration.
- Addresses clinical validation, regulatory, and ethical challenges of wearable and nearable systems.
- Presents case studies and applications in smart health monitoring, sleep analysis, cardiac, and respiratory assessment.
- Provides a comprehensive reference for graduate students, researchers, and professionals in biomedical and health informatics.

This book bridges the gap between theoretical foundations and practical applications in healthcare and may prove a useful resource for researchers, practitioners, and professionals working in biomedical engineering, signal processing, and intelligent health systems.

Advances in Wearables and Nearables for Healthcare Applications

Edited by
Ganesh R. Naik

CRC Press
Taylor & Francis Group
Boca Raton London New York

CRC Press is an imprint of the
Taylor & Francis Group, an **informa** business

Designed cover image: Shutterstock

First edition published 2027
by CRC Press
2385 NW Executive Center Drive, Suite 320, Boca Raton FL 33431

and by CRC Press
4 Park Square, Milton Park, Abingdon, Oxon, OX14 4RN

CRC Press is an imprint of Taylor & Francis Group, LLC

ISBN: 9781032796543 (hbk)
ISBN: 9781032815756 (pbk)
ISBN: 9781003500445 (ebk)

DOI: 10.1201/9781003500445

Typeset in Times
by Newgen Publishing UK

Contents

Preface

The rapid evolution of wearable and nearable technologies has transformed the landscape of modern healthcare, enabling continuous, noninvasive, and personalized monitoring of physiological and behavioral parameters. Advances in sensor miniaturization, low-power electronics, wireless communication, and intelligent data analytics have collectively driven the adoption of these technologies across clinical, home-based, and mobile health environments. Wearables and nearables now play a pivotal role in preventive healthcare, early disease detection, rehabilitation, and long-term health management, bridging the gap between patients, clinicians, and digital health ecosystems.

This edited book, *Advances in Wearables and Nearables for Healthcare Applications,* presents a comprehensive overview of contemporary research, methodologies, and real-world implementations in this rapidly expanding domain. The book brings together contributions from researchers and practitioners across engineering, computer science, medicine, and health sciences, highlighting how wearable and nearable systems are reshaping healthcare delivery through continuous sensing, intelligent interpretation, and cloud-enabled decision support.

The chapters in this book are organized to reflect both foundational principles and emerging applications. Early chapters focus on the design and development of wearable sensing systems, addressing physiological signal acquisition, multimodal data fusion, and challenges related to noise, motion artifacts, and real-world variability. Subsequent chapters explore advanced analytical frameworks, including machine learning (ML), deep learning (DL), and explainable artificial intelligence (AI), demonstrating their effectiveness in extracting clinically relevant insights from complex wearable data. Several contributions are dedicated to critical healthcare applications, including sleep apnea detection, stress and mental health assessment, neurological disorder monitoring, maternal and child health, and infectious disease severity assessment. Collectively, these chapters illustrate the growing maturity of wearable and nearable technologies from experimental prototypes to deployable healthcare solutions.

A distinguishing feature of this volume is its emphasis on robustness, interpretability, and translational impact. Beyond algorithmic performance, the chapters address practical considerations, including system reliability, user comfort, data privacy, cloud integration, and human-in-the-loop frameworks. By presenting interdisciplinary perspectives and case studies, the book underscores the importance of designing wearable healthcare systems that are not only technologically advanced but also clinically meaningful and user centric.

This book is intended for a broad audience, including researchers, academicians, graduate students, clinicians, and industry professionals working in biomedical engineering, healthcare technology, data science, and digital health. It is my hope that this volume will serve as a valuable reference for understanding current advancements, inspire future research directions, and foster innovation in the development of next-generation wearable and nearable healthcare systems.

I would like to express my sincere gratitude to all contributing authors for their high-quality scholarly contributions and collaborative spirit. I also acknowledge the support of reviewers and publishers whose efforts have helped shape this volume. Their collective dedication has made this book a meaningful contribution to the growing field of wearable healthcare technologies.

Ganesh R. Naik
January 2026

About the Editor

Ganesh R. Naik Dr. Ganesh R. Naik is a globally recognized biomedical engineer and signal processing expert, ranked in the top 2% of researchers by Stanford University. He holds a PhD from RMIT University and is currently an Associate Professor in Computer Science and IT at Torrens University Australia. A prolific researcher, he has edited 18 books and authored over 175 papers. Dr. Naik is an associate editor for several prestigious journals, including the Institute of Electrical and Electronics Engineers (IEEE) ACCESS. His career includes significant research roles at Flinders University, Western Sydney University, and the University of Technology Sydney, where he contributed to advancements in sleep health and wearable technologies. He has received numerous fellowships, including from the Royal Academy of Engineering UK, the Government of Australia, and Germany's Baden–Württemberg Scholarship.

Contributors

Brindha A.
SRM Institute of Science and Technology
Kattankulathur, Tamil Nadu
India

Vitor Emmanuel Andrade
Faculdade Área 1
Salvador, Bahia
Brazil

Sridhar P. Arjunan
RMIT University,
Melbourne, Victoria
Australia

Aditya Asopa
Anthriq Pvt Ltd.
Koramangala, Bengaluru
India

Maria Inês Barbosa
Universidade Católica Portuguesa
Escola Superior de Biotecnologia, Porto
Portugal

Francisco Sulivan Bastos Mota
Instituto da Primeira Infância – IPREDE
Fortaleza
Brasil

Patrícia Batista
Universidade Católica Portuguesa
Escola Superior de Biotecnologia, Porto
Portugal

Francisco Nauber Bernardo Gois
Controladoria e Ouvidoria Geral do Estado do Ceará
Fortaleza, Cear
Brazil

Soumya Bhattacharjee
Anthriq Pvt Ltd.
Koramangala, Bengaluru
India

Bruno Catarino Bispo
Federal University of Santa Catarina
Florianópolis, Santa Catarina
Bazil

Victor Hugo C. de Albuquerque
Universidade Federal do Ceará
Presidente Kennedy, Fortaleza – CE
Brazil

Adriel de Oliveira
Universidade Federal do Ceará
Presidente Kennedy, Fortaleza – CE
Brazil

N. Deepa
Centre for Health Innovations
Manav Rachna International Institute of Research and Studies
Faridabad, Haryana
India

Sara Mohan George
M.S. Ramaiah Institute of Technology
Department of Electronics & Communication Engineering
M S R Nagar, Mathikere, Bengaluru
Karnataka
India

R. Girija
Centre for Health Innovations,
Department of Computer Science and Engineering
School of Engineering and Technology

Manav Rachna International Institute of Research and Studies
Faridabad
India

Camila Guerra
Instituto da Primeira Infância – IPREDE
Fortaleza
Brasil

S. L. Jayalakshmi
Pondicherry University
Department of Computer Science, School of Engineering and Technology
Chinna Kalapet, Puducherry
India

S. L. Jothi Lakshmi
Amrita Vishwa Vidyapeetham
Amrita School of Computing
Department of Artificial Intelligence and Data Science
Nagercoil, Tamil Nadu
India

Fayaz Pathan Khan
Neurostellar Pvt Ltd.
IIT Madras Campus
Chennai
India

Arpita Kulkarni
BNM Institute of Technology
Banashankari, Bengaluru
Karnataka
India

Camila Ferreira Leite
Universidade Federal do Ceará
Presidente Kennedy, Fortaleza – CE
Brazil

Vrinda M.
Neurostellar Pvt Ltd.
IIT Madras Campus
Chennai
India

João Paulo Madeiro
Universidade Federal do Ceará
Presidente Kennedy, Fortaleza – CE
Brazil

Roney Malaguti
Stratio Automotive
Coimbra, Portugal
Brazil

João Alexandre Lobo Marques
University of Saint Joseph
Laboratory of Applied Neurosciences
Macau Special Administrative Region (SAR)
China

Jyoti R. Munavalli
BNM Institute of Technology
Banashankari, Bengaluru
Karnataka
India

Ganesh R. Naik
Torrens University
School of Technology, Business Vertical
Adelaide
Australia

Paulo Cezar Nascimento Filho
Lê Sante Clinic
Fortaleza
Brazil

Arnaldo Aires Peixoto Jr.
Universidade Federal do Ceará
Presidente Kennedy, Fortaleza – CE
Brazil

Daniel Pordeus
Petrobras: Brazilian Energy
Brazil

Karthik Raghavendran
Neurostellar Pvt Ltd.
IIT Madras Campus
Chennai
India

Pedro Ribeiro
Faculty of Biotechnology Universidade Católica Portuguesa
Porto
Portugal

Pedro Miguel Rodrigues
Universidade Católica Portuguesa
Faculty of Biotechnology
Porto
Portugal

Arun Sasidharan
National Institute of Mental Health and Neuro Sciences (NIMHANS)
Centre for Consciousness Studies
Neurophysiology
Bengaluru
India

Shruthi S. Sharma
Siddaganga Medical College and Research Institute
Tumkur
India

Manoel Alves Sobreira-Neto
Universidade Federal do Ceará
Presidente Kennedy, Fortaleza – CE
Brazil

Piyush Swami
SAMOVAR, Télécom SudParis
Institut Polytechnique de Paris
Palaiseau
France

Karthik Venkataraman
Neurostellar Pvt Ltd.
IIT Madras Campus
Chennai
India

Varsha Vijayan
Neurostellar Pvt Ltd.
IIT Madras Campus
Chennai, India

Laíla Zacarias
Universidade Federal do Ceará
Presidente Kennedy, Fortaleza – CE
Brazil

1 Sleep Apnea Detection Using Wearable Sensors

Principles, Methods and Challenges

Sara Mohan George

1.1 INTRODUCTION

Sleep apnea is a common sleep disorder characterized by recurrent episodes of partial or complete breathing cessation during sleep. These respiratory interruptions, termed apnea and hypopnea, occur when the airway becomes blocked or when the brain fails to signal the respiratory muscles properly. An apnea is defined as a complete pause in breathing lasting at least ten seconds, while a hypopnea represents a significant reduction in airflow accompanied by oxygen desaturation or arousal from sleep (John et al. 2021) (Franklin and Lindberg 2015). The severity of sleep apnea is quantified using the apnea-hypopnea index (AHI), which measures the average number of apneas and hypopneas per hour of sleep.

Three primary forms of sleep apnea are clinically recognized. Obstructive sleep apnea (OSA), the most common type, occurs when the throat muscles relax during sleep, causing the upper airway to collapse and block airflow despite continued respiratory effort. Central sleep apnea (CSA) results from the brain's failure to transmit proper signals to the respiratory muscles, leading to temporary cessation of breathing effort. Mixed sleep apnea combines features of both obstructive and central forms, typically beginning with central apnea followed by obstructive components. The clinical consequences of untreated sleep apnea extend well beyond disrupted sleep. The repeated cycles of oxygen desaturation and arousal trigger a cascade of physiological disturbances that affect multiple organ systems. Sleep apnea has been strongly associated with cardiovascular complications, including hypertension, stroke, coronary artery disease, and heart failure. The condition also contributes to excessive daytime sleepiness, cognitive impairment, metabolic dysfunction, and increased risk of traffic accidents. These serious health implications highlight the importance of timely detection and treatment. Current epidemiological data reveal a concerning picture, that sleep apnea affects a substantial proportion of adults worldwide, with prevalence rates higher in men than women and showing an upward trend in recent studies. More alarmingly, many affected individuals remain undiagnosed and untreated, creating a significant public health challenge.

DOI: 10.1201/9781003500445-1

Polysomnography (PSG) remains the gold standard for diagnosing sleep apnea. This comprehensive sleep study simultaneously records multiple physiological parameters, including electroencephalography (EEG), electrocardiography (ECG), electromyography (EMG), electrooculography (EOG), nasal airflow, and blood oxygen saturation (SpO_2). However, PSG requires patients to spend one or more nights in a specialized sleep laboratory under clinical supervision, with multiple sensors and wires attached to their bodies. This approach is not only costly and time-consuming but also uncomfortable for patients, often affecting their natural sleep patterns and potentially leading to inaccurate results (Paul et al. 2022). The limited availability of sleep laboratories, combined with the substantial number of patients requiring evaluation, makes PSG impractical for widespread screening and long-term monitoring. Despite being one of the most prevalent sleep disorders affecting modern populations, sleep apnea remains critically underdiagnosed, with over 80% of patients remaining undiagnosed and untreated (Wang et al. 2025), creating a significant public health challenge.

The emergence of wearable sensor technology has opened new possibilities for detecting sleep apnea. These devices offer several compelling advantages over traditional PSG. First, they enable patients to sleep in their own homes in familiar environments, potentially capturing more representative sleep data. Second, wearable devices can continuously collect data over extended periods, enabling longitudinal monitoring of disease progression, and capturing sleep patterns across multiple nights in the patient's natural sleep environment (Hayano et al. 2020). Third, these devices significantly reduce the cost and improve accessibility of sleep monitoring, potentially enabling earlier detection and intervention.

Recent years have witnessed remarkable progress in applying artificial intelligence (AI) and machine learning (ML) techniques to analyze data from wearable sensors for sleep apnea detection. This chapter examines the current state of wearable sensor-based sleep apnea detection, exploring the underlying principles, methodological approaches, and practical challenges. The study examines the various types of physiological signals utilized, the preprocessing techniques employed, the ML and deep learning (DL) models developed, and the performance characteristics achieved in recent studies.

1.2 PHYSIOLOGICAL SIGNALS AND WEARABLE SENSOR TECHNOLOGIES

1.2.1 Types of Physiological Signals

The detection of sleep apnea through wearable sensors relies on capturing specific physiological signals that reflect respiratory and cardiovascular changes during apneic events. Research has identified several key signals that can be reliably measured using wearable devices.

Photoplethysmography (PPG) is one of the widely used signals for wearable-based sleep apnea detection (Hayano et al. 2020) (Jiang et al. 2023) (Zahra and Siamak 2025). PPG is a noninvasive optical technique that measures changes in blood volume in the microvascular bed by analyzing variations in light intensity passing through or reflected by tissue. The technique involves emitting red ($\lambda = 660$ nm) and infrared (IR, $\lambda = 880$ nm) light and using a photodiode sensor to capture the reflected signals. PPG sensors can be easily integrated into wrist-worn devices, rings, and patches, making them highly accessible for continuous monitoring. Beyond basic heart rate measurement, PPG signals provide valuable information about heart rate variability (HRV), respiratory rate, and SpO_2 levels (Hayano et al. 2020).

SpO_2 is another important signal for sleep apnea detection (Jiang et al. 2023) (Osa-Sanchez et al. 2025) (Hoang and Liang 2025). During apneic events, the cessation or reduction of airflow results in decreased oxygen levels in the blood, which can be detected by pulse oximetry. SpO_2 measurements perform better than other signals in certain classification tasks related to sleep apnea (Osa-Sanchez et al. 2025). The oxygen desaturation index (ODI), which quantifies the frequency of desaturation events, has been widely used as an important marker for sleep apnea severity (Jiang et al. 2023) (Hoang and Liang 2025). However, it is important to note that oxygen desaturation typically shows a 10-40-second delay following an apneic event, which poses challenges for real-time detection (Hoang and Liang 2025).

ECG signals have been investigated for sleep apnea detection (John et al. 2021) (Osa-Sanchez et al. 2025). ECG records the electrical activity of the heart, capturing P waves, QRS complexes (i.e., Q, R and S waves), and T waves for each heartbeat. Apneic events manifest in ECG signals through characteristic changes such as bradycardia followed by tachycardia and variations in R-R intervals. HRV derived from ECG shows a strong correlation with sleep apnea, making it a valuable indicator. Single-lead ECG can be recorded using portable, noninvasive wearable devices, including soft patches that provide wireless recording capabilities (Jiang et al. 2023).

Respiratory signals provide direct measurements of breathing patterns, which are fundamentally altered during sleep apnea (Osa-Sanchez et al. 2025). These signals can be acquired through various methods, including nasal airflow sensors, thoracic and abdominal motion sensors, respiratory effort belts, and chest or abdominal accelerometers. Apnea is characterized by the cessation of airflow, whereas hypopnea is characterized by a reduction in breathing amplitude. Modern wearable devices employ innovative approaches such as flexible respiratory sensors that can be positioned near the nostrils to capture airflow signals during sleep.

Accelerometer-based measurements offer the capability to monitor body position and respiratory movements, including tracheal movements (Hayano et al. 2020) (Jiang et al. 2023) (Osa-Sanchez et al. 2025). Accelerometers detect changes in gravitational forces across different axes when integrated into portable devices, providing essential data for activity tracking, fall detection, and sleep pattern monitoring. Body position monitoring is particularly relevant for addressing positional sleep apnea, which worsens in certain postures such as the supine position. Three-axis accelerometers placed at the suprasternal notch can detect tracheal respiratory movements, providing valuable information on respiratory effort cycles that aid in estimating sleep apnea severity.

1.2.2 Wearable Device Platforms

Studies have demonstrated practical implementation of sleep apnea detection across various wearable device platforms, each offering distinct advantages and trade-offs in terms of comfort, signal quality, and user acceptance.

Wrist-worn devices represent the most widely adopted platform for continuous health monitoring. Commercial smartwatches and fitness trackers from manufacturers such as Fitbit, Apple, Samsung, and Huawei have integrated PPG sensors, accelerometers, and, in some cases, SpO_2 sensors (John et al. 2021) (Osa-Sanchez et al. 2025). These devices benefit from high user acceptance due to their similarity to traditional watches and the ability to integrate multiple functions beyond sleep monitoring. Studies have achieved accuracies ranging from 90% to 95% using wrist-worn PPG data for sleep apnea detection (John et al. 2021) (Zahra and Siamak 2025) (Osa-Sanchez et al. 2025) (Hoang and Liang 2025).

Ring-based sensors have gained attention for their compact and discreet form factor. Smart rings can measure PPG and SpO_2 signals with potentially higher accuracy than wrist-worn devices, due to the thinner skin on the finger. The Belun Ring, for example, has been validated for sleep apnea detection and sleep stage classification, demonstrating moderate to substantial agreement with PSG-derived AHI values, with accuracies ranging from 0.85 to 0.91 (Osa-Sanchez et al. 2025). However, rings may not accurately measure all sleep stages and may cause discomfort during prolonged overnight wear.

Adhesive patches offer several advantages for the acquisition of physiological signals. These flexible, thin devices can be applied directly to specific body locations, ensuring stable skin contact and high-quality signal acquisition. Patches can integrate multiple sensors, including ECG electrodes, PPG sensors, accelerometers, and even EEG electrodes. Studies have employed patches on various body locations, including the chest for bioimpedance and ECG measurement, the forehead for EEG and EOG, the chin for EMG, and the sternum for combined ECG, PPG, and seismocardiography (SCG) (Paul et al. 2022) (Osa-Sanchez et al. 2025). The soft sternal patch, for instance, achieved 100% sensitivity and 95% precision in detecting apnea and hypopnea (Osa-Sanchez et al. 2025). According to a systematic review of 28 studies, adhesive patches were the most commonly used wearable device type, appearing in approximately 46% of the studies, primarily because they can record multiple signal types simultaneously and offer superior signal quality compared to other wearable formats. Despite their excellent signal quality, patches face challenges to long-term user acceptance due to potential skin irritation and the need for regular replacement.

Chest bands and straps provide a balance between signal quality and user comfort (Paul et al. 2022) (Osa-Sanchez et al. 2025). These devices can measure respiratory effort through bioimpedance or inductive plethysmography, capture ECG signals, and monitor body position through integrated accelerometers. Chest bands are particularly effective for measuring breathing patterns and detecting respiratory events. However, they may be less comfortable for extended overnight use compared to wrist-worn devices, and proper positioning is critical for accurate measurements.

Headband and forehead devices acquire EEG signals, which are valuable for comprehensive sleep staging. Wearable EEG systems equipped with dry frontopolar electrodes have been developed to streamline sleep staging processes (Osa-Sanchez et al. 2025). While these devices can provide high-quality neurophysiological data, they may be less comfortable than other wearable options and typically require more careful placement to ensure adequate signal quality.

Selecting an appropriate wearable platform involves balancing multiple factors, including signal quality requirements, user comfort and acceptance, cost considerations, and the specific application context. For clinical validation studies, patches and chest bands may be preferred due to their superior signal quality. For long-term home monitoring and screening applications, wrist-worn devices and rings offer advantages in user acceptance and compliance with continuous wear. Table 1.1 summarizes the commonly used wearable device platforms for sleep apnea detection, highlighting the typical sensors, body placement, key advantages, and primary limitations.

1.3 SIGNAL PREPROCESSING AND FEATURE ENGINEERING

The raw signals acquired from wearable sensors require substantial preprocessing before they can be effectively utilized for sleep apnea detection. This section examines the critical preprocessing steps and feature extraction techniques that have proven effective in recent research. Figure 1.1 illustrates the typical signal preprocessing and feature engineering steps applied to wearable physiological data prior to sleep apnea classification.

1.3.1 Preprocessing Techniques

Data quality assessment and cleaning are the basis for effective signal processing. Studies typically implement multiple quality control stages. For SpO_2 signals, readings below 60% or above 100% are commonly removed as these values represent physiological outliers or measurement errors (Jiang et al. 2023) (Hoang and Liang 2025). Missing data handling strategies vary depending on the extent of data loss; segments with more than 10% artifact content are often excluded from analysis to ensure data integrity.

Filtering is an important preprocessing step for removing noise and artifacts while preserving physiologically relevant signal components. For ECG signals, band-pass filtering is commonly applied to eliminate baseline wander, powerline interference (50-60 Hz), and high-frequency noise from muscle activity. The specific filter parameters depend on the signal type and application. For example, third-order Butterworth filters have been employed for various physiological signals. PPG signals may require additional preprocessing steps, including removal of motion artifacts, which represent a significant challenge in wearable sensing.

Segmentation and windowing strategies determine the temporal resolution of analysis (John et al. 2021) (Paul et al. 2022) (Jiang et al. 2023) (Osa-Sanchez et al. 2025). Different approaches serve different purposes. For epoch-wise analysis, common segment lengths include 30 seconds (the standard PSG epoch length), 60 seconds (one-minute segments aligned with apnea annotations), and 11 seconds with a ten-second overlap (enabling per-second resolution). The choice of segmentation strategy

TABLE 1.1
Wearable Devices for Sleep Apnea Detection

Device Type	Typical Sensors	Body Placement	Key Advantages	Main Limitations	Primary Signals Captured
Wrist-worn Devices (Smartwatches/Fitness Trackers)	PPG, Accelerometer, SpO_2 sensor	Wrist (radial artery)	- High user acceptance - Comfortable for long-term wear - Multiple health metrics - Similar to regular watches - Noninvasive	- Motion artifacts during movement - Lower signal quality than patches - Device-specific variations - Gap in performance between devices	- Heart rate - HRV - SpO_2 - Sleep stages - Activity levels
Adhesive Patches	ECG electrodes, PPG sensors, Accelerometers, SCG sensors, EEG electrodes, EMG electrodes	Chest, Forehead, Chin, Sternum, Suprasternal notch	- Stable skin contact - High signal quality - Multiple sensors in one device - Flexible placement options - Direct physiological measurement	- Potential skin irritation - Needs regular replacement - Lower long-term acceptance - Single-use in many cases - User discomfort	- Electrocardiogram - PPG - SCG - Brain activity (EEG) - Muscle activity (EMG) - Eye movements (EOG)
Smart Rings	PPG sensor, SpO_2 sensor, Accelerometer	Finger	- Discreet and compact - Thinner skin improves signal - Comfortable design - Less obtrusive than watches - Good accuracy for heart rate	- May cause discomfort overnight - Limited to certain measurements - Cannot capture all sleep stages accurately - Smaller battery capacity	- Pulse rate - SpO_2 - Movement patterns - Sleep-wake patterns

Chest Bands/ Straps	ECG electrodes, Bioimpedance sensors, Inductive plethysmography, Accelerometers	Chest (around thorax)	- Direct respiratory measurement - Good breathing pattern detection - Reusable and washable - Balances quality and comfort - Effective for respiratory effort	- Less comfortable than wrist devices - May shift during sleep - Requires proper positioning - More intrusive than wrist wear	- Respiratory effort - Breathing patterns - Electrocardiogram - Body position - Thoracic movements
Headband/ Forehead Devices	EEG sensors (dry electrodes), EOG sensors	Forehead/Head	- Brain activity monitoring - Comprehensive sleep staging - Can detect arousals - Noninvasive EEG recording - Neurophysiological data	- Less comfortable for sleep - Requires careful placement - Higher cost - May slip during the night - More complex setup	- Brain waves (EEG) - Eye movements (EOG) - Sleep architecture - Neurophysiological signals - Arousal events
Specialized Respiratory Patches	Temperature sensors, Accelerometers, Flexible respiratory sensors, Piezoelectric sensors	Near nostrils, Chest, Suprasternal notch, Diaphragm	- Direct airflow measurement - Captures breathing dynamics - Flexible and thin design - Specific respiratory focus - High sensitivity to breathing	- Requires adhesion near the face - May detach during the night - Needs specific positioning - Replacement after use - Limited to respiratory signals	- Nasal airflow - Temperature changes (breathing) - Tracheal movements - Diaphragm motion - Respiratory rhythm

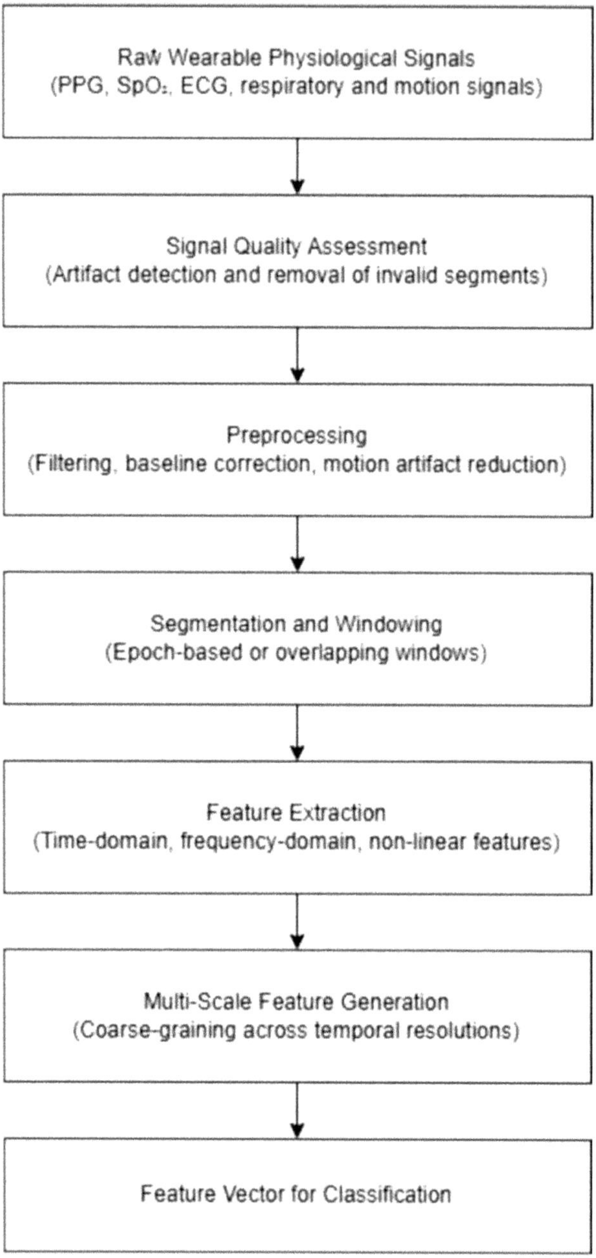

FIGURE 1.1 Signal Preprocessing and Feature Engineering Pipeline for Wearable-Based Sleep Apnea Detection.

significantly impacts the ability to detect individual events versus assessing overall severity. Studies aiming for high-resolution detection have employed 11-second windows to achieve one-second resolution, recognizing that apnea events must last at least ten seconds by definition (John et al. 2021).

Feature extraction transforms preprocessed signals into meaningful quantitative measures that capture relevant patterns for sleep apnea detection. The sophistication and diversity of features have evolved considerably in recent research.

1.3.2 Time-Domain Features

Time-domain features provide statistical characterizations of signal behavior. For HRV analysis derived from either ECG or PPG signals, standard measures include SDNN (i.e., standard deviation of normal-to-normal intervals), RMSSD (i.e., root mean square of successive differences), and various percentile-based metrics (Hayano et al. 2020). These features capture both the overall variability and the dynamic changes in heart rate that accompany apneic events. For SpO_2 signals, time-domain features include mean, maximum, minimum, and standard deviation values, which reflect the overall oxygenation level and its stability (Hoang and Liang 2025).

1.3.3 Frequency-Domain Features

Spectral analysis of physiological signals reveals periodic patterns and frequency components associated with sleep apnea. Power spectral density estimation identifies the distribution of signal energy across frequency bands. For HRV analysis, the low-frequency (0.04-0.15 Hz) and high-frequency (0.14-0.40 Hz) bands reflect different aspects of autonomic nervous system activity (Hayano et al. 2020). The LF/HF (low-frequency/high-frequency) ratio has been proposed as an indicator of sympathovagal balance, though its interpretation in the context of sleep apnea requires careful consideration.

1.3.4 Nonlinear Features

Nonlinear features have demonstrated particular promise for sleep apnea detection, especially when working with lower-resolution data. Entropy measures quantify signal complexity and regularity, with multiple variants showing effectiveness in sleep apnea detection. Sample entropy (SampEn) and fuzzy entropy (FuzzEn) both showed correlations with AHI exceeding 0.80, maintaining strong relationships even at coarse time scales up to 600 seconds (Hoang and Liang 2025). Approximate entropy (ApEn) showed a correlation of 0.85 with AHI and maintained a correlation above 0.5 even at a 120-second timescale.

Additional nonlinear measures include permutation entropy, which showed a correlation of 0.86 with AHI, and the central tendency measure (CTM), which maintained correlations above 0.7 across multiple time scales. Lempel-Ziv complexity quantifies the rate of new pattern generation in a signal and has shown utility for sleep apnea detection, though its correlation with AHI decreases substantially at longer timescales (Hoang and Liang 2025).

1.3.5 Oximetry-Specific Biomarkers

The ODI is one of the most clinically established markers of sleep apnea, defined as the average number of desaturation episodes per hour. A desaturation episode is typically defined as a decrease in mean oxygen saturation of ≥3% (over the last 120 seconds) lasting for at least ten seconds. At the original one-second resolution, ODI exhibits a strong correlation with AHI ($\rho = 0.77$), but this correlation weakens substantially at lower resolutions, dropping to 0.25 at 60-second resolution (Hoang and Liang 2025).

Other oximetry biomarkers include the cumulative time spent below specific SpO_2 thresholds, the area under the desaturation curve (normalized by recording time), and various indices characterizing the depth and duration of desaturation events. The percentage of recording time with SpO_2 at least 2% below the median correlated with AHI at the two-second timescale, with a correlation coefficient of 0.54 (Hoang and Liang 2025).

1.3.6 Multiscale Feature Engineering

Recent research involves extracting features at multiple temporal scales through coarse-graining procedures. This approach creates multiple representations of the original signal by averaging data points within nonoverlapping windows of increasing length, ranging from one second to 600 seconds (Hoang and Liang 2025). Remarkably, certain nonlinear features maintain strong correlations with AHI even at very coarse resolutions. Nine features, including CTM, FuzzEn, SampEn, complex entropy, increment entropy, Kolmogorov entropy, permutation entropy, Shannon entropy, and average magnitude of change, maintained correlations with AHI above 0.4 across all timescales up to 60 seconds. Complex entropy demonstrated particularly remarkable performance, reaching a correlation coefficient of -0.86 with AHI at the ten-second timescale and maintaining a correlation of -0.75 at 60 seconds. This finding has important implications for wearable device applications, where power efficiency often requires lower sampling rates and data storage at coarser temporal resolutions.

The multiscale approach offers additional benefits beyond computational efficiency. It functions as a low-pass averaging filter, reducing the impact of high-frequency noise and transient fluctuations and potentially revealing underlying patterns more effectively than single-scale analysis. Some features that show weak correlations at the original fine-grained resolution achieve substantially stronger correlations after coarse graining. For example, the zero-crossing rate reached a correlation of 0.61 with AHI at the 20-second timescale, whereas it showed essentially no correlation at one-second resolution (Zahra and Siamak 2025).

1.4 MACHINE LEARNING AND DEEP LEARNING APPROACHES

The application of AI to sleep apnea detection has evolved from traditional ML methods to sophisticated DL architectures. This section examines the landscape of computational approaches, their performance characteristics, and practical considerations for implementation.

1.4.1 Traditional Machine Learning Methods

Traditional ML algorithms continue to play an important role in sleep apnea detection, particularly when interpretability and computational efficiency are priorities. These methods typically operate on hand-crafted features extracted from preprocessed physiological signals.

Random forest (RF) classifiers have demonstrated consistent performance across multiple studies. The algorithm constructs multiple decision trees using bootstrap sampling and aggregates their predictions through majority voting, which helps reduce overfitting and improve generalization. In one study using PPG and SpO_2 signals from a wearable ring device, RF achieved 93.88% accuracy, 91.8% specificity, and 89.93% sensitivity. Another investigation using longer observation windows (WIN-61) reported an accuracy of 95% and an F1-score of 94%. The algorithm's ability to handle high-dimensional feature spaces and provide feature importance rankings makes it particularly valuable for understanding which physiological signals contribute most to detection performance. RF also showed strong performance in the systematic review analysis, being one of the most frequently employed algorithms across 28 studies, with consistent results across different device types and signal modalities (Osa-Sanchez et al. 2025).

Support Vector Machines (SVMs) identify optimal hyperplanes to separate different classes in high-dimensional feature spaces. While SVM has shown reasonable performance, with accuracy rates around 88–91% reported across different studies, it generally performs slightly below ensemble methods like RF in recent comparative analyses (Osa-Sanchez et al. 2025). The algorithm's effectiveness depends significantly on kernel selection and hyperparameter tuning.

Gradient boosting methods, including XGBoost and CatBoost, have demonstrated strong performance in sleep apnea classification tasks (Osa-Sanchez et al. 2025) (Hoang and Liang 2025). CatBoost particularly distinguished itself, achieving the highest performance among traditional ML methods in several studies, with accuracy exceeding 93% for severe sleep apnea detection (AHI ≥30) (Hoang and Liang 2025). The algorithm's ability to handle categorical features and its resistance to overfitting make it well-suited for medical applications.

K-Nearest Neighbors (KNN) achieved a notable 95% accuracy in some studies when applied to sleep apnea diagnosis using wearable device data. The performance, however, can be sensitive to the choice of distance metric and the k parameter, requiring careful validation.

The performance of traditional ML methods varies considerably depending on the specific features employed, the quality and quantity of the training data, and the complexity of the classification task. For binary classification, distinguishing between normal subjects and from those with any degree of sleep apnea (AHI ≥5), these methods typically achieve accuracies ranging from 85% to 95% (John et al. 2021) (Osa-Sanchez et al. 2025) (Hoang and Liang 2025).

1.4.2 Deep Learning Architectures

DL approaches have increasingly dominated sleep apnea detection research due to their ability to automatically learn relevant features from raw or minimally processed signals, eliminating the need for extensive hand-crafted feature engineering.

Convolutional neural networks (CNNs) have emerged as a primary architecture for analyzing physiological signals (John et al. 2021) (Paul et al. 2022) (Zahra and Siamak 2025) (Osa-Sanchez et al. 2025). CNNs excel at extracting hierarchical features through successive convolutional and pooling layers. For sleep apnea detection, one-dimensional (1D) CNNs are typically used to process time-series signals. The architecture proposed by John et al. used three convolutional layers with three, 50, and 30 filters, achieving 99.56% accuracy and 96.05% sensitivity on the University College Dublin Sleep Apnea Database (UCDDB) dataset when applied to 11-second ECG windows at one-second resolution. The model demonstrated high performance even after pruning to 80% sparsity, maintaining 97.34% accuracy and 86.48% sensitivity (John et al. 2021).

A simplified CNN architecture called SomnNET, designed specifically for smartwatch integration, achieved 97.08% accuracy in detecting sleep apnea events from SpO_2 signals. The network's architecture emphasized efficiency while maintaining performance, making it suitable for resource-constrained wearable devices. After model pruning with 80% sparsity, the network still achieved 89.75% accuracy (Osa-Sanchez et al. 2025).

More complex CNN variants have incorporated multiscale processing capabilities. The one-dimensional multiscale bidirectional temporal convolutional neural network (1D-MsBiTCNet) model integrated multiscale feature extraction with bidirectional temporal convolutional networks, achieving 82.76% accuracy for per-segment detection and 97.83% accuracy for detecting severe sleep apnea syndrome (Osa-Sanchez et al. 2025). This architecture demonstrated the value of capturing features at multiple temporal scales within the network design itself.

Recurrent neural networks (RNNs) and their variants handle the temporal dependencies inherent in physiological signals. Long short-term memory (LSTM) networks have been widely adopted due to their ability to capture long-range dependencies while avoiding the vanishing gradient problem (Paul et al. 2022) (Jiang et al. 2023).

Several studies have employed LSTM for sleep apnea detection with promising results. An LSTM-based model applied to hybrid physiological signals (ECG and breathing patterns) achieved an average recognition rate of 84–85% for sleep apnea-hypopnea syndrome classification (Paul et al. 2022). When combined with MobileNet V1 architecture, an LSTM model analyzing ECG signals achieved 90.29% accuracy,

90.01% sensitivity, and 90.72% specificity (Osa-Sanchez et al. 2025). The combination of CNN and LSTM layers has proven particularly effective, with one study reporting F1-scores ranging from 12% to 71% for event-by-event detection across different sleep apnea severity groups.

Hybrid architectures combining multiple neural network types have shown considerable promise. The integration of CNN layers for spatial feature extraction with LSTM layers for temporal modeling enables comprehensive analysis of physiological signals. One study employing this approach to analyze tracheal movements achieved 81% sensitivity, 87% specificity, and 84% overall accuracy in sleep apnea diagnosis (Jiang et al. 2023).

Transfer learning (TL) approaches have addressed the challenge of limited training data by leveraging knowledge from pretrained models. ResNet architectures, originally developed for image classification, have been adapted for sleep apnea detection from ECG signals. ResNet18 demonstrated superior performance among several ResNet variants, achieving an average Cohen's kappa coefficient of 0.57 and Pearson's correlation coefficient of 0.87 between PSG-derived AHI and estimated AHI. The model also achieved area under the precision-recall curve (AUPR) values ranging from 0.65 to 0.91 across different datasets (Zahra and Siamak 2025). TL using TinySleepNet, a lightweight model optimized for single-channel EEG sleep staging, has been investigated for sleep apnea detection. The model's 1.3 million parameters and architecture, which combines CNN and LSTM layers, achieved robust generalizability across diverse datasets, with Cohen's kappa values ranging from 0.77 to 0.82 (Osa-Sanchez et al. 2025).

A particularly innovative approach combining hardware design with algorithmic sophistication is the two-stage detection strategy implemented with dual-modal sensing (Wang et al. 2025). This system integrates a self-powered piezoelectric nanogenerator (PENG) with a PPG sensor, using a biomimetic fingertip structure to optimize signal acquisition. In the first stage, the energy-efficient PENG performs continuous preliminary screening with 93.41% sensitivity and consumes negligible power. When suspicious events are detected, the system activates the PPG sensor for precise diagnosis in the second stage. The high-accuracy configuration, utilizing a Vision Transformer-based (ViT-based) DL model, achieved 99.59% accuracy with 99.73% specificity and 99.45% sensitivity, while the energy-optimized two-stage approach maintained 94.95% accuracy with approximately 23% reduction in power consumption compared to continuous PPG operation. This dual-modal approach demonstrates how intelligent system design can balance diagnostic accuracy with practical constraints of battery-powered wearable devices, potentially enabling truly continuous, long-term sleep apnea monitoring in home settings.

1.4.3 Federated and Edge Computing Approaches

Recent research has begun exploring deployment strategies that balance model performance with the practical constraints of wearable devices. Hyperdimensional computing (HDC) frameworks have been proposed for energy-efficient sleep apnea detection on resource-constrained processors. One implementation achieved 70.17%

accuracy while demonstrating significantly lower memory footprint, reduced latency, and energy savings on ARM Cortex-M4 processors (Osa-Sanchez et al. 2025). Though accuracy is lower than that of state-of-the-art approaches, these methods enable continuous on-device processing without requiring constant data transmission to cloud servers.

1.4.4 Performance Comparison and Model Selection

The choice between traditional ML and DL approaches, involves multiple considerations beyond raw accuracy. DL models generally achieve higher performance, with accuracies frequently exceeding 95% for well-designed architectures on high-quality datasets (John et al. 2021) (Paul et al. 2022) (Osa-Sanchez et al. 2025). However, they require more training data, computational resources, and expertise to develop and optimize.

Traditional ML methods offer several advantages despite somewhat lower peak performance. They provide better interpretability, which is crucial in clinical contexts where understanding the basis for predictions can inform treatment decisions (Osa-Sanchez et al. 2025). They require less training data and computational resources, making them more accessible for research groups with limited resources. Furthermore, they often demonstrate more stable performance across different datasets and patient populations.

For wearable device applications, additional constraints apply. Energy efficiency becomes paramount for battery-powered devices intended for overnight or multi-day use. Model size and inference time must be minimized to enable real-time processing on resource-constrained hardware. The multiscale feature engineering approach, when combined with efficient algorithms such as CatBoost, offers an attractive balance by achieving strong performance (exceeding 93% accuracy for severe sleep apnea detection) while maintaining computational efficiency (Hoang and Liang 2025).

The integration of model pruning, quantization, and knowledge distillation techniques has enabled the deployment of sophisticated models on wearable devices. Pruned CNNs maintaining 80% sparsity have achieved accuracies above 89% while substantially reducing computational requirements (Osa-Sanchez et al. 2025). Quantization to eight-bit precision has reduced energy consumption from 2.18 μJ to 1.80 μJ per inference while maintaining performance above 94% accuracy (John et al. 2021).

1.5 CLINICAL VALIDATION AND PERFORMANCE EVALUATION

The translation of wearable sensor-based sleep apnea detection from research prototypes to clinical applications requires rigorous validation using standardized evaluation frameworks and diverse patient populations.

1.5.1 Evaluation Metrics and Protocols

Sleep apnea detection systems are evaluated using multiple complementary metrics that capture different aspects of performance. Sensitivity (also called recall) measures the proportion of true apnea cases correctly identified, reflecting the system's ability to detect individuals who have the condition. Specificity quantifies the proportion of true negative cases correctly identified, indicating the system's ability to rule out the condition in healthy individuals. Accuracy represents the overall proportion of correct classifications. However, accuracy alone can be misleading when dealing with imbalanced datasets where one class substantially outnumbers the other (Hoang and Liang 2025).

The Matthews correlation coefficient (MCC) provides a balanced measure that accounts for class imbalance, with values ranging from -1 to +1 (Hoang and Liang 2025). An MCC of zero indicates performance no better than random, while values approaching one indicate perfect classification. The F1-score represents the harmonic mean of precision and sensitivity, providing a single metric that balances these two important characteristics (John et al. 2021) (Jiang et al. 2023) (Osa-Sanchez et al. 2025).

For clinical applications, the area under the receiver operating characteristic curve (AUC, also called ROC AUC) offers valuable insights into classification performance across different decision thresholds. AUC values above 0.9 generally indicate excellent discrimination ability, while values between 0.8 and 0.9 suggest good performance (Zahra and Siamak 2025).

Classification tasks in sleep apnea research typically use standardized AHI thresholds defined by clinical guidelines. Binary classification with AHI ≥5 distinguishes normal subjects from those with any degree of sleep apnea. The AHI threshold of ≥15 separates individuals with mild or no symptoms from those with moderate to severe sleep apnea, who require closer medical attention. Classification at AHI ≥30 identifies severe cases that typically require immediate treatment. Multiclass classification schemes categorize patients into four severity levels: normal (AHI < 5), mild (5 ≤ AHI < 15), moderate (15 ≤ AHI < 30), and severe (AHI ≥ 30) (Hoang and Liang 2025). Table 1.2 summarizes these clinical classifications, along with their typical symptoms and treatment implications, according to the American Academy of Sleep Medicine (AASM) 2015 guidelines.

1.5.2 Performance Across Classification Tasks

Recent studies have demonstrated varying performance across specific classification tasks and dataset characteristics. For the challenging task of distinguishing normal subjects from any degree of sleep apnea (AHI ≥5), where class imbalance is typically most pronounced, achieved accuracies range from 73% to 90%. The CatBoost model achieved 89.63% accuracy, 92.27% precision, 96.06% sensitivity, and 0.51 MCC on this task. Notably, multiscale feature engineering improved performance, particularly for models that initially showed bias toward the majority class, with the Bayes model improving from 67.17% to 73.59% accuracy (Hoang and Liang 2025).

For the clinically important threshold of AHI ≥15, separating mild from moderate-severe cases, recent systems have achieved more balanced performance across classes. Accuracies in this category typically range from 86% to 87%, with sensitivities of 84% to 85% and specificities of 84% to 87%. The CatBoost model again

TABLE 1.2
Apnea-Hypopnea Index Severity Classifications and Clinical Implications

AHI Category	AHI Range (events/hour)	Clinical Significance	Typical Symptoms	Treatment Recommendations
Normal	< 5	No clinically significant sleep apnea	Minimal or no symptoms	Lifestyle modifications, sleep hygiene
Mild	5–14	Mild sleep disruption	Occasional daytime sleepiness, snoring	Weight loss, positional therapy, and oral appliances
Moderate	15–29	Moderate health risk	Daytime sleepiness, morning headaches	CPAP therapy, consider medical evaluation
Severe	≥ 30	High cardiovascular risk	Severe daytime sleepiness, witnessed apneas	CPAP therapy mandatory, comprehensive medical evaluation

demonstrated strong performance with 87.17% accuracy, 87.59% precision, 85.42% sensitivity, and 0.74 MCC (Hoang and Liang 2025).

Classification of severe sleep apnea (AHI ≥30) is an important clinical application for identifying patients who require urgent treatment. Recent studies report accuracies ranging from 90% to 93% for this task. The CatBoost model achieved 93.47% accuracy, 84.37% precision, 77.50% sensitivity, and an MCC of 0.77, demonstrating strong performance for this clinically critical application. Multiclass classification into four severity categories is the most challenging scenario due to ambiguity at class boundaries and unbalanced class distributions. Recent studies report accuracies of 57–70% for this task. The CatBoost model achieved the best performance with 70.46% accuracy, 71.88% precision, 67.64% sensitivity, and 0.58 MCC. Misclassification occurs most frequently between adjacent severity categories, particularly between normal and mild apnea groups (Hoang and Liang 2025).

1.5.3 Dataset Considerations

The choice of dataset significantly impacts model development and validation. The Sleep Heart Health Study (SHHS) represents one of the largest publicly available sleep datasets, with over 5,700 overnight recordings. This dataset offers diverse ages, genders, and apnea severities. However, careful preprocessing is essential; one study retained 4,664 recordings after quality filtering. The dataset exhibits class imbalance, with 86.40% of subjects having some degree of sleep apnea (AHI ≥5) (Hoang and Liang 2025).

The UCDDB dataset, while smaller with 25 recordings, has been widely used for algorithm development and provides high-quality polysomnographic data with detailed annotations. Studies using this dataset have reported excellent performance, with accuracies exceeding 99% for some models (John et al. 2021). However, the limited sample size raises concerns about generalizability to broader populations.

Recent research has increasingly emphasized the importance of validation across multiple datasets to assess generalizability (Zahra and Siamak 2025) (Osa-Sanchez et al. 2025). TL approaches have demonstrated that models can maintain reasonable performance on new datasets, though typically with some degradation relative to within-dataset validation (Osa-Sanchez et al. 2025).

1.6 CHALLENGES AND LIMITATIONS

Despite significant progress in wearable sensor-based sleep apnea detection, several substantial challenges continue to limit clinical adoption and effectiveness.

1.6.1 Signal Quality and Reliability

Motion artifacts are among the most persistent challenges in wearable sensing. Movement during sleep can disrupt sensor contact with the skin, introducing noise and gaps in physiological recordings (Osa-Sanchez et al. 2025). While preprocessing techniques can mitigate some artifacts, excessive movement may render segments of data unusable. Studies commonly exclude recordings with more than 10–20% artifact content, which may bias results toward subjects with less restless sleep (John et al. 2021). Signal resolution trade-offs pose a fundamental challenge for wearable devices. Consumer devices often store data at resolutions lower than those of research-grade equipment to conserve battery life and reduce storage requirements. For example, many smartwatches record PPG at one-minute intervals rather than continuously at high frequency. This reduced resolution limits the ability to detect short-duration events and fine-grained temporal patterns. Research has shown that traditional biomarkers, such as ODI, lose much of their correlation with AHI when derived from low-resolution data, with correlation dropping from 0.77 at one-second resolution to 0.25 at 60-second resolution (Hoang and Liang 2025).

Inter-device variability complicates the development of generalizable algorithms. Different manufacturers employ varied sensor configurations, signal processing algorithms, and data formats. Models trained on data from one device may not perform well when applied to another device, even if both measure the same physiological signals (Osa-Sanchez et al. 2025). This issue highlights the need for robust, device-agnostic approaches or careful device-specific calibration.

1.6.2 Data Imbalance and Bias

Class imbalance affects most sleep apnea datasets, particularly at the AHI ≥5 threshold, where healthy subjects comprise only 13–14% of typical study populations. This imbalance can lead models to exhibit bias toward the majority class (apnea patients), achieving high overall accuracy while failing to correctly identify healthy individuals.

The Bayes model, for instance, initially classified nearly all subjects as having apnea, achieving 67% accuracy but demonstrating poor discrimination. While techniques such as multiscale feature engineering, class weighting, and oversampling can partially address this issue, the fundamental challenge of limited healthy subject data remains.

Population diversity in training data affects model generalizability. Many datasets contain predominantly older adults or individuals already suspected of having sleep disorders. Models trained on such populations may not perform well when applied to younger, healthier individuals or different demographic groups. The SHHS dataset, while large, has a mean age of 66 years and includes relatively few subjects under 40 (Osa-Sanchez et al. 2025).

1.6.3 Feature Selection and Model Interpretability

The curse of dimensionality arises when extracting numerous features from multiple signal types and timescales. With 106 features extracted at each of 23 timescales, some studies work with feature spaces exceeding 2,000 dimensions. While feature selection and dimensionality reduction techniques help address this issue, determining the optimal feature subset remains challenging and may vary across different populations and device types. Model interpretability presents particular concerns for clinical applications. DL models that achieve the highest accuracies often function as "black boxes," making it difficult to understand which signal characteristics drive their predictions. This opacity can hinder clinical adoption, as healthcare providers may be reluctant to trust recommendations they cannot easily explain to patients. Traditional ML methods offer better interpretability, but typically achieve somewhat lower performance (Osa-Sanchez et al. 2025) (Hoang and Liang 2025).

1.6.4 Computational and Energy Constraints

Resource limitations of wearable devices constrain the complexity of algorithms that can be deployed for on-device processing. Battery capacity, processing power, and memory all impose practical limits. The energy consumption of continuous signal processing and analysis must be minimized to enable overnight or multi-day monitoring without recharging. Model compression techniques like pruning and quantization help address these constraints but typically result in some performance degradation. One study reduced energy consumption from 2.55 μJ to 0.52 μJ per inference through 80% model pruning, but accuracy decreased from 99.56% to 97.34% (John et al. 2021).

Real-time processing requirements add another layer of complexity. While classification of overall sleep apnea severity can be performed retrospectively, some applications may require real-time or near-real-time detection of apneic events to trigger interventions. The delayed response of SpO_2 to respiratory events complicates real-time detection, as meaningful oxygen desaturation may not occur until 10-40 seconds after an apneic event begins (Hoang and Liang 2025).

1.6.5 Validation and Regulatory Challenges

Limited clinical validation remains a significant gap. While many studies report excellent performance on research datasets, few have conducted prospective clinical trials comparing wearable device-based detection to PSG in real-world settings. The performance achieved under carefully controlled research conditions may not transfer directly to diverse clinical populations and home-monitoring scenarios.

Regulatory approval pathways for AI-based medical devices continue to evolve. Wearable sleep apnea detection systems have not yet received widespread Food and Drug Administration (FDA) approval as diagnostic tools. Obtaining regulatory approval requires demonstrating safety, effectiveness, and consistency across diverse populations, which is a substantial undertaking requiring extensive clinical validation. Longitudinal validation has been limited. Most studies evaluate single-night recordings, but the longitudinal stability of wearable device measurements and algorithms over weeks or months of repeated use has not been thoroughly characterized. Changes in sensor performance over time, variations in device placement, and evolution of the underlying condition could all affect long-term accuracy.

1.6.6 Clinical and Practical Considerations

Definition variability affects cross-study comparisons. Different scoring rules for apnea and hypopnea have evolved over time, with the AASM 2015 guidelines differing from earlier standards. Studies using different definitions or datasets, or scoring criteria, may not be directly comparable.

Phenotype diversity in sleep apnea presents a challenge. While most research focuses on OSA, which accounts for the majority of cases, central and mixed sleep apnea have different physiological signatures that may require different detection approaches (John et al. 2021). Furthermore, positional sleep apnea (worse in the supine position) and REM-related sleep (rapid-eye-movement-related-sleep) apnea represent subtypes that may benefit from specialized algorithms. User compliance with wearable devices for long-term monitoring remains uncertain. While devices are designed to be comfortable and unobtrusive, sustained nightly use over extended periods may prove challenging for some users. Skin irritation from adhesive patches, discomfort from chest bands, or simply forgetting to wear wrist devices could all limit real-world effectiveness.

1.7 FUTURE DIRECTIONS AND OPPORTUNITIES

Despite current challenges, several promising avenues exist for advancing wearable sensor-based sleep apnea detection.

Multimodal sensor fusion represents a key opportunity. Combining complementary signals like PPG, SpO_2, accelerometry, and acoustic measurements may provide more robust detection than any single modality (Paul et al. 2022) (Jiang et al. 2023). Sophisticated fusion algorithms that appropriately weight different signals based on their quality and relevance could enhance both accuracy and reliability.

Advanced materials and sensor technologies promise improved signal quality and user comfort. Flexible, skin-conformable electronics enable better sensor-skin contact while maintaining comfort. Dry electrodes eliminate the need for conductive gels, simplifying device application and improving long-term wearability. Miniaturization of components enables less obtrusive devices that users are more likely to wear consistently.

Edge computing capabilities in next-generation wearable devices will enable more sophisticated on-device processing. As processing power increases and energy efficiency improves, it becomes feasible to deploy more complex algorithms locally, reducing latency and enabling real-time applications while preserving privacy.

Personalized models adapted to individual patients may improve performance compared to population-level models. Patient-specific models derived from generic models have achieved strong performance while requiring fewer parameters and less computational resources (John et al. 2021). TL and meta-learning approaches could enable efficient adaptation to individual characteristics.

Multiscale and multiresolution analysis techniques show promise for handling data from diverse devices with varying sampling rates. Research has demonstrated that nonlinear features such as complex entropy and SampEn maintain strong correlations with sleep apnea severity even when computed from coarsely-sampled data (Zahra and Siamak 2025) (Hoang and Liang 2025). This finding suggests that effective screening may be possible using lower-resolution data than previously assumed, potentially enabling broader deployment of detection algorithms across diverse consumer devices.

Explainable AI methods could address the interpretability challenges of DL models. Techniques like attention mechanisms, gradient-based visualization, and rule extraction may help elucidate which signal characteristics drive model predictions, increasing clinical trust and adoption (Osa-Sanchez et al. 2025).

Longitudinal monitoring applications represent a significant opportunity. Rather than replacing PSG for initial diagnosis, wearable devices could excel at tracking disease progression, monitoring treatment effectiveness, and detecting changes that warrant clinical re-evaluation (Wang et al. 2025). Continuous monitoring over weeks or months could provide insights into how sleep apnea severity varies with factors like weight changes, alcohol consumption, medication use, and sleeping position.

Screening and triage applications may be the most immediately viable use case. Wearable devices could identify individuals at high risk of sleep apnea who should undergo formal PSG evaluation, thereby addressing the current situation in which over 80% of patients remain undiagnosed (Paul et al. 2022). Effective screening could substantially increase the efficiency of sleep medicine clinics by focusing PSG resources on individuals most likely to have clinically significant sleep apnea.

Treatment guidance represents another valuable application. For patients using continuous positive airway pressure (CPAP) therapy, wearable devices could monitor treatment adherence and effectiveness, alerting patients and clinicians to problems (Wang et al. 2025). Similarly, monitoring could help optimize oral appliance therapy or track outcomes following surgical interventions.

Large-scale prospective studies are needed to validate the performance of wearable devices across diverse populations in real-world settings. Such studies should include adequate representation of different age groups, ethnic backgrounds, body types, and comorbid conditions. They should also compare not just diagnostic accuracy but also clinical outcomes and cost-effectiveness.

Standardization efforts would enable cross-study comparisons and clinical adoption. Standardized protocols for data collection, preprocessing, and feature extraction would enable more meaningful comparisons between different approaches. Agreement on reporting standards for model performance, including specification of confidence intervals and performance across different patient subgroups, would improve research quality.

Open datasets and benchmarks would accelerate algorithm development. While the SHHS and similar datasets have proven valuable, additional large, diverse, and well-annotated datasets with simultaneous PSG and wearable device recordings would benefit the research community (Hoang and Liang 2025). Benchmark challenges with standardized evaluation protocols could help identify the most promising approaches. Regulatory science research is needed to establish appropriate validation frameworks for AI-based wearable medical devices. This includes determining appropriate endpoints, defining acceptable performance thresholds for different applications, and establishing post-market surveillance approaches (Osa-Sanchez et al. 2025).

1.8 CONCLUSION

Wearable sensor-based sleep apnea detection has evolved substantially in recent years, progressing from proof-of-concept studies to systems approaching clinical viability. Current research has demonstrated that diverse physiological signals, including PPG, SpO_2, ECG, and respiratory effort, can be reliably captured using wearable devices and analyzed to detect sleep apnea with accuracy often exceeding 90%.

Significant methodological advances have shaped this progress. Multiscale feature engineering has shown that effective detection does not necessarily require the highest temporal resolution, as certain nonlinear features maintain strong correlations with sleep apnea severity even when computed from coarsely sampled data. This finding has important implications for consumer wearable devices, where battery life and storage constraints favor lower sampling rates. DL architectures, particularly CNNs and LSTMs, have achieved performance that approaches or exceeds that of traditional ML methods while reducing the need for manual feature engineering. Model compression techniques, including pruning and quantization, have enabled the deployment of sophisticated models on resource-constrained wearable hardware.

Significant challenges remain before wearable devices can serve as primary diagnostic tools or be widely adopted for large-scale screening. Signal quality issues, including motion artifacts, variable device placement, and inter-device differences, continue to affect reliability. Class imbalance in training datasets and limited diversity in study populations raise concerns about model generalizability. The interpretability limitations of high-performing DL models present barriers to clinical adoption. Regulatory approval pathways remain uncertain, and comprehensive prospective validation across diverse clinical settings remains limited.

The most promising near-term applications likely involve screening and longitudinal monitoring rather than definitive diagnosis. Wearable devices could identify individuals at high-risk who should undergo formal PSG evaluation, potentially addressing the critical problem that over 80% of sleep apnea patients remain undiagnosed. For diagnosed patients, continuous home monitoring could track treatment effectiveness, detect changes requiring clinical attention, and provide insights into how lifestyle factors influence sleep apnea severity.

Future advancements will depend on coordinated efforts across multiple domains. Technological advances in sensor design, materials, and edge computing will improve signal quality and enable more sophisticated on-device analysis. Methodological innovations in personalized modeling, multimodal fusion, and explainable AI will enhance both performance and clinical interpretability. Large-scale prospective validation studies across diverse populations will establish real-world effectiveness and identify appropriate use cases. Collaborative efforts to standardize data collection, processing, and reporting will accelerate progress and enable regulatory approval.

The integration of wearable sensor technology with AI has created unprecedented opportunities for transforming sleep apnea detection from an expensive, laboratory-based process to an accessible, home-based capability. While substantial work remains to fully realize this potential, the foundation has been established for wearable devices to play an increasingly important role in addressing this widespread and underdiagnosed condition. Success will ultimately be measured not by algorithmic sophistication but by improved patient outcomes, which include earlier detection, better monitoring, more effective treatment, and ultimately, reduced cardiovascular complications and improved quality of life for the millions affected by sleep apnea.

REFERENCES

Franklin, K. A., and Lindberg, E. Obstructive sleep apnea is a common disorder in the population—a review on the epidemiology of sleep apnea. *Journal of Thoracic Disease*, 7(8), 1311–1322, 2015.

Hayano, J., Yamamoto, H., Nonaka, I., et al. Quantitative detection of sleep apnea with wearable watch device. *PLoS ONE*, 15(11), e0237279, 2020.

Hoang, N. H., and Liang, Z. Detection and severity classification of sleep apnea using continuous wearable SpO_2 signals: A multi-scale feature approach. *Sensors*, 25, 1698, 2025.

Jiang, X., Ren, Y., Wu, H., Li, Y., and Liu, F. Convolutional neural network based on photoplethysmography signals for sleep apnea syndrome detection. *Frontiers in Neuroscience*, 17, 1222715, 2023.

John, A., Cardiff, B., and John, D. A 1D-CNN based deep learning technique for sleep apnea detection in IoT sensors. *arXiv preprint arXiv:2105.00528v1*, 2021.

Osa-Sanchez, A., Ramos-Martinez-de-Soria, J., Mendez-Zorrilla, A., Oleagordia Ruiz, I., and Garcia-Zapirain, B. Wearable sensors and artificial intelligence for sleep apnea detection: A systematic review. *Journal of Medical Systems*, 49, 66, 2025.

Paul, T., Hassan, O., Alaboud, K., et al. ECG and SpO_2 signal-based real-time sleep apnea detection using feed-forward artificial neural network. *AMIA Joint Summits Translational Science Proceedings*, 379–385, 2022.

Wang, J., Xue, J., Zou, Y., et al. A dual-modal wearable pulse detection system integrated with deep learning for high-accuracy and low-power sleep apnea monitoring. *Advanced Science*, 12(24), 2501750, 2025.

Zahra, M., and Siamak, M., SleepLiteCNN: Energy-efficient sleep apnea subtype classification with 1-second resolution using single-lead ECG. arXiv *preprint arXiv:2508.02718v1*, 2025.

2 Deep Learning-Driven Classification Techniques for Wearable and Nearable Health Devices

R. Girija, S.L. Jayalakshmi, and S.L. Jothi Lakshmi

2.1 INTRODUCTION

Wearable devices (smartwatches, fitness trackers, and health-monitoring bands) and nearable technologies embedded in smart environments have changed the process of collecting and analyzing data on human activity and health. The continuous acquisition of signals from motion and physiological sensors delivers helpful information for daily activity recognition and gesture detection, as well as for medical diagnostics and sports performance monitoring. Lightweight models, edge processing, and federated learning (FL) models are becoming popular to overcome the limitations of lightweight and embedded devices. Besides, explainability has a crucial role in safety-related fields like healthcare, where the ability to gain insight into decision processes is just as significant as precision. Although much has been done, there are still a number of issues, such as personalization, regulatory acceptance, energy efficiency, and ethical issues, that require tackling to support sustainable adoption. Figure 2.1 summarizes this chapter.

2.2 BACKGROUND AND MOTIVATION

The recent development of wearable or nearable sensors is poised to change health and human activity monitoring, but processing this type of data is associated with latency, energy consumption, and privacy concerns. The ability of deep learning (DL) models to run on physical hardware can provide inference at a scale of a split second and eliminate the need for an internet connection, while ensuring sensitive data is not stored in the cloud and is not lost. Signal fusion can be achieved by combining signals from accelerometers, electrocardiographs (ECGs), and electroencephalographs (EEGs) to improve accuracy and robustness across diverse environments. The strategy will enable the delivery of real-time, personalized analytics not only in the healthcare sphere but also in sports, while ensuring user privacy and battery life.

DOI: 10.1201/9781003500445-2

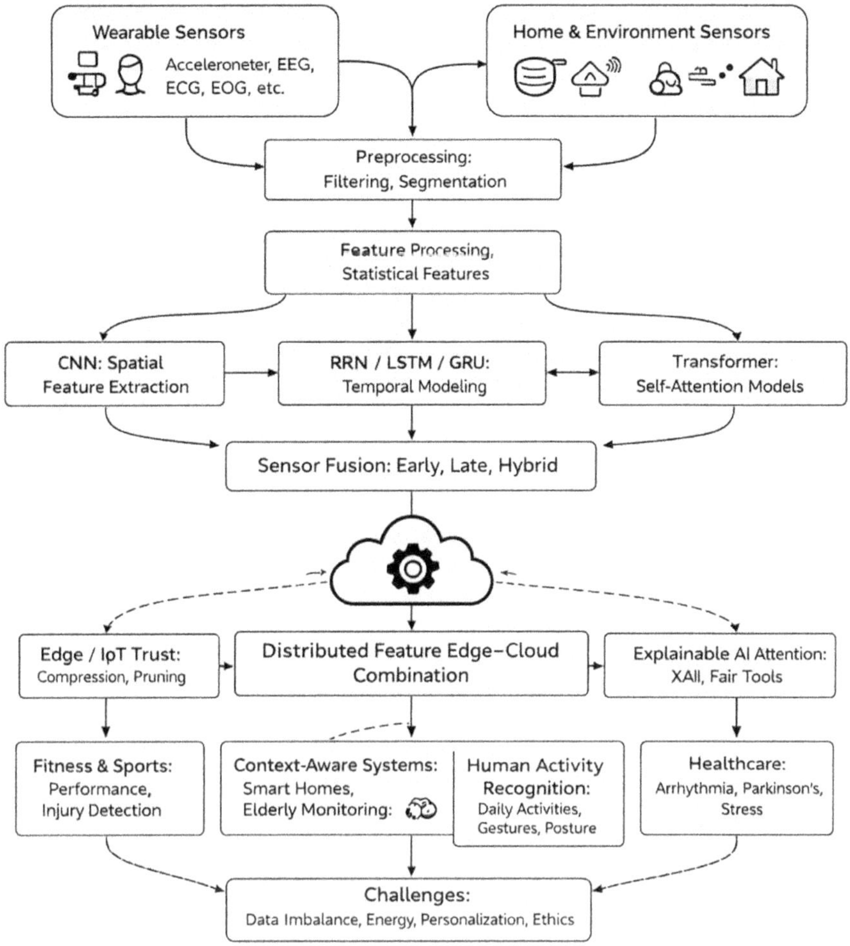

FIGURE 2.1 Overview of the Chapter.

2.2.1 Deep Learning Architectures for Wearable Sensor Data Classification

Wearable and nearable sensors, such as accelerometers, gyroscopes, EEG, ECG, and electromyography (EMG), currently generate rich, continuous data streams that are key to activity and health monitoring. DL models such as convolutional neural networks (CNNs), recurrent neural networks (RNNs), long short-term memory (LSTM), gated recurrent units (GRUs), and transformers can automatically learn complex temporal and spatial features from this data and achieve highly accurate, efficient classification on devices with limited resources. Karako (2024) noted that the market for wearable health devices has been booming over the last few years due to the need to monitor health status in real time through sensors, including ECG, photoplethysmography (PPG), and motion detectors.

The tiny body movements generated by each heartbeat and each breath are captured by wearable devices that use BCG. By observing these mechanical cues, they approximate heart rate, breathing rate, and minute-to-minute positional or sleep-related variations. Wearables based on ballistocardiography (BCG) can monitor sleep quality and how the body functions when resting. Alterations in the BCG pattern may also indicate stress, fatigue, or changes in cardiovascular workload. Altogether, BCG in wearables is a convenient and consistent way to track health and well-being daily. This data is used to recognize activities, detect anomalies, and predict early-stage diseases using DL. Although most research focuses on short-term outcomes, long-term observation of user behavior and physiology can provide more precise health-related information, as illustrated in Figure 2.2. It is essential to combine wearable data and electronic health records to enable individualized disease prediction and lifestyle guidance. Those systems would be able to change preventive care and greatly enhance the quality of life.

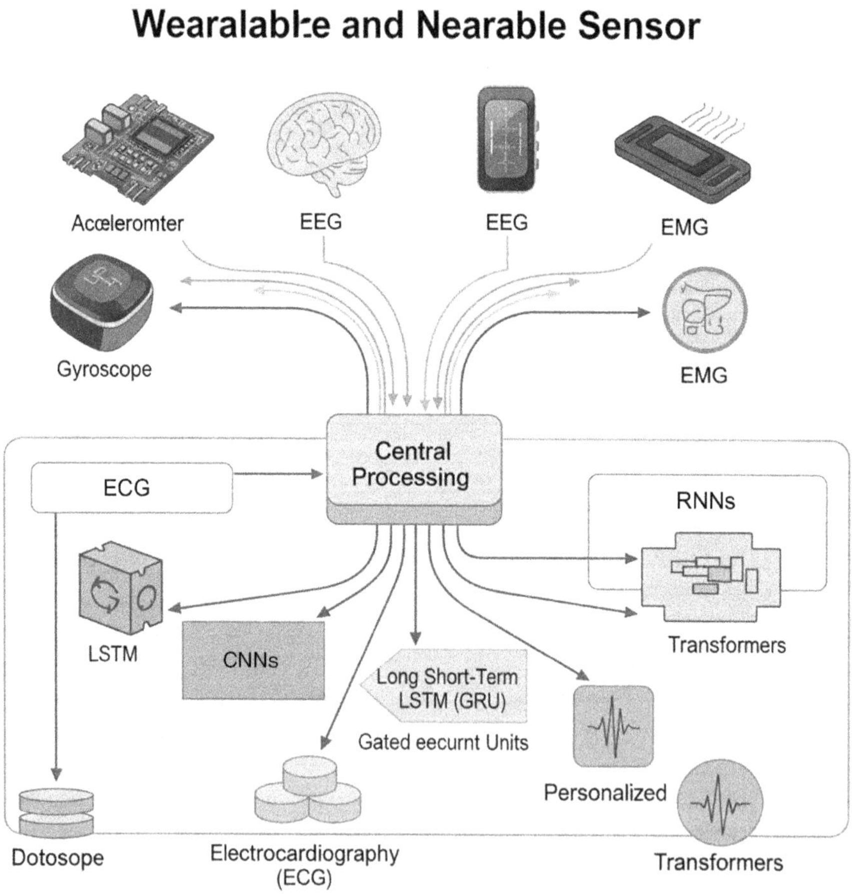

FIGURE 2.2 Deep Learning Architectures for Wearable Sensor Data Classification.

2.2.2 Human Activity Recognition Using Wearables and Nearables

Wearable and nearable devices provide continuous streams of motion and physiological data despite practical challenges such as user variability, noisy readings, and uneven sensor placement. Real-world human activity can be detected using this information. Benchmark datasets, such as University of California, Irvine – human activity recognition (UCI-HAR), OPPORTUNITY activity recognition, wireless sensor data mining (WISDM), physical activity monitoring dataset (PAMAP2), and Mobile Health (MHealth), enable researchers to evaluate and compare approaches efficiently by providing a standardized environment for accurate testing. Rani et al. (2023) elaborated that human activity recognition (HAR) based on EMG has been on a roll due to its application in clinical diagnosis, rehabilitation, and motion intention recognition like in Figure 2.3. Recent papers point to the fact that artificial intelligence (AI) has improved the classification of EMG-based activities, and much has been done on preprocessing to improve signal quality such as filtering, normalization and removal of noise. Both time- and frequency-based feature extraction techniques remain at the core of the study of muscle activity patterns. Machine learning (ML) and DL methods have also been used to enhance their own classification performance, and each has unique strengths and weaknesses. Integration of hardware and software is also highlighted to enable real-time monitoring. Future research directions and open issues are identified by current research and offer opportunities for more robust EMG-driven HAR systems. As explained by Alqudah and Moussavi (2025), HAR with wearables and nearables has emerged as a mainstream research field for monitoring and understanding human behavior. These machines can continuously monitor daily activity, gestures, and postures with great precision, without being intrusive. Physiological sensors such as EMG, gyroscopes, and accelerometers are used in wearable devices to collect motion and physiological data, while nearable devices monitor the surrounding environment. Combined, they offer useful insights for use in the fields of healthcare, fitness, rehabilitation, and human-computer interaction. Such integration not only facilitates real-time tracking but also enables individual feedback and improved quality of life.

2.2.3 Multimodal Sensor Fusion for Classification

Researchers have shown that wearable inertial measurement unit (IMU) sensors (e.g., accelerometers), in combination with in-home location systems (e.g., real-time location system or RTLS) and environmental sensors, can significantly improve HAR, achieving 86% accuracy and high F1-scores in daily living conditions. Other smart home applications combine accelerometer motion data with visual or ambient sensor data at the feature and decision levels using CNN+SVM (i.e., convolutional neural network + Support Vector Machine) models and ensemble architectures to achieve more reliable, context-informed activity recognition across modalities. Lara and Labrador (2013) gave a detailed overview and assessment of the DL methodologies in biomedical signal processing and demonstrated advancements in network designs, including CNNs, RNNs, Transformers, and hybrid designs. It discusses preprocessing and feature extraction techniques and demonstrates their

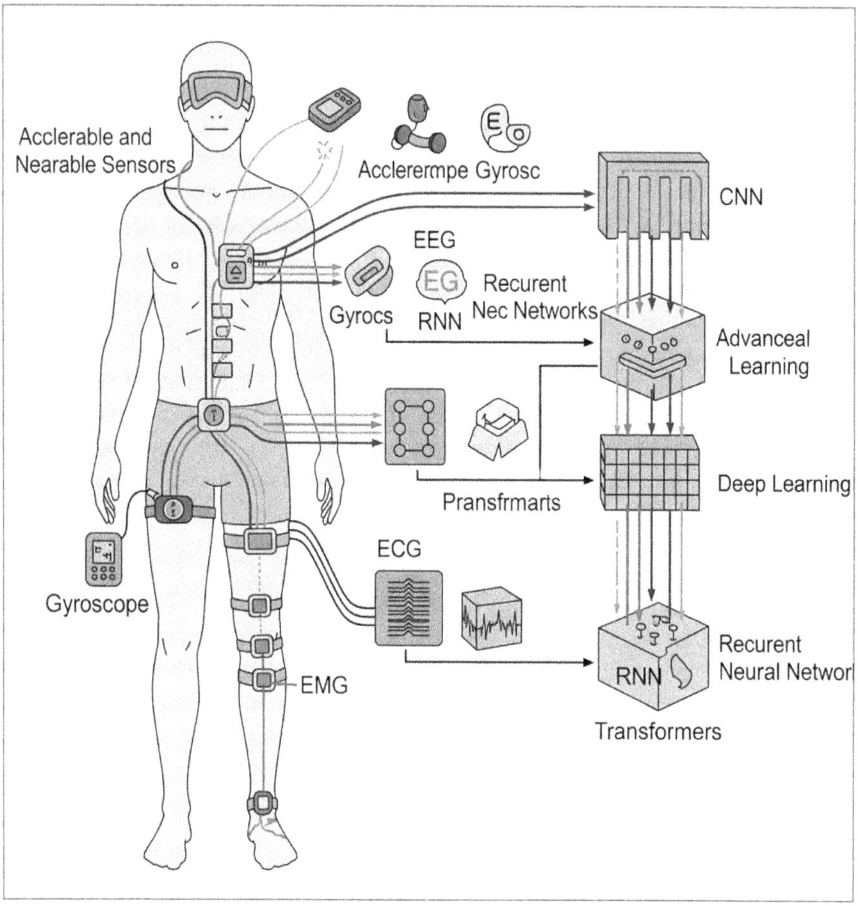

FIGURE 2.3 Human Activity Recognition Using Wearables and Nearables.

impact on accuracy, robustness, and efficiency in arrhythmia classification, seizure detection, and anomaly segmentation. Experimental findings support the superiority of DL over conventional methodologies, as it is more accurate, operates in real-time, and is more robust to noise in ECG, EEG, and EMG signals. Precision, recall, F1-score, the area under the receiver operating characteristic curve (AUC, also called ROC AUC), and computational complexity are also benchmarked in the study. The most important issues are resolved through synthetic data generation, interpretability tools, and privacy-protecting solutions such as FL. In general, the paper provides a systematic taxonomy, combines the new paradigms, and relates technical advances with scalability in clinical context and compliance with regulation, making the process of deploying reliable biomedical AI systems feasible, as illustrated in Figure 2.4. Hoang, et al. (2025) investigated the role of AI in changing the wearables or smartwatches, fitness bands, smart clothing, and eye wear. By integrating ML and DL into the Internet of Things (IoT), devices enable more

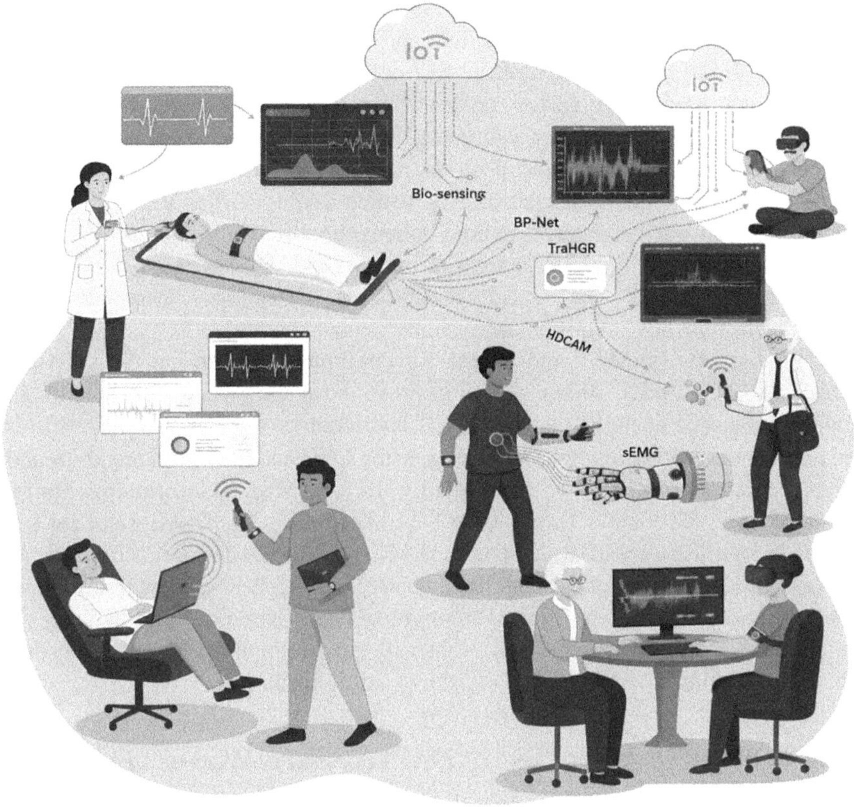

FIGURE 2.4 Multimodal Sensor Fusion for Classification.

sophisticated capabilities in activity recognition, health tracking, and personalized feedback. Methods based on CNNs and RNNs have been used for stress detection from heart rate variability and for real-time muscular control and exercise suggestions. Other meteorological aspects, such as accuracy, precision, and sampling rate, which determine AI performance in wearables, are also discussed in the work. It shows the impact of algorithmic decisions on efficiency and appropriateness in real-time operation on resource-constrained devices. Lastly, privacy and security concerns are also considered in the research, and the implementation of AI-based wearable technologies is kept as safe as possible in the real world. According to Jeong et al. (2022), noninvasive digital biomarkers are taking a central stage in digital healthcare because they are easy to measure and rely on raw data, and recent progress in DL enables their analysis through representation learning that discovers features and supports supervised prediction. The clinical applications express the ability to apply various DL methods to all types of data. Meanwhile, concurrent analysis of multidimensional data has become a strong approach that may yield more detailed biomarkers. It has been found that integrating heterogeneous sources via dimensionality reduction and multimodal integration not only improves performance but also leverages the complementarity of the various data streams. These integrative biomarkers are especially useful in situations where one or more signals need to be considered jointly, as they capture the fine details and interactions among signals; thus, they can be detected earlier, predict disease symptoms more accurately, and ultimately lead to better patient treatment. Zabihi (2023) clarified the wearable technologies, which are a promising post-smartphone platform that has found use in healthcare, robotic prosthesis control, Augmented Reality/Virtual Reality (AR/VR), human-machine interaction, and remote patient support. Their popularity is driven by the development of flexible electronics, the IoT, and cloud systems, as well as the growing needs of tech-savvy consumers and elderly customers. Wearable devices in healthcare typically record noninvasive biosignals, including ECG, PPG, surface electromyography (sEMG), and others, for continuous monitoring. This dissertation aims to develop DL structures that improve the accuracy and efficiency of such devices. First, one of the models (BP-Net) is offered for subject-specific, cuff-less, and continuous blood pressure monitoring, using ECG and PPG measurements and a combined dataset from MIMIC-I and MIMIC-III (i.e., Medical Information Mart for Intensive Care). Second, a Transformer-based hybrid model, Transformer for hand gesture recognition (TraHGR), enhances sEMG-based hand gesture recognition performance and can be used for prosthetic control and AR/VR. Lastly, it is proposed to use a light CNN attention hybrid, hierarchical depth-wise convolution along with the attention mechanism (HDCAM), that will provide both accuracy and resource efficiency, making it viable for real-world wearable scenarios.

2.2.4 Healthcare Applications of Deep Learning in Wearable Disease Monitoring

Wearable DL models that use CNNs and hybrid architectures are excellent at identifying cardiac abnormalities, such as arrhythmias, and often deliver real-time performance and high diagnostic accuracy (e.g., > 90%). Multimodal sensor and DL fusion improves accuracy and user comfort by enabling early, noninvasive seizure forecasting for neurological conditions such as epilepsy. While awaiting regulatory approval for clinical use, AI applied to continuous wearable data enables proactive detection of glucose patterns and health insights during the monitoring of metabolic illnesses like diabetes. Hurley et al. (2019) described that cardiovascular disorders cause nearly one in three deaths in the United States. Most decisions rely heavily on short hospital stays, missing the broader picture of patient health. Intelligent sensing and analytics for longitudinal monitoring can help gain deeper insight into disease patterns and support risk forecasting. The field has three requirements: strong sensing in the presence of noisy or missing observations, more sophisticated analytics to monitor persistent risk, and explainable, personalized ML for clinical decision-making. Addressing these gaps provides great opportunities to change the cardiovascular care as populations grow older because of increased life expectancy and decreasing birth rates; these groups are exposed to the challenges of injuries, diminished mobility, and mental health problems that affect the quality of life. Ni et al. (2024) clarified that in aging populations, the factors are injuries, diminished mobility, and mental health issues that affect the quality of life. One of the most important technologies adopted to support healthy aging is wearable sensor-based human activity recognition (WSHAR). Nevertheless, the available surveys primarily focus on single-sensor or DL methods, ignoring the fact that human interactions are multisensory. Multimodal ML, which combines diverse data, provides a path towards more intelligent and robust WSHAR systems. This survey presents a survey of recent sensor modalities, DL techniques, multimodal techniques, and visual, non-visual, and non-visual-only systems. It further relates computer vision and natural language processing (NLP) to WSHAR lessons and identifies open issues and research opportunities to be developed in the future.

Maqbool et al. (2025) explained how generative AI approaches such as GANs and VAEs can be used to make wearable devices more personalized, offer personalized recommendations, be smarter, and be more human-computer interactive. Current devices like Muse headbands, OrCam MyEye, and Garmin demonstrate their capabilities in stress management, visual support, and sports statistics. These AI-enabled wearables have potential in healthcare, sports, and smart cities, but there are still a few issues, especially in data privacy, regulatory compliance, energy use, and clinical uptake. These concerns, combined with advances in DL and HAR, will help make smart wearables more widely accepted and more innovative. Despite rapid technological changes, Saad et al. (2024) stated that disease outbreaks are among the primary concerns worldwide, and healthcare professionals must focus on their prevention and management. In the current hectic schedule, it is hard to stay healthy, which is where smart health monitoring systems are needed. ML and wearable devices have become potent tools for monitoring vital signs, tracking daytime activity, and enabling early diagnosis in the elderly. The medical sensor technology of the last five years has accelerated innovation in new wearable applications. Nevertheless, studies on implementing ML in these devices are rather scarce. In this paper, the current advances in ML-based healthcare wearables are listed and reviewed, and the challenges to their broader use are outlined. According to Fei et al. (2021), health is a major determinant of quality of life, and there is increased interest in devices that can monitor human health in real-time and quickly. This paper presents a systematic review of data mining and ML applications in wearable health monitoring (WHM). It includes older ML methods such as neural networks, SVMs, Kriging models, and principal component analysis, as well as more modern techniques such as DL. The review finds that DL outperforms traditional techniques in feature extraction and classification accuracy. To provide more specific information, the classifier performance is addressed within the frames of detection, monitoring, identification, and reliability. Since sensor data in WHM are time series, the research will also provide information on the use of DL in particular health areas. It identifies future directions for enhancing DL-based algorithms in wearable health applications. Table 2.1 presents a comparative analysis of various DL architectures—such as CNN, LSTM, and hybrid CNN-LSTM models—demonstrating that hybrid networks generally yield the highest recognition accuracy in wearable sensor tasks. For example, CNN-LSTM consistently outperforms standalone models and alternatives like CNN-GRU, achieving up to ~95.9% average accuracy on activity datasets

TABLE 2.1
Comparative Analysis of Deep Learning-Based Algorithms in Wearable Applications

Ref.	Focus	Methods/ Tech.	Applications	Research Gaps
Karako (2024)	Wearables + DL	DL integration in health	Preventive healthcare, disease monitoring	Lack of long-term clinical trials, privacy-preserving DL has not matured, and limited personalization for diverse populations.
Rani et al. (2023)	sEMG + AI for HAR	ML + DL on EMG	Activity recognition, rehabilitation	Robust real-time EMG processing is missing, high noise sensitivity is present, and datasets are not standardized.
Alqudah and Moussavi (2025)	Biomedical signals + DL	CNN, RNN, hybrid DL	ECG, EEG, EMG diagnosis	The explainability of DL, generalization across datasets, and multimodal integration remain underdeveloped.
Lara and Labrador (2013)	ML/DL in IoT wearables	Edge AI, DL	Smart health monitoring	Edge devices face latency and energy bottlenecks, no unified framework for IoT security + AI.
Hoang (2025)	Digital biomarkers	DL on noninvasive data	Chronic disease tracking	Lack of clinically validated datasets, limited regulatory frameworks, and reproducibility concerns.
Jeong et al. (2022)	Hybrid wearable signal processing	DNN + hybrid models	Noise removal + learning	Scalability issues, hybrid methods are still theoretical, and there are few real-world deployments.
Zabihi (2023)	HAR with wearables	Classical ML	Activity recognition	Small, homogeneous datasets, battery/sensor limitations, and a lack of temporal modeling.
Hurley et al. (2019)	Cardiovascular sensing	Sensor + analytics	CVD monitoring	Multimodal fusion has not matured, long-term monitoring reliability is weak, and integration into clinical workflows is lacking.

TABLE 2.1 (Continued)
Comparative Analysis of Deep Learning-Based Algorithms in Wearable Applications

Ref.	Focus	Methods/ Tech.	Applications	Research Gaps
Ni et al. (2024)	Multimodal HAR	DL + multiple sensors	Complex action recognition	Dataset diversity is low, TL remains underexplored, and the temporal dynamics of multimodal data are insufficiently understood.
Maqbool et al. (2025)	Generative AI + wearables	GenAI integration	Data augmentation, synthetic sensing	Trustworthiness of GenAI output remains untested, ethical/ interpretability concerns persist, and hardware support for real-time GenAI is lacking.
Saad et al. (2024)	ML + wearables in healthcare	Classical + DL	General healthcare	No standards for interoperability, fragmented data pipelines, and an absence of scalable deployment strategies.
Fei et al. (2021)	ML/DL for WHM	CNN, RNN, SVM	Health monitoring	Computational cost is high, edge deployment is limited, and cross-domain evaluation is lacking.

2.3 DEEP LEARNING FOR FITNESS AND SPORTS ANALYTICS

2.3.1 Edge Artificial Intelligence, TinyML, and Federated Privacy-Preserving Wearables

The rise in the use of wearable devices and health apps has been a major influence on sports health monitoring (SHM), especially among individuals who engage in frequent physical exercise. Proper evaluation of sport performance is essential for high performance, and automated sport-specific movement recognition can fill gaps in manual assessment. Sports-related fitness and analytics can usually have a long-term impact on the health, sport performance, and financial well-being of the athletes, as is depicted in Figure 2.5. Wearable technologies and analytical tools are an excellent solution to identify the risks of injuries and preventative strategies. These devices may measure vital functional capabilities before vigorous exercise, thereby improving the management of sports injuries. Preventing and forecasting sports injuries is essential

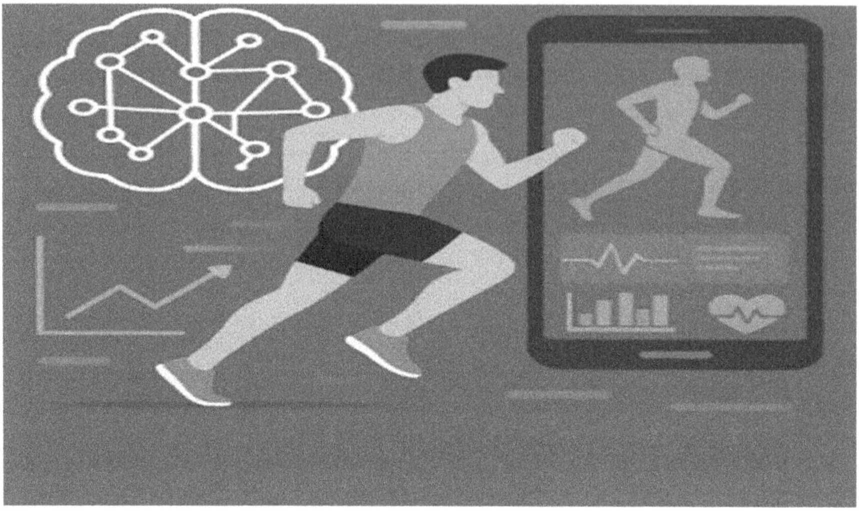

FIGURE 2.5 Deep Learning for Fitness and Sports Analytics.

to safeguard athletes' health and maintain high performance. DL offers new tools for analyzing complicated data and detecting concealed patterns of injury.

2.3.2 Deep Learning for Fitness and Sports Analytics

The article by Souaifi et al. (2024) explores the use of AI in sports biomechanics to enhance performance and minimize injury risk. Seven hundred and thirty-three relevant studies were identified in five major databases, including publications from 2015 to 2024. Recent studies indicate a distinct drift in assessment approaches based on ML, specifically CNNs and computer vision. These technologies have demonstrated excellent capabilities for analyzing athletes' techniques and tracking motion with high precision. There is also the application of AI systems to predict and reduce the risk of recurring injuries. Random forests (RF) have been successfully applied to predict injury probability. Meanwhile, new analytical tools are being developed to help coaches make sense of this information in a way that athletes can respond to. However, despite these developments, certain problems remain. Also, it remains difficult to consolidate information across platforms, and athletes and trainers want AI systems to provide clearer explanations. The other problem is the explanation of how these technologies are applied in daily training scenarios. With the advanced sensors in wearables, which are becoming increasingly widespread, as noted by Kovoor et al. (2024) and Zadeh et al. (2021), among others, wearables are revolutionizing sport science not only in performance tracking but also in injury prevention. Wearable systems can also measure a wide range of variables, such as heart rate, muscle movements, and movement kinematics. The information is automatically handled so that the athletes can get feedback immediately. Models built on this information can warn of potential danger, and even minor gait or biomechanical alterations can suggest the emergence of soft-tissue or heat-related injury. It has also been proven that athletes respond more positively to increasing their training loads than to repeating high-intensity training when they are not in optimal condition. The article by Sadr et al. (2025) compares various DL architectures, including CNNs, RNNs, and LSTM. LSTM performed well at predicting complex injuries across a range of sporting situations. In a similar vein, the study by Alzahrani and Ullah (2024) analyzed wearable devices, including IMUs, surface EMG sensors, and pressure sensors, to provide more detailed information on sports physiotherapy. The mean heart rate was 76.5 bpm, the mean joint motion was 112.3 o, and the muscle activity was approximately 43.2. There were significant differences among sportsmen, which evidences the principle of individual monitoring and treatment. Wearable-based sessions yielded better results than those without wearables. These findings encourage the incorporation of devices into physiotherapy, where real-time biomechanical and physiological monitoring can personalize care for each athlete. Chao et al. (2024) proposed an IoT-based framework backed by big data analytics and CNNs to enhance sports health management. Wearable data was used to prevent injuries and enhance athletic performance.

2.3.3 Edge Artificial Intelligence and TinyML for Wearable or Nearable Classification

Alajlan and Ibrahim (2022) examined a field called TinyML. They identified the need to use ML on low-power IoT edge devices for real-time decision-making without relying on cloud computing. TinyML is used in applications across healthcare, smart homes, and industry to reduce latency, save bandwidth, and enhance privacy. Their paper also discussed embedding DL models on microcontrollers and emphasized lightweight design, energy efficiency, and low memory requirements. The main issues of model compression, pruning, and quantization were tackled, and illustrations were presented in the areas of predictive maintenance, health monitoring, and sensing. In the future, the research identified hybrid edge-cloud solutions, hardware accelerators, and TinyML systems as promising areas of interest. Channar et al. (2025) intended to conduct a review of the role of edge AI in real-time health tracking using wearable IoT devices. Edge computing lowers latency, safeguards privacy, and reduces bandwidth by processing data at the edge rather than transmitting it to remote servers. The advantages are faster reaction times for matters such as glucose monitoring, heart-rate analysis, and respiratory tracking. Nevertheless, drawbacks run sophisticated models on small devices were noted as well. The chapter emphasizes algorithmic trade-offs and the optimization of accuracy, energy consumption, and performance. Ethical factors, especially privacy and impartiality (i.e., fairness), were considered, and the next steps are adaptive learning, hardware accelerators, and further development of TinyML, as demonstrated in Figure 2.6.

2.3.4 Federated and Privacy-Preserving Deep Learning in Wearables

Wang et al. (2025) propose a FL-based privacy-preserving method for healthcare analytics. As wearable and IoT devices generate various streams of data, centralized approaches raise concerns about data leakage. In FL, model training does not involve directly sharing sensitive information, which ensures confidentiality. The accuracy

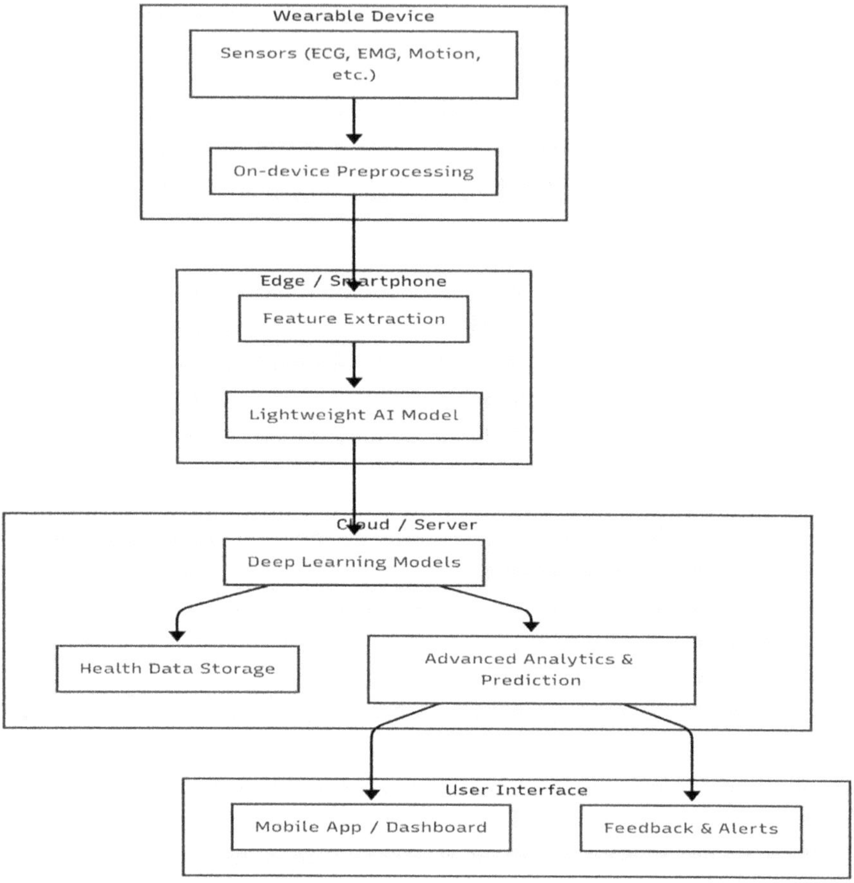

FIGURE 2.6 Edge Artificial Intelligence and TinyML for Wearable or Nearable Classification.

and robustness of the tests were found to be higher than those of the conventional methods, but communication overhead and device variability were higher and remain a challenge. Similarly, Deepak et al. (2024) examined privacy-conscious DL methods for wearable health data, including encryption, anonymization, and FL. Findings showed that accuracy, although there are still some issues with computation and scalability.

2.3.4.1 Context-Aware Classification on Nearable Environments

Lastly, Mouhim and Lachhab (2025) have introduced a framework, which combines IoT, analytics, and big data platforms to design context-aware systems. Data from IoT devices was constantly processed in real-time, enabling intelligent responses, predictions, and resource management. The framework was confirmed for healthcare, industrial, and smart city applications, demonstrating increased responsiveness and adaptability. Nevertheless, other problems, such as interoperability, privacy, and power consumption, were cited as critical issues before full-scale implementation.

Akbari et al. (2021) proposed a framework to identify complex activities of daily living (ADLs). Noisy data, variability in undertaking activities, and multi-user scenarios are also considered in the framework. Findings verify that the technique can provide strong, highly precise recognition of complex ADLs.

Table 2.2 summarizes the major areas of focus, such as real-time tracking of workload, injury prevention, and rehabilitation throughout sports, and demonstrates it through such approaches as the use of accelerometers, global positioning system (GPS) integration, and DL analytics. It also has a special practical use in fatigue management and biomechanical risk prediction, and it points out serious gaps, such as a lack of device reliability, interpretation difficulties, and a lack of longitudinal and large-scale field studies.

2.4 NEXT-GENERATION DEEP LEARNING FOR WEARABLES AND NEARABLES: ADAPTATION, EXPLAINABILITY, AND FUTURE CHALLENGES

2.4.1 Transfer Learning and Domain Adaptation for Wearable Data

The article by Dhekane and Ploetz (2025) is a detailed survey of transfer learning (TL) techniques for sensor-based HAR. The article categorizes various transfer cases (e.g., cross-subject, cross-device, cross-dataset recognition) and connects them with the respective strategies (e.g., feature adaptation and model fine-tuning). It also describes the limitations of existing benchmarks, explains the challenges, including sensor heterogeneity and negative transfer, and outlines a roadmap that prioritizes reproducibility, interpretability, and efficiency when deploying HAR in the real-world. In Kazemi et al. (2025), a TL architecture for respiration rate estimation based on smartwatch PPG and accelerometers is presented. The proposed model combines big-picture pretraining with multiple domain-adaptation methods. This will enable it to make consistently precise forecasts, regardless of the machine user or the location of the sensors. Significant improvements were observed in estimation accuracy across different motion scenarios. Better still, the trade-offs between local device processing and cloud processing are also considered in this study. In the end, there is still a long way to go toward achieving the aim of deploying everyday consumer wearables to support continuous respiratory monitoring, but this work represents a significant step in the right direction. The researchers Jeong et al. (2025) developed a customized health prediction model that incorporates TL and what they term strategic overfitting. They refine the general population models with a little user-specific data rather than general population models. This individual touch improves near-term forecasting accuracy while carefully considering overfitting risks. When they applied it to wearable health data, they found significant promise in custom-made tracking and prompt issue identification. Nonetheless, the work has also mentioned that there is still a need to determine how to eliminate privacy concerns and ensure transparency in operations. The central argument of the article by Dai et al. (2025) is that we can employ Wi-Fi channel state information (CSI) to perform cross-domain gesture recognition. Their method was based on meta-TL, enabling the model to learn rapidly with minimal calibration information.

TABLE 2.2
Overview of Literature on Wearable Sensor-Based Sports Injury Monitoring: Focus, Techniques, Applications, and Research Gaps

Ref.	Focus	Techniques Used	Applications	Research Gaps
Souaifi et al. (2025)	AI in sports biomechanics – wearables, motion analysis, injury prevention	Scoping review, survey of AI + wearable methods	Sports biomechanics, injury prevention	Limited integration of AI with real-time biomechanical feedback; need for longitudinal studies
Kovoor, et al. (2024)	Sensor-enhanced wearables for injury prevention	Automated analytics, sensor fusion	Sports injury monitoring and prevention	Lack of large-scale trials; interoperability challenges between devices
Zadeh et al. (2021)	Predicting sports injuries using wearables + data analysis	Predictive modeling, ML	Injury prediction in athletes	Small datasets; difficulty in generalizing models across sports
Sadr et al. (2025)	Injury prediction using DL	CNNs, RNNs for time-series	Enhanced performance and safety in athletics	Model explainability: need for real-time deployment
Alzahrani and Ullah (2024)	Biomechanical analytics with wearables for precision health	AI-based biomechanical analysis	Precision monitoring in sports	Limited personalization of models; challenges in validation
Chao et al. (2024)	IoT-enabled health monitoring of students in sports	Big data analytics, CNN	Health monitoring for college students	Energy efficiency in IoT: generalization across diverse populations
Alajlan and Ibrahim (2022)	TinyML on IoT edge devices	TinyML, lightweight DL	Ultra-low-power edge AI	Limited model complexity due to device constraints
Channar et al. (2025)	Edge AI for low-latency wearable IoT health monitoring	Edge computing, AI frameworks	Real-time wearable IoT	Scalability, privacy, and standardization issues
Wang et al. (2025)	Privacy-preserving multimodal data fusion for healthcare	FL, heterogeneous data fusion	Smart healthcare with wearables	High communication overhead; heterogeneous device compatibility
Deepak et al. (2024)	Privacy-preserving DL for wearable health data	Privacy-preserving DL, secure analytics	Wearable health data utilization	Trade-off between privacy and model accuracy
Mouhim and Lachhab (2025)	Context awareness using IoT, AI, and big data	IoT integration, AI, big data analytics	Smart healthcare, sports, and daily monitoring	Data quality, scalability, and context adaptability
Akbari et al. (2024)	Context detection from nearables and passive sensing	Data-driven context detection, passive sensing, ML	Activity recognition, healthcare monitoring	High variability in daily living contexts; energy-efficient deployment

These findings were remarkable, with remarkable flexibility across various rooms, hardware, and user directions, and were more effective than conventional fine-tuning approaches. This shows the opportunities of RF-based sensing as a versatile, affordable gesture recognition method.

2.4.2 Explainable Deep Learning for Wearable Classification

DL that can be explained for Wearable Classification. Li et al. (2025) examined the concept of unsupervised multitarget TL that aims to enhance activity detection using wearable devices in the case of sensor-body position variation. Their approach learns a common representation across multiple unlabeled target positions, enabling constructive transfer of knowledge from a labeled source position. This approach demonstrates better recognition performance across a variety of sensor locations and reduces reliance on position-specific labeled datasets. The chapter presents scalable solutions for practical wearable activity recognition. The article by Kazemi et al. (2025) is an extensive survey of the security and privacy issues related to the use of the Internet of Medical Things (IoMT). The article discusses the application of DL and ML algorithms to overcome vulnerabilities, including data breaches, adversarial attacks, and unauthorized access in the IoMT ecosystems. It also mentions the drawbacks of current methods, such as scalability, computational complexity, and interpretability. The research finds barriers by synthesizing solutions derived recently. Regulatory compliance, interoperability, and energy-efficient implementation. The authors end with a prospective view of the fact that explainable AI, FL, and lightweight models should be used in order to provide robust, secure, and privacy-saving IoMT applications. Xu et al. (2025) provide the role of wearable technologies in Industry 5.0, with the focus on their use in the interaction of humans and machines and safety. The article presents an overview of new wearable devices such as AR glasses, smart protective equipment, and physiological monitors, and suggests that these may be used to increase productivity and safety in the industrial environment. Clusters like interoperability, privacy, and ergonomically design are also discussed, and suggestions on how wearable analytics can be integrated into real-time industrial procedures are made. Yeong et al. (2025) survey multi-sensor fusion approaches in autonomous vehicles and evaluate the role of explainable AI (XAI) in enhancing system transparency. The review analyses the strategy for integrating light detection and ranging (LiDAR), radar, camera, and inertial data and discusses XAI as a means of providing interpretation for perception and decision-making modules. The authors note the lack of evaluation metrics, and they request the new frameworks in which the fusion accuracy and the quality of the explanation are evaluated simultaneously, and the role of trust in autonomous vehicle systems is vital. A side-by-side comparison of the current methods, including TL to adapt models across domains, TinyML techniques to deploy models to low-power devices, and FL to keep privacy under device, limits is provided in Table 2.3. It also identifies some critical issues, such as the high cost of communication and the other constraints of the model on limited hardware, and the generalization of the model that is required to be robust across different users and environments.

TABLE 2.3
Comparative Overview of Methods and Gaps in Transfer Learning, TinyML, and Privacy-Aware Wearable Systems

Ref.	Focus	Techniques Used	Applications	Research Gaps
Dhekane and Ploetz (2025)	TL in sensor-based human activity recognition	Feature adaptation, domain adaptation, fine-tuning	HAR	Limited generalization across diverse sensors; need for benchmark datasets
Kazemi et al. (2025)	Respiration rate estimation via smartwatch sensors	TL, sensor fusion (PPG + accelerometer)	WHM	Handling motion artifacts, improving real-time robustness
Jeong et al. (2025)	Personalized health prediction using wearable data	TL, strategic overfitting	Personalized healthcare	Balancing personalization versus generalization; limited long-term evaluation
Dai et al. (2025)	Cross-domain gesture recognition using Wi-Fi signals	Meta-TL, CSI analysis	Gesture recognition, HCI	Scalability across environments; limited real-world validation
Li et al. (2025)	Cross-body-position activity recognition	Multitarget unsupervised TL	Wearable HAR	Lack of labeled data for all positions; domain shift issues
Xu et al. (2025)	Role of wearables in Industry 5.0 for safety and HMI	Literature synthesis, comparative analysis	Industrial safety, human-machine interaction	Need for interoperability, real-world pilot studies
Yeong et al. (2025)	Multi-sensor fusion and XAI in autonomous vehicles	Sensor fusion (camera, radar, LiDAR), XAI models	Autonomous vehicles	Lack of explainability standards; computational efficiency concerns

2.4.3 Challenges and Future Directions

Difficulty of applying interpretable methods on resource-constrained IoT devices. Balancing effectiveness with the understandability of security models. Meeting ethical and regulatory transparency requirements in practice, as emphasized by Sharma et al. (2025), highlighted key hands-on challenges, including the lack of standardized evaluation frameworks for assessing quantum explainability and hardware constraints that limit the real-world deployment of quantum-enhanced vision models. Ensuring interpretability as a foundation for trust in quantum vision systems by Khan et al. (2025). Ethical concerns in deploying intelligent health technologies. Regulatory compliance when handling sensitive health data. Privacy risks in digital well-being and patient monitoring systems. Building and maintaining patient trust while adopting innovative solutions by Dhinakaran et al. (2025). Regulatory hurdles in implementing telehealth and wearable solutions. Data quality concerns affect the reliability of monitoring outcomes. Patient privacy issues in handling sensitive health information. Lack of standardized clinical validation for new technologies. Interoperability gaps across devices and platforms (Stan et al., 2025). Table 2.4 summarizes the main conclusions from all the references that use DL techniques.

The personalized and adaptive models moving forward should be improved to address individual differences in physiology and behavior, leveraging both the model's adaptive and personalized capabilities. Increasing energy efficiency at the edge through methods such as model compression and energy harvesting will extend device battery life while maintaining real-time performance. Scalability Privacy-aware FL systems will guarantee collaborative model learning among machines without centralizing sensitive information to overcome critical privacy and legislative issues. Lastly, it is important to promote cross-domain robustness and interpretability via TL and transparency tools to enable models to be applicable across users, devices, and environments and be considered trustworthy.

2.5 CONCLUSION

Wearable and nearable technologies have become effective tools for measuring health and fitness and for activity recognition. Their applicability has been extended to clinical decision support and smart environments due to the use of developed classification methods. Multimodal integration, FL, and lightweight deployment are moving forward, and explainable models are bridging technical advancement with the trustworthiness of the real-world. Nevertheless, constraints associated with sensor data inconsistency, user heterogeneity, and computational limitations remain debatable. These gaps should be addressed to provide a scalable, reliable, and acceptable solution in real-life situations.

TABLE 2.4
Summary of Studies on Machine Learning and Deep Learning for Wearable IoT Devices

Focus Area	Key Studies (Refs)	Devices / Sensors	DL/ML Approaches	Key Results / Findings
Activity and Motion Recognition	Rani et al. (2023), Lara and Labrador (2013), Hoang (2025), Ni et al. (2024), Akbari et al. (2021), Dhekane and Ploetz (2025), Dai et al. (2025), Li et al. (2025)	Accelerometer, gyroscope, IMUs, Wi-Fi, CSI	CNN, LSTM, Hybrid Models, TL	Achieved >95% accuracy in HAR; TL improves cross-domain and cross-body recognition; Wi-Fi-based gesture recognition is feasible.
Cardiac and Cardiovascular Health	Hurley et al. (2019), Saad et al. (2024), Fei, et al. (2021)	ECG, PPG, smartwatches	CNN, RNN, GNN	Cardiovascular disorder detection with **95–98% sensitivity**; edge deployment for real-time monitoring; survey identifies challenges in scaling.
Sleep and Respiratory Monitoring	Jeong et al. (2022), Kazemi et al. (2025)	Smartwatches, PPG, accelerometers	TL, Attention Models	Respiration rate estimation with **<5% error**; sleep stage classification >90% accuracy.
Mental Health, Stress and Emotion	Jeong et al. (2022), Dhinakaran et al. (2025)	HRV, EDA, multimodal wearable data	Multimodal Fusion Networks	AI-powered emotion/stress detection shows >90% accuracy; integration with wellness tech emphasized.
Sports and Injury Prevention	Souaifi et al. (2025), Kovoor et al. (2024), Zadeh (2021), Sadr (2025), Alzahrani and Ullah (2024), Chao et al. (2024)	Wearables, motion sensors, IoT devices	CNN, RNN, Edge AI	Sports biomechanics studies show that AI can detect early injury risk, and IoT-CNN models can monitor athlete health in real time.
Diabetes, Glucose, and Chronic Disease Management	Hoang et al. (2025), Saad et al. (2024),Fei et al. (2021), Wang et al. (2025)	Smart patches, CGM, IoT devices	FL, Transformers	Predictive glucose modeling supports **personalized treatment**; FL ensures privacy without performance loss.

Context-Aware Systems and Nearables	Hoang et al. (2025), Akbari et al. (2021), Xu et al. (2025)	Nearable IoT sensors, smart environments	Context-Aware AI, Graph Learning	Nearable devices improve ADL recognition, Industry 5.0 safety, and context detection at >90% precision.
Privacy and Security in Wearables	Wang et al. (2025), Deepak et al. (2024), Sharma et al. (2025), Dhinakaran et al. (2025)	Wearables, IoT devices	FL, Privacy-Preserving DL, XAI	Privacy-preserving FL is deployed for multimodal sensor fusion; explainable AI (XAI) enhances trust and adoption.
Edge and TinyML Deployments	Alajlan and Ibrahim (2022), Channar et al. (2025), Xu et al. (2025)	Edge devices, low-power IoT nodes	TinyML, Edge AI	Ultra-low-power inference (< 1 mW) is feasible; edge AI reduces latency, enabling continuous health monitoring.
Explainable AI (XAI) and Trust	Yeong et al. (2025), Sharma et al. (2025), Khan et al. (2025)	Multi-sensor systems	XAI, Quantum ML	XAI improves interpretability for clinicians and is gaining a growing role in safety-critical wearable deployments.
Future Directions and Systematic Reviews	Karako (2024), Alqudah and Moussavi (2025), Hoang, et al. (2025), Stan et al. (2025)	-	DL, ML, Generative AI	Reviews show that multimodal sensing, FL, edge deployment, and generative AI are emerging pillars in WHM.

REFERENCES

Akbari, A., Barton, A. R., Gazal, S., et al. (2024). Pervasive findings of directional selection realize the promise of ancient DNA to elucidate human adaptation. *bioRxiv* 2024.09.14.613021. https://doi.org/10.1101/2024.09.14.613021

Akbari, A., Grimsley, R., & Jafari, R. (2021). Data-driven context detection leveraging passively sensed nearables for recognizing complex activities of daily living. *ACM Transactions on Computing for Healthcare*, 2(2), 1–22.

Alajlan, N. N., & Ibrahim, D. M. (2022). TinyML: Enabling inference deep learning models on ultra-low-power IoT edge devices for AI applications. *Micromachines*, 13(6), 851.

Alqudah, A. M., & Moussavi, Z. (2025). A review of deep learning for biomedical signals: Current applications, advancements, future prospects, interpretation, and challenges. *Computers, Materials & Continua*, 83(3), 1–89.

Alzahrani, A., & Ullah, A. (2024). Advanced biomechanical analytics: Wearable technologies for precision health monitoring in sports performance. *Digital Health*, 10, 20552076241256745.

Channar, N. A., Koondhar, M. Y., Shaikh, S., Issani, F. N., Dahri, N. N., Maher, Z. A., & Ghulam, A. (2025). A review on edge ai for low-latency health monitoring in wearable iot devices: Challenges and future directions. *Spectrum of Engineering Sciences*, 3(7), 1424–1435.

Chao, Z., Yi, L., Min, L., & Long, Y. Y. (2024). IoT-enabled prediction model for health monitoring of college students in sports using big data analytics and convolutional neural network. *Mobile Networks and Applications*, 1–18.

Dai, P., Zhou, J., Ma, J., Zhang, H., & Wu, X. (2025). *Meta-Transfer Learning based Cross-Domain Gesture Recognition using WiFi Channel State Information*. IEEE Transactions on Consumer Electronics.

Deepak, G., Sharma, P., Jayachitra, S., Chepur, J., Srihari, T., & Judgi, T. (2024). Privacy-preserving deep learning approaches for effective utilization of wearable health data. *Measurement: Sensors*, 33, 101238.

Dhekane, S. G., & Ploetz, T. (2025). Transfer learning in sensor-based human activity recognition: A survey. *ACM Computing Surveys*, 57(8), 1–39.

Dhinakaran, D., Raja, S. E., Jasmine, J. J., Kumar, P. V., & Ramani, R. (2025). The future of well-being: AI-powered health management with privacy at its core. *Wellness Management Powered by AI Technologies*, 363–402.

Fei, C., Liu, R., Li, Z., Wang, T., & Baig, F. N. (2021). Machine and deep learning algorithms for wearable health monitoring. In: Manocha, A. K., Jain, S., Singh, M., Paul, S. (eds) *Computational Intelligence in Healthcare. Health Information Science*. Springer. https://doi.org/10.1007/978-3-030-68723-6_6

Hoang, M. L. (2025). *A Comprehensive Review of Machine Learning, and Deep Learning in Wearable IoT Devices*. IEEE Access.

Hurley, N. C., Spatz, E. S., Krumholz, H. M., Jafari, R., & Mortazavi, B. J. (2019). A survey of challenges and opportunities in sensing and analytics for cardiovascular disorders. *arXiv preprint arXiv*:1908.06170.

Jeong, H., Jeong, Y. W., Park, Y., Kim, K., Park, J., & Kang, D. R. (2022). Applications of deep learning methods in digital biomarker research using noninvasive sensing data. *Digital Health*, 8, 20552076221136642.

Jeong, I., Kong, S., Kim, Y., Kim, Y., Kim, B., Ahn, S. J., ... & Lee, H. (2025). Personalized health prediction AI models using transfer learning and strategic overfitting on wearable device data. *Journal of Medical Systems*, 49(1), 1–12.

Karako, K. (2024). Integration of wearable devices and deep learning: New possibilities for health management and disease prevention. *BioScience Trends*, 18(3), 201–205.

Kazemi, K., Azimi, I., Liljeberg, P., & Rahmani, A. M. (2025). Respiration rate estimation via smartwatch-based photoplethysmography and accelerometer data: A transfer learning approach. *Proceedings of the ACM on Interactive, Mobile, Wearable and Ubiquitous Technologies*, 9(1), 1–24.

Khan, A. I., Al Badi, A., & Alqahtani, M. (2025). Explainable artificial intelligence for computer vision and quantum machine learning. *Procedia Computer Science*, 258, 3723–3730.

Kovoor, M., Durairaj, M., Karyakarte, M. S., Hussain, M. Z., Ashraf, M., & Maguluri, L. P. (2024). Sensor-enhanced wearables and automated analytics for injury prevention in sports. *Measurement: Sensors*, 32, 101054.

Lara, O. D., & Labrador, M. A. (2013). A survey on human activity recognition using wearable sensors. *IEEE Communications Surveys & Tutorials*, 15(3), 1192–1209, doi: 10.1109/SURV.2012.110112.00192.

Li, J., Kang, P., & Shull, P. B. (2025). Multi-target unsupervised transfer learning improves wearable-sensor cross-body-position activity recognition via inter-target shared representation. *IEEE Sensors Journal*, 25(5), 9101–9112. doi: 10.1109/JSEN.2025.3528441.

Maqbool, K. Z., Ali, A., Asghar, S., Majeed, M., & Khamparia, A. (2025). Challenges and opportunities in integrating generative AI with wearable devices. *Artificial Intelligence in Microbial Research: Bridging the Gap,* 45, 385–398. https://doi.org/10.1007/978-981-96-3448-4_17

Mouhim, S. A. N. A. A., & Lachhab, F. A. D. W. A. (2025). *Towards a Context Awareness System using IoT, AI, and Big Data Technologies*. IEEE Access.

Ni, J., Tang, H., Haque, S. T., Yan, Y., & Ngu, A. H. (2024). A survey on multimodal wearable sensor-based human action recognition. *arXiv preprint arXiv*:2404.15349.

Rani, G. J., Hashmi, M. F., & Gupta, A. (2023). Surface electromyography and artificial intelligence for human activity recognition—A systematic review on methods, emerging trends applications, challenges, and future implementation. *IEEE Access*, 11, 105140–105169.

Saad, H. S., Zaki, J. F. W., & Abdelsalam, M. M. (2024). Employing of machine learning and wearable devices in healthcare system: Tasks and challenges. *Neural Comput & Applic*, 36, 17829–17849. https://doi.org/10.1007/s00521-024-10197-z

Sadr, M. M., Khani, M., & Tootkaleh, S. M. (2025). Predicting athletic injuries with deep learning: Evaluating CNNs and RNNs for enhanced performance and Safety. *Biomedical Signal Processing and Control*, 105, 107692.

Sharma, A., Sharma, N., & Jain, A. (2025). XAI-driven approaches for ensuring security and data protection in IoT. In *The Next Generation Innovation in IoT and Cloud Computing with Applications* (pp. 110–130). CRC Press. https://doi.org/10.1201/9781003406723

Souaifi, M., Dhahbi, W., Jebabli, N., Ceylan, H. İ., Boujabli, M., Muntean, R. I., & Dergaa, I. (2025). Artificial intelligence in sports biomechanics: A scoping review on wearable technology, motion analysis, and injury prevention. *Bioengineering*, 12(8), 887.

Stan, I. E., D'Auria, D., & Napoletano, P. (2025). A systematic literature review of innovations, challenges, and future directions in telemonitoring and wearable health technologies. *IEEE Journal of Biomedical and Health Informatics*, 30(3), 2630–2645. doi: 10.1109/JBHI.2025.3598056

Wang, J., Quasim, M. T., & Yi, B. (2025). Privacy-preserving heterogeneous multi-modal sensor data fusion via federated learning for smart healthcare. *Information Fusion*, 120, 103084.

Xu, J., Lee, K., Dias, I., Ranaweera, C., & Sinha, R. (2025). Wearable technologies for enhancing human-machine interaction and safety in industry 5.0: A review. *IEEE Sensors Journal*, 26(10), 14270–14280. doi: 10.1109/JSEN.2025.3595122

Yeong, D. J., Panduru, K., & Walsh, J. (2025). Exploring the unseen: A survey of multi-sensor fusion and the role of explainable ai (xai) in autonomous vehicles. *Sensors*, 25(3), 856.

Zabihi, S. (2023). Hybrid wearable signal processing/learning via deep neural networks (Doctoral dissertation, Concordia University).

Zadeh, A., Taylor, D., Bertsos, M., Tillman, T., Nosoudi, N., & Bruce, S. (2021). Predictin sports injuries with wearable technology and data analysis. *Information Systems Frontiers*, 23(4), 1023–1037.

3 Wearable Devices and Deep Learning for Tremor Monitoring, Parkinson's Disease Management, and Rehabilitation

Brindha A., Sridhar P. Arjunan, and N. Deepa

3.1 INTRODUCTION

Parkinson's disease (PD) is a progressive neurological disorder characterized by motor symptoms including tremors, rigidity, bradykinesia, and postural instability. Ongoing monitoring of tremors and related motor impairments plays a critical role in enabling early diagnosis, tailoring treatment plans, and supporting effective rehabilitation. Wearable devices have established themselves as valuable tools in this context, providing real-time, noninvasive, and continuous physiological data collection in everyday settings. This chapter examines how wearable sensor technologies, including inertial measurement units (IMUs), surface electromyography (sEMG), and gyroscopes, scan be used to detect and quantify tremors in people living with PD. It also explores how deep learning (DL) approaches, particularly convolutional neural networks (CNNs) and hybrid models, can be applied to analyze and classify the complex signals generated by these devices. Rehabilitation applications are considered as well, with attention to feedback-driven systems designed to support motor training and optimize therapeutic outcomes. Together, wearable technology and DL offer promising avenues for advancing the monitoring, assessment, and management of tremors and other motor symptoms in PD.

3.2 OVERVIEW OF PARKINSON'S DISEASE AND MOTOR SYMPTOMS

Parkinson's disease or PD is a chronic, progressive neurological condition that mostly affects mobility. It is the second most prevalent neurological illness after Alzheimer's (Hauser et al., 2006). PD is defined by the progressive loss of dopamine-producing

DOI: 10.1201/9781003500445-3

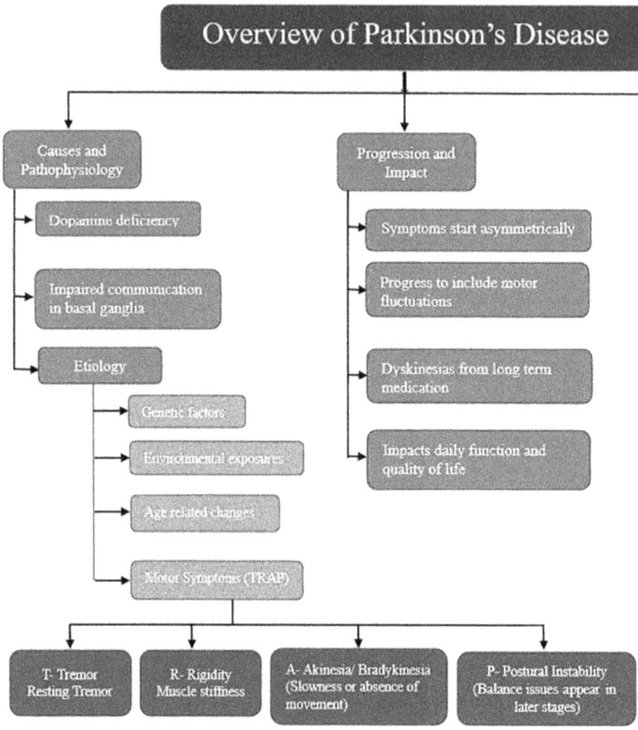

FIGURE 3.1 Overview of Parkinson's Disease.

neurons in the substantia nigra, a brain area critical for motor control. The pathophysiology, progression, and motor symptoms are detailed in Figure 3.1.

3.2.1 Progression and Impact of Motor Symptoms in Parkinson's Disease

- Motor symptoms typically begin asymmetrically and progress over time (Mahoney et al., 2007).
- As the disease advances, motor complications such as motor fluctuations and dyskinesias (involuntary movements) can occur, often as side effects of long-term dopaminergic therapy.
- Motor symptoms significantly impact daily functioning and quality of life.

3.2.2 Role of Wearable Technologies in Neurodegenerative Disorders

Wearable technologies are transforming the management of neurodegenerative disorders (NDDs) by providing continuous, objective, and remote monitoring of symptoms, which are often challenging to track with traditional clinical methods. These devices offer a valuable complement to clinic-based assessments, providing real-world data that can lead to earlier diagnosis, more personalized treatment, and improved quality of life for patients, as shown in Table 3.1.

TABLE 3.1
Breakdown of the Role of Wearable Technologies in Neurodegenerative Disorders

Role of Wearable Sensors	Applications	Procedure for Using Wearable Sensors
Continuous and Objective Monitoring	Beyond Clinic Visits (Mazzetta et al., 2019)	Traditional clinical assessments offer only a snapshot of a patient's condition. Wearables provide 24/7 insights into how a disorder impacts daily life, capturing symptom variability that might be missed in brief appointments.
	Objective Measurements (AlMahadin et al., 2020)	Wearables provide quantitative data on various parameters (e.g., movement, tremors, gait, balance, sleep patterns, heart rate, blood pressure, brain activity), reducing reliance on subjective patient-reported symptoms.
Early Detection and Diagnosis	Subtle Symptom Recognition (Lang et al., 2011)	Wearables can detect subtle changes in physiological and behavioural data (e.g., walking speed, stride length, keyboard dynamics, voice patterns, eye movements) that may signal the early onset of NDDs, even years before clinical diagnosis.
	Predictive Models (Prakash et al., 2016)	The data collected from wearables can be used with ML and DL approaches to develop predictive models that support clinicians in making informed decisions about diagnosis and treatment.
Disease Progression Monitoring and Management	Personalized Treatment Plans (Murman et al., 2012)	Wearable real-time data help healthcare professionals detect small changes in symptom severity and treatment response, enabling rapid adjustments to drug doses or other therapeutic measures.
	Tracking Motor Symptoms (Perumal et al., 2016)	For conditions such as PD and Huntington's disease (HD), wearables (e.g., smart bracelets, wristbands, and smart insoles) can measure tremor, bradykinesia (slowed movement), gait abnormalities, and motor fluctuations.
	Monitoring Non-Motor Symptoms (Goetz et al.,2008)	Non-motor symptoms, including cognitive abnormalities and sleep disruptions, can be monitored using wearable technology.
	Fall Detection (Silva de Lima et al., 2020)	Some devices can detect hard falls and notify family members or emergency responders if the individual does not get up.
Research and Clinical Trials	Large-Scale Data Collection. (Izmailova et al., 2018)	Wearables enable the collection of vast amounts of data from diverse populations, accelerating biomarker discovery and supporting remote participation in clinical trials.
	Reducing Reliance on Clinic Visits. (Espay et al., 2016)	Wearables can reduce the need for frequent, expensive in-person clinic visits.

3.2.3 Challenges

Despite their significant potential, challenges remain. These include patient acceptance and comfort, data security and privacy, the need for standardized evaluation frameworks, and the financial stability of device companies. Many commercial wearables lack Food and Drug Administration (FDA) approval, and more high-quality data is needed to confirm their clinical effectiveness for various neurological conditions. However, the future of wearables in neurology is promising. Continued advancements in artificial intelligence (AI), biosensors, flexible electronics, and integration with telemedicine and brain-computer interfaces (BCIs) are expected to make these technologies even more user-friendly, accessible, and integral to the diagnosis, monitoring, and personalized management of NDDs.

3.3 UNDERSTANDING TREMORS IN PARKINSON'S DISEASE

3.3.1 Pathophysiology of Tremors

PD tremors are a hallmark motor symptom, often presenting as a "resting tremor" – rhythmic shaking at rest that typically diminishes with voluntary movement. Understanding the pathophysiology of these tremors is complex, involving dysfunction in multiple brain circuits and neurotransmitter systems, primarily dopamine. The primary pathological event in PD is the progressive degeneration of dopaminergic neurons in the substantia nigra pars compacta (SNpc). These neurons project to the striatum and release dopamine. The core issue is the degeneration of dopamine-producing neurons, primarily affecting the basal ganglia's ability to regulate movement. This leads to the generation of abnormal oscillatory activity within the basal ganglia and its interaction with the cerebello-thalamo-cortical loop. While dopamine depletion is a central factor, the variable response of tremors to dopaminergic medications and the involvement of other neurotransmitters and brain regions highlight the multifaceted nature of PD tremor pathophysiology. Ongoing research continues to unravel the precise mechanisms underlying the development of more targeted and effective treatments (Patel et al., 2009).

Clinical assessment of PD is a multifaceted process that primarily relies on a neurologist's evaluation of the patient's symptoms and medical history. There is no single definitive diagnostic test for PD, so a comprehensive approach is essential for accurate diagnosis, monitoring disease progression, and guiding treatment. Clinical assessment in PD is an ongoing process. Regular follow-up appointments are crucial to monitor symptom progression, adjust medications, and address emerging challenges, ensuring personalized care for individuals living with PD (Skinner et al., 2016).

3.3.2 Clinical Assessment Methods

Figure 3.2 presents a hierarchical overview of the key clinical assessment methods employed in the diagnosis and monitoring of PD, organized across four principal categories: (1) diagnosis and general assessment, (2) standardized rating scales,

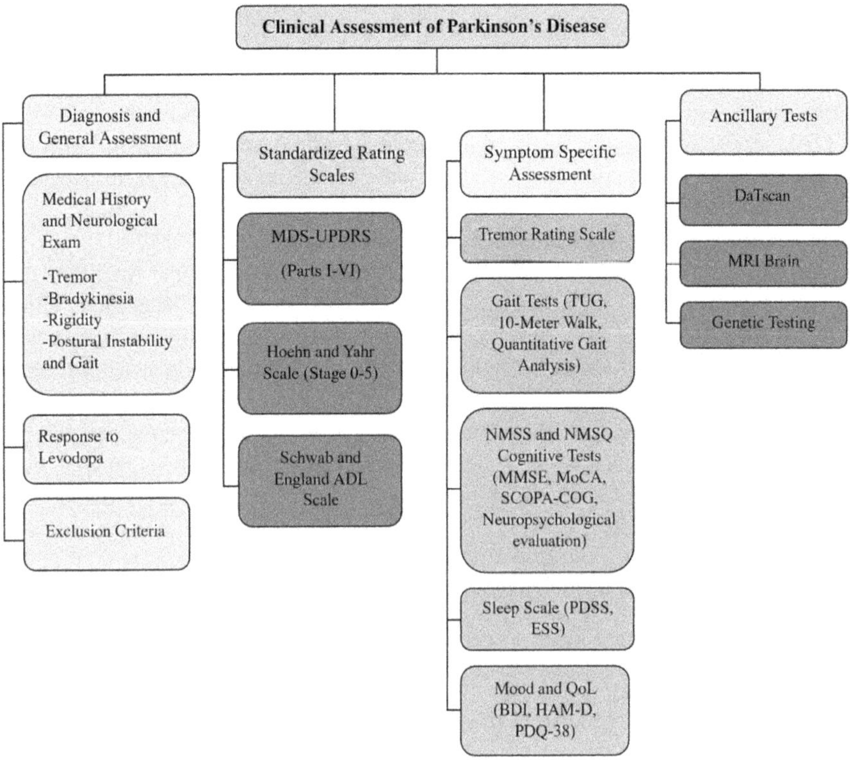

FIGURE 3.2 The Key Clinical Assessment Methods Used in Parkinson's Disease. (Van Den Eeden SK et al., 2003.)

(3) symptom specific assessment, and (4) ancillary tests. The first category, diagnosis and general assessment, forms the foundational step in the clinical evaluation of PD. It encompasses a thorough medical history and neurological examination, during which clinicians assess the four cardinal motor features of the disease: tremor, bradykinesia, rigidity, and postural instability and gait. This category also includes an evaluation of the patient's response to levodopa (a key diagnostic indicator) as well as the application of exclusion criteria to rule out alternative neurological conditions. The second category, standardized rating scales, provides structured and validated tools for quantifying disease severity and functional impairment. The Movement Disorder Society-Unified Parkinson's Disease Rating Scale (MDS-UPDRS, Parts I–VI) offers a comprehensive, multi-domain assessment spanning non-motor experiences, motor experiences, and motor complications. The Hoehn and Yahr Scale (Stage 0–5) categorizes overall disease progression from no signs of disease to severe disability, while the Schwab and England activities of daily living (ADL) Scale measures the degree of patient independence in performing everyday tasks. The third category, symptom specific assessment, captures a broader range of motor and non-motor manifestations through targeted evaluation tools. The tremor rating scale quantifies tremor severity, while gait function is assessed using the timed up and go (TUG) test,

the 10-meter walk test, and quantitative gait analysis. Non-motor symptom burden is evaluated through the non-motor symptoms scale (NMSS) and non-motor symptoms questionnaire (NMSQ), complemented by cognitive assessments including the mini-mental state examination (MMSE), the Montreal cognitive assessment (MoCA), SCOPA-COG, and broader neuropsychological evaluation. Sleep disturbances are assessed via the Parkinson's disease sleep scale (PDSS) and the Epworth sleepiness scale (ESS), while mood and quality of life are evaluated using the Beck depression inventory (BDI), the Hamilton depression rating scale (HAM-D), and the Parkinson's disease questionnaire (PDQ-38). The fourth category, Ancillary tests, encompasses objective diagnostic investigations used to support or confirm clinical findings. These include DaTscan imaging for dopaminergic pathway visualization, MRI (i.e., magnetic resonance imaging) brain imaging to exclude structural abnormalities, and genetic testing to identify disease-associated mutations. Collectively, Figure 3.2 illustrates the multidimensional nature of PD assessment, underscoring the need for both standardized and individualized evaluation approaches that span motor function, cognition, sleep, mood, and quality of life, all of which are relevant to the development and validation of wearable-based monitoring and DL systems discussed throughout this chapter.

3.3.3 Limitations of Conventional Diagnostic Tools

While conventional diagnostic tools for PD are the cornerstone of clinical practice, they come with several significant limitations (Miller et al., 2015):

- **Lack of a Definitive Biomarker for Early Diagnosis:**
  - *Clinical Diagnosis Relies on Motor Symptoms*: The presence of the cardinal motor symptoms—bradykinesia, stiffness, rest tremor, and postural instability—is currently the main clinical basis for diagnosing PD. The problem is that these symptoms usually do not appear until the substantia nigra has already sustained a substantial loss of dopaminergic neurons (50–70%).
  - *Late Diagnosis:* This means that by the time a diagnosis is made, the disease has often been progressing for many years, limiting the window for neuroprotective interventions that could slow or halt the progression.
  - *Lack of Diagnostic Test*: Unlike many other diseases, there isn't a simple blood test, imaging scan, or other lab test that can definitively diagnose PD in its early stages or even later. This reliance on clinical judgment inherently introduces variability.
- **Subjectivity and Variability in Clinical Assessment:**
  - *Rater Dependence:* The neurological examination and the use of rating scales like the MDS-UPDRS rely heavily on the clinician's experience, interpretation, and subjective observation. This can lead to inter-rater variability, meaning different neurologists might assign slightly different scores for the same patient.

    - *Fluctuating Symptoms*: PD symptoms can fluctuate throughout the day, depending on medication timing, stress, and other factors. A brief clinic visit may capture only a snapshot of the patient's condition, potentially missing the full spectrum of their symptoms and their impact on daily life.
    - *"On" vs. "Off" States:* The effectiveness of medication (e.g., levodopa) can vary, and patients experience "on" (good motor control) and "off" (poor motor control) periods. Assessments in the clinic may not fully capture these fluctuations, leading to an incomplete picture of the patient's functional status.
    - *Patient Recall Bias:* Patients may not accurately recall or consistently report the frequency and severity of their symptoms, especially nonmotor symptoms like sleep disturbances, pain, or mood changes.
- **Challenges in Differential Diagnosis:**
    - *Overlap with Other Conditions:* PD symptoms can mimic those of other conditions, such as drug-induced parkinsonism, essential tremor, or atypical parkinsonian syndromes (e.g., progressive supranuclear palsy, multiple system atrophy, corticobasal syndrome). Differentiating these conditions, especially in the early stages, can be very challenging, even for experienced movement disorder specialists.
    - *High Misdiagnosis Rates*: Studies have shown that misdiagnosis of PD can occur in a significant percentage of cases, sometimes as high as one in four, especially in the early stages. This can lead to inappropriate treatment and missed opportunities for condition-specific management.
    - *DaTscan Limitations:* While a DaTscan (dopamine transporter scan) can help differentiate PD from conditions like essential tremor by showing reduced dopamine transporters, it has limitations:
        - Cannot differentiate PD from other Parkinsonian syndromes: DaTscans will be abnormal in other conditions with a loss of dopamine neurons (e.g., atypical Parkinsonism), so they cannot definitively diagnose PD.
        - Not a diagnostic tool for early PD symptoms: Once motor symptoms are evident, the accuracy of the DaTscan and clinical exam are often similar. It's not typically used for routine diagnosis but rather to support a suspicious diagnosis or rule out mimics.
        - False Negatives/Positives: Like any test, DaTscan has a small percentage of false negatives (a person has PD, but the scan is normal) and false positives (a person doesn't have PD, but the scan is abnormal).
- **Difficulty in Assessing Nonmotor Symptoms:**
    - *Underestimation:* Nonmotor symptoms (e.g., loss of smell, depression, anxiety, constipation, sleep disorders, cognitive impairment) are common in PD and often precede motor symptoms by years. However, they are frequently overlooked or underestimated during routine clinical assessments because they are not as readily observable or quantifiable.
    - *Impact on Quality of Life*: These nonmotor symptoms significantly impact a patient's quality of life but are harder to assess objectively and track over time using conventional methods.

- **Limited Monitoring of Disease Progression and Treatment Efficacy:**
  - *Episodic Assessment:* Clinic visits provide only episodic assessments, making it challenging to capture subtle changes in symptoms, treatment response, or the impact of medication fluctuations over prolonged periods in the patient's natural environment.
  - *Lack of Real-World Data:* Conventional tools don't provide continuous, real-world data on how symptoms affect daily activities, limiting the ability to personalize treatment strategies based on the individual patient's true needs and fluctuations.

These limitations highlight the critical need for objective, continuous, and remote monitoring tools, which wearable technologies are proving invaluable in filling.

3.4 WEARABLE SENSOR TECHNOLOGIES

3.4.1 Types of Wearable Sensors

3.4.1.1 Accelerometer

Kubota et al. (2016) describe a novel method for detecting tremors using accelerometer data collected in real-world settings. The proposed method uses a deep multiple-instance learning approach that combines feature extraction and a pooling scheme inspired by the attention mechanism to identify key segments in the data. The authors argue that the proposed method has several advantages over existing tremor-detection methods. First, it does not require specialized equipment or laboratory conditions, making it more suitable for real-world applications. Second, it can identify key segments in the data, which may provide valuable insights into the underlying mechanisms of tremors. Finally, the approach is based on DL, which has shown promising results in a variety of medical applications. Overall, the paper provides a novel approach to tremor detection that has the potential to be useful for monitoring and managing PD in real-world settings.

Papadopoulos et al. (2019) developed a novel device (wearable accelerometers) to detect tremors at home. An accelerometer measures linear acceleration (change in velocity over time) along one or multiple axes (typically three: X, Y, and Z for forward/backward, side-to-side, and up/down movement). When the device accelerates, the mass moves, and this displacement is converted into an electrical signal. They can also detect the static force of gravity, allowing them to determine tilt and orientation. It measures parameters such as linear acceleration (e.g., changes in speed during walking or running), vibration and shock, Tilt and orientation relative to gravity, and activity levels (steps, movement intensity). These features are classified using a DL approach. An evaluation of the strategy using a dataset of 12 individuals with PD revealed that, in terms of binary classification accuracy, the proposed method outperformed several cutting-edge techniques. Thus, the paper provides an efficient approach to home-based tremor detection that could be useful for diagnosing PD severity.

3.4.1.2 Inertial Measurement Units Sensors

Benba et al. (2016) examined the feasibility of monitoring and assessing resting tremors in patients with PD using consumer smartwatches. The suggested approach comprises a tremor detector, a context classifier that determines resting durations, and a module that evaluates the magnitude and consistency of resting tremors. The study involved ten PD patients who wore a smartwatch on their non-dominant wrist for seven consecutive days. Data from the smartwatch accelerometer were collected and analyzed to identify resting periods and tremors. The proposed method demonstrated high sensitivity and specificity in detecting resting tremors and in differentiating PD patients from healthy subjects. The method presented in the study has the potential to be used for long-term monitoring of PD patients, which is essential for evaluating disease progression and treatment efficacy. The results of this study could pave the way for the development of low-cost, noninvasive wearable technologies for early detection and monitoring of PD.

Devices and solutions for the evaluation, ongoing monitoring, and diagnosis of tremors in neurological disorders were covered by Vescio et al (2021). It highlights the limitations of current tremor assessment methods and presents various technological approaches for tremor monitoring, including wearable sensors, mobile applications, and machine learning (ML) algorithms. The paper emphasizes the need for noninvasive, cost-effective tremor-monitoring solutions for patients with neurological disorders, such as PD. Overall, the paper provides an overview of the current state of the art in tremor monitoring technology and highlights the potential of these technologies for improving the quality of life of patients with neurological disorders

3.4.2 Data Acquisition and Transmission

Wearable sensors based on IMU technology are increasingly being explored for continuous, real-time monitoring of such motor symptoms. An IMU typically includes accelerometers, gyroscopes, and, sometimes, magnetometers, which can collectively capture complex movement data. Wearable sensors are tiny, sophisticated devices that capture various physiological and kinetic data from the wearer. They are crucial for monitoring health, tracking activity, and aiding in diagnosing and managing conditions such as NDDs. In this research, an IMU sensor has been developed to identify PD in the resting tremor stage. This sensor data is classified using an ML algorithm that incorporates additional parameters, such as recovery rate, L-dopa dose, and heart rate, to improve diagnostic accuracy. An Android app that allows users to add patient details and send them to a Flask REST API (i.e., application programming interface) was also developed. The ML model is deployed in Flask, and the app displays a tremor frequency graph and other statistics, including the maximum tremor frequency and duration. The system overview is as follows: Data is collected from patients using an MPU-6050 accelerometer and other sensors. This data is then processed using the ML algorithm. The analysis results are made available to users through an Android app that communicates with a Flask API. Users can add patient details and view the analysis results, including the tremor frequency graph and other statistics, as shown in Figure 3.3.

The frequency at which data points are collected. For tremors, a sufficiently high sampling rate (e.g., 50–200 Hz or higher) is crucial to accurately capture the characteristic tremor frequency (typically 4–6 Hz in PD). A sampling rate that is too low can lead to aliasing and the loss of important information. The precision of the measurements (e.g., 16-bit or 24-bit resolution). Higher resolution provides more detail and reduces quantization noise. Once data is acquired, it must be transmitted from the wearable sensor to a receiving device (e.g., a smartphone, tablet, dedicated gateway, or cloud server) for storage, processing, and analysis.

3.4.3 Preprocessing of Tremor Signals

The data preprocessing plays a critical role in preparing the dataset for ML algorithms to effectively analyze and predict tremor frequency in PD patients. Start by examining the dataset for any missing values, outliers, or inconsistent entries. The degree of missing data will determine whether incomplete records are filled in or whether methods such as mean imputation or interpolation are used. One way to deal with outliers is to eliminate them or use statistical techniques such as the Z-score or the interquartile range (IQR) to identify and address them. It is crucial to align the other features on a common scale to avoid biasing model training towards certain parameters. Features with varying scales can be normalized using techniques such as min-max scaling (to [0,1]) or standardization (to zero mean and unit variance).

The most relevant features are selected from the dataset that contribute significantly to predicting tremor frequency. Removing irrelevant or redundant features has improved model performance and reduced complexity, as shown in Table 3.2a and Table 3.2b. The preprocessed dataset is split into training and testing sets. The training set is used to train the ML model, while the testing set is kept separate to evaluate the model's performance on unseen data. By carefully preprocessing the data, we ensure the ML model receives clean, consistent, and properly formatted data, leading to accurate predictions and reliable insights into tremor frequency in PD patients, as shown in Figures 3.4 and 3.5.

There are several potential areas for future enhancement of the proposed system. Firstly, the current system focuses only on hand tremors, while PD can also cause other motor symptoms such as gait disturbances and bradykinesia. Thus, adding additional sensors to capture these symptoms could improve the system's overall diagnostic accuracy. Secondly, integrating the system with cloud-based data storage and analysis could provide real-time monitoring and early detection of disease progression. Finally, incorporating patient-specific data and feedback into the ML model could improve its performance and lead to personalized treatment plans.

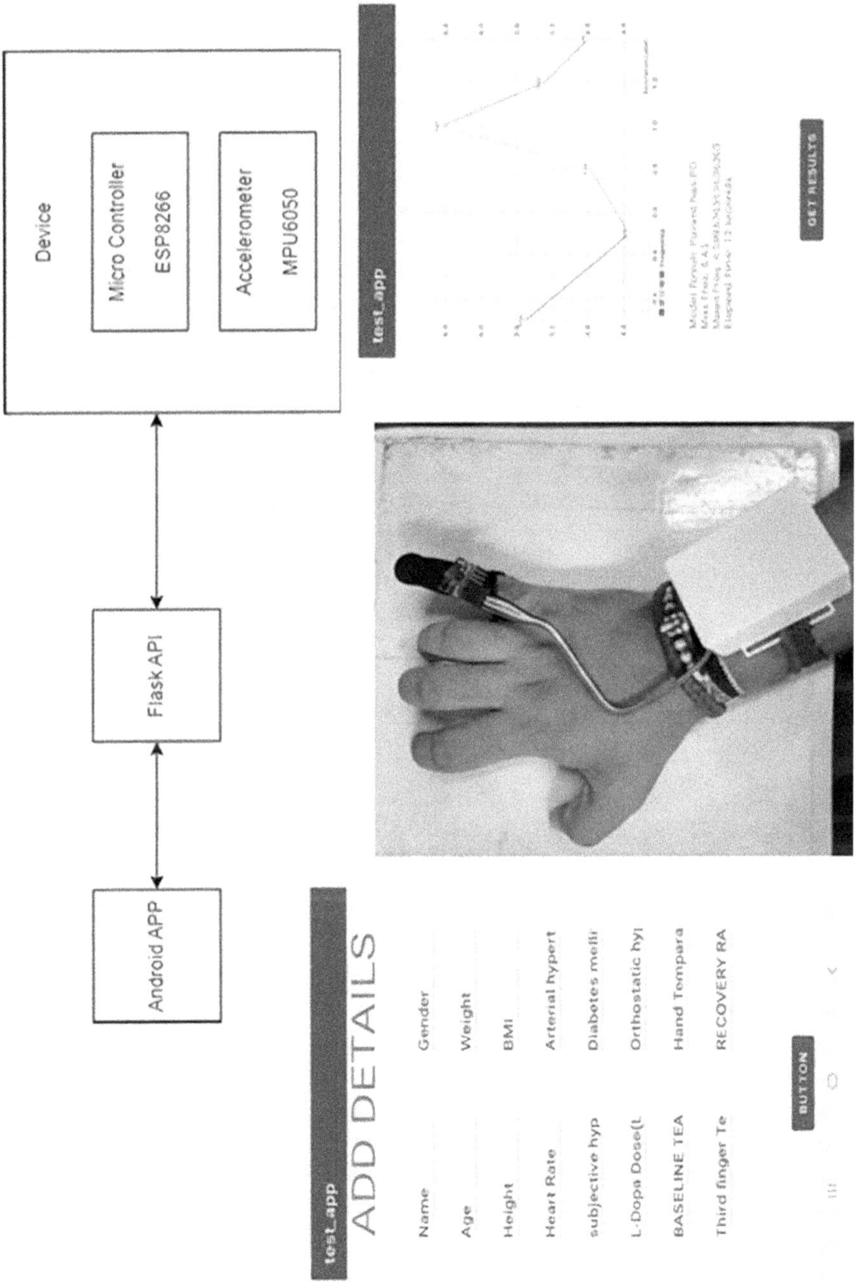

FIGURE 3.3 The Wearable Sensor and Android APP.

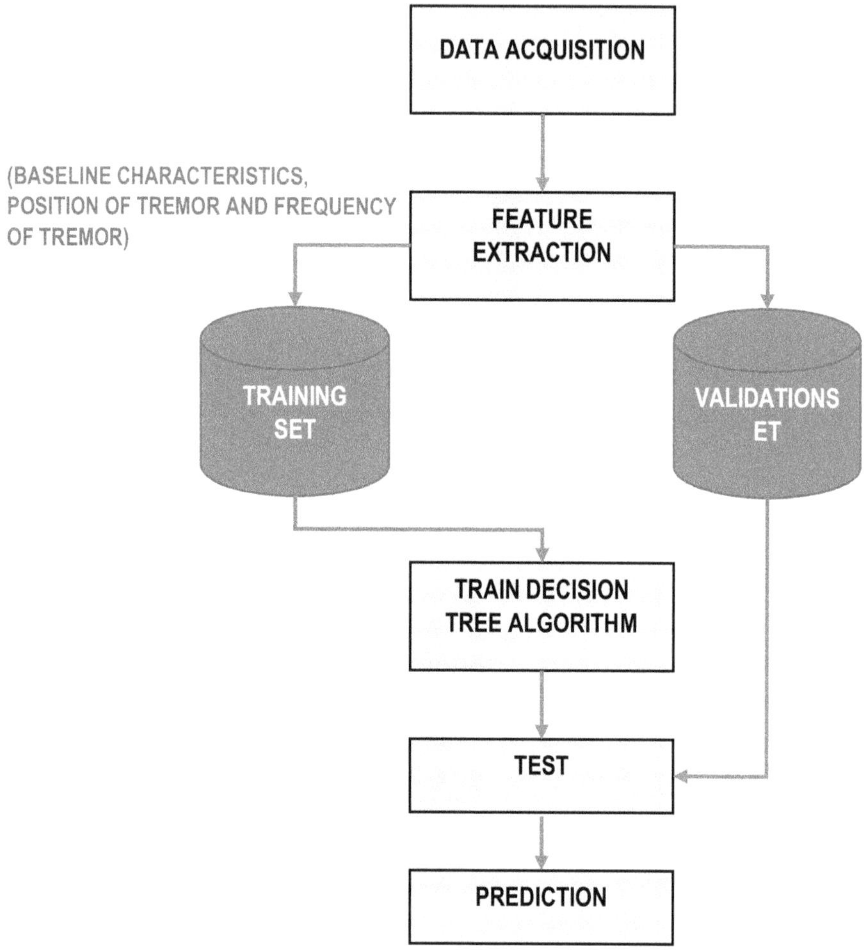

FIGURE 3.4 Various Steps Involved in the Classification of Tremor.

3.5 DEEP LEARNING FOR TREMOR DETECTION AND CLASSIFICATION

3.5.1 Wearable Sensors and Artificial Intelligence

Wearable electronics and AI are transforming the monitoring of chronic illnesses by enabling continuous, objective assessment outside of clinical environments (Luis-Martínez et al., 2020). Traditional approaches to monitoring PD are often limited by the lack of real-time, objective data and the impracticality of frequent hospital visits. In contrast, (Rodríguez-Martín et al., 2022) emphasize that wearable sensors offer a promising alternative by facilitating continuous monitoring in natural living conditions, an essential component for effective disease assessment and personalized care.

TABLE 3.2a
Statistical Representation of Parkinson's Disease Features

Statistic	Age	Weight in Kgs	Height in Meters	BMI	Heart Rate (Supine)	Tremor Frequency	Dose (LEDD) mg/day	Baseline Temperature	Hand Temperature	Third Finger Temperature	Recovery Rate
Count	60	60	60	60	60	60	60	60	60	60	60
Mean	58.17	72.07	1.70	25.02	68.00	4.54	87.50	35.93	30.68	30.51	40.45
Standard Deviation (std)	10.57	7.46	0.07	2.74	5.29	3.80	154.49	1.78	1.52	1.60	13.99
Min	21.00	60.00	1.54	18.73	60.00	0.00	0.00	34.10	27.10	27.10	14.40
25%	54.00	66.00	1.64	22.99	63.75	0.00	0.00	35.00	29.33	29.45	33.01
50%	59.50	72.00	1.71	24.68	66.00	4.98	0.00	35.80	30.40	30.70	38.36
75%	65.00	77.50	1.75	26.88	72.00	7.28	150.00	36.33	31.43	31.73	43.37
Max	80.00	85.00	1.82	30.48	81.00	11.57	600.00	47.00	33.00	33.80	92.16

TABLE 3.2b
Types of Classifiers and Classification Metrics

Classifier	Accuracy	Recall	Precision
Support Vector Classifier (SVC)	77%	79%	73%
Decision Tree	100%	100%	100%
Random Forest (RF)	95.8%	96.7%	95.2%
K-Nearest Neighbors (KNN)	83%	90.09%	83.33%

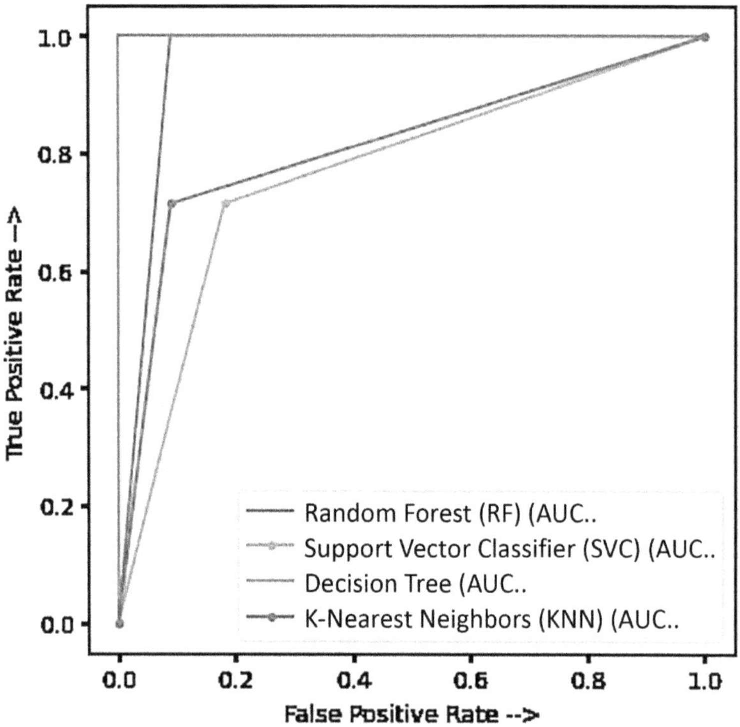

FIGURE 3.5 Classification of Tremor frequency with Machine Learning.

Although wearable sensors provide a low-cost and scalable method for data collection, the raw sensor data they generate is often complex and voluminous, requiring advanced analytical methods to extract clinically meaningful information. AI techniques, particularly data mining and ML, have been widely applied to manage what is known as "Big Data." ML algorithms offer semi-automated solutions for interpreting sensor outputs, uncovering latent patterns and trends that can inform diagnosis and disease progression.

While traditional ML techniques have achieved success in detecting PD motor symptoms such as tremors, these approaches rely heavily on manual feature extraction.

This requirement for handcrafted features limits the adaptability and scalability of ML-based monitoring solutions (Mei et al., 2021). Designing and selecting optimal features is not only time-consuming but also requires domain expertise, hindering widespread clinical integration.

DL, a subfield of ML, has emerged as a transformative solution in this context. DL algorithms surpass traditional methods by automatically learning hierarchical feature representations directly from raw data, thereby eliminating the need for manual feature engineering. This end-to-end capability makes DL particularly suitable for wearable-based remote health monitoring systems, enabling faster development and deployment (Tanveer et al., 2022).

3.5.2 Learning Architectures for Tremor Analysis

To objectively monitor PD symptoms, both motor and non-motor, various DL models have been developed to analyze large volumes of wearable sensor data. DL architectures, composed of multiple processing layers, are particularly well-suited for the noninvasive, cost-effective analysis of high-dimensional sensor data because they can learn complex data representations at progressively higher levels of abstraction.

Among the DL architectures, CNNs have been most widely adopted. CNNs eliminate the need for extensive feature engineering by learning directly from raw input signals. These networks typically include convolutional layers for feature extraction, pooling layers (e.g., max or average pooling) to reduce spatial dimensions, and fully connected layers for final classification or regression.

To capture temporal relationships in sensor signals, recurrent neural networks (RNNs), in particular long short-term memory (LSTM) networks, have been used. These are frequently used in conjunction with thick layers to forecast output. Variants including gated recurrent units (GRUs), bidirectional LSTM, and convolutional recurrent neural networks (CRNNs) have also been investigated.

3.5.3 Model Training, Validation, and Evaluation Metrics

Evaluating the performance of DL models for tremor detection and classification is critical to ensure clinical relevance and generalizability. For classification tasks, performance is measured using metrics such as True Positives (TP), False Positives (FP), False Negatives (FN), and True Negatives (TN). From these, Sensitivity (Recall) and Specificity quantify the model's ability to correctly detect tremors and non-tremor states, respectively. Accuracy measures overall correctness, while the F1-score balances precision and recall, especially valuable for imbalanced datasets. Area under the receiver operating characteristic curve (AUROC) indicates class separation ability, and equal error rate (EER) denotes the point at which sensitivity and specificity are equal.

For regression models, which aim to quantify tremor severity, performance is evaluated using Pearson's correlation coefficient (r) to assess the linear relationship between true and predicted values. Mean absolute error (MAE) and root mean square error (RMSE) quantify the magnitude of prediction errors, with RMSE placing a greater penalty on large deviations.

Validation strategies include leave-one-subject-out (LOSO), which tests model generalization across unseen subjects, making it ideal for subject-independent models. K-fold Cross-Validation (CV) and hold-out methods may be subject-independent or subject-dependent, depending on the data split. Random Shuffle (RS) validations mix data from different individuals, increasing the risk of overfitting and reducing model generalizability.

3.5.4 Deep Learning for Tremor Detection and Classification in Literature

Recent studies have increasingly adopted DL models for tremor detection due to their ability to process raw sensor data without manual preprocessing.

For instance, Varghese et al. (2021) used an artificial neural network (ANN) on wrist-based accelerometer data from 260 participants, achieving 82.3% accuracy and 90.5% sensitivity via nested cross-validation. Papadopoulos et al. (2020) implemented a CNN on raw hand accelerometer signals with LOSO validation, yielding moderate sensitivity (61.2%) but high specificity (85.0%). San-Segundo et al. (2020) achieved a strong area under the curve (AUC) of 0.884 using CNNs on engineered features, with a high correlation ($\rho = 0.9$) between predictions and clinical assessments. To further enhance performance, Sigcha et al. (2021) developed a multitask CNN using raw and FFT-transformed wrist accelerometer data. Their model achieved an AUC of 0.936, with balanced sensitivity and specificity (86.1%) and a near-perfect correlation ($r = 0.969$).

Kim et al. (2018) combined wrist accelerometer and gyroscope data and applied CNNs to FFT features. The model achieved 85% accuracy and a correlation of 0.93 under K-fold (random split) validation. Phokaewvarangkul et al. (2021) used LSTM on raw gyroscope data from 20 subjects, obtaining 86.5% accuracy and a correlation of 0.77. Despite a small sample, Lauraitis et al. (2020a) achieved outstanding results (accuracy, sensitivity, specificity >95%) using an ensemble of LSTM models on touchscreen-derived data.

Together, these studies confirm the efficacy of DL (particularly CNNs, LSTMs, and their combinations) in tremor detection from wearable data. Subject-independent validation methods, such as LOSO, remain critical for robust model evaluation. Despite challenges such as dataset size and subject variability, DL offers a viable pathway to developing scalable, automated tremor-monitoring systems with significant potential for clinical integration in the management of PD and essential tremor.

3.6 APPLICATIONS IN REHABILITATION

The integration of wearable devices and DL technologies into rehabilitation presents transformative opportunities for individuals with PD. These innovations have the potential to support continuous monitoring, real-time feedback, personalized therapy, and motor recovery. PD rehabilitation aims to improve motor functions, mitigate the impact of tremors, and maintain the quality of life. Using wearable technologies and intelligent algorithms, clinicians can track patient progress, detect abnormalities, and dynamically adjust treatment protocols.

Wearable sensors that give a wealth of kinematic and physiological data include electromyography (EMG) patches, IMUs, and smart fabrics. This data, when combined with DL models, may be used to identify tremor patterns, therapeutic response, and minor motor deficits. The spatiotemporal dynamics of PD-related motion abnormalities are better captured by DL architectures such as CNNs, RNNs, and LSTM networks (Sama et al., 2017; Um et al., 2017).

3.6.1 Wearables for Real-Time Feedback and Biofeedback Systems

Real-time feedback is a key element in effective rehabilitation. Wearables enable immediate insights into a patient's performance, allowing both patients and clinicians to adjust interventions based on objective data. Devices equipped with IMUs, such as accelerometers and gyroscopes, are widely used for motion tracking and tremor assessment. When integrated with smartphone apps or cloud-based platforms, they offer instant feedback through visual, auditory, or haptic cues (Del Din et al., 2016).

Biofeedback systems aim to train individuals to gain voluntary control over physiological processes. In the context of PD, biofeedback has been utilized to enhance gait, posture, and hand movements. For example, vibrotactile feedback systems can alert patients when their tremor amplitude exceeds a threshold, promoting compensatory strategies (Pham et al., 2018). Additionally, EMG-based systems can detect anomalies in muscle activity and inform corrective actions during exercises.

DL enhances these systems by enabling adaptive feedback mechanisms. Through pattern recognition and predictive analytics, models can tailor feedback based on symptom progression or user behavior. For instance, an LSTM-based tremor detection model can continuously learn from new data and adjust feedback thresholds accordingly (Eskofier et al., 2016).

3.6.2 Rehabilitation Protocols and Assistive Technologies

Wearable technology plays a significant role in delivering structured rehabilitation protocols. In PD management, these protocols often focus on repetitive motor training, balance exercises, and strength development. Wearables assist by quantifying adherence and performance metrics, thereby fostering more consistent, measurable rehabilitation efforts (Mirelman et al., 2016).

Advanced assistive technologies incorporate wearables into exoskeletons, robotic limbs, and smart walkers. These tools are often augmented by AI to support dynamic adjustments based on patient input. For example, robotic gait trainers combined with inertial sensors and AI algorithms can personalize therapy sessions by analyzing patient-specific walking patterns (Sale et al., 2021).

Moreover, virtual and augmented reality systems integrated with wearables are gaining traction in PD rehabilitation. These immersive environments can simulate real-world challenges and measure user responses, enhancing cognitive-motor interaction. DL models are used to interpret motion data and optimize virtual scenarios in real-time, ensuring that the training remains relevant and engaging (Stamate et al., 2020).

Home-based rehabilitation is enabled by the scalability of wearable regimens, which eliminate the need for regular clinician visits. Patients with restricted mobility or those living in distant places can especially benefit from this. Wearables with cloud connectivity enable medical professionals to monitor patient compliance and conduct remote interventions as needed (López et al., 2020).

3.6.3 Case Studies and Clinical Trials

Clinical trials and case studies offer valuable insights into the real-world efficacy of wearable technologies in PD rehabilitation. Numerous studies have shown that wearable-enabled interventions improve motor outcomes, enhance adherence, and increase patient satisfaction.

For instance, a randomized controlled trial conducted by Rodríguez-Molinero et al. (2015) involved 50 PD patients using a wearable gait monitor during their rehabilitation. The study found that patients receiving real-time feedback showed significant improvements in gait regularity and stride length compared to the control group.

Another notable study by Griffiths et al. (2020) tested a wearable tremor-suppression device powered by a ML algorithm. The system successfully distinguished between voluntary and involuntary movements and applied counteracting forces in real time. Participants reported reduced tremor severity and greater ease in daily activities.

In a large-scale clinical study, the Parkinson@Home initiative deployed wearable sensors and DL analytics to over 300 PD patients across Europe. The project demonstrated the feasibility of remote symptom tracking and algorithm-based treatment recommendations, highlighting the potential for scalable, data-driven PD management (Dorsey et al., 2020).

Case reports also illustrate personalized interventions. For example, a 68-year-old patient underwent a 12-week wearable-assisted rehabilitation program using EMG sensors and a CNN-based classifier to optimize upper limb exercises. Post-intervention assessments revealed a notable reduction in tremor amplitude and an increase in motor coordination (Lee et al., 2019).

These findings underscore the importance of interdisciplinary collaboration among clinicians, engineers, and data scientists to develop robust, user-centric rehabilitation solutions. However, challenges remain in standardizing protocols, ensuring data privacy, and achieving regulatory compliance. Future research should focus on longitudinal studies, cross-population validation, and the integration of multimodal data streams.

3.7 CONCLUSION

PD remains a major global health challenge, characterized by progressive motor dysfunction, particularly tremors that significantly affect the quality of life of affected individuals. Traditional diagnostic and monitoring methods, while clinically valuable, often lack the sensitivity and real-time capabilities required for continuous assessment and early intervention. This chapter examined the convergence of wearable sensor technologies and DL algorithms as a promising approach for enhancing the detection, monitoring, and rehabilitation of tremors in individuals with PD.

Wearable devices (ranging from wrist-worn IMUs to sEMG systems) offer a practical, low-cost, and noninvasive means for real-time symptom tracking in naturalistic settings. These devices enable longitudinal monitoring of motor symptoms outside clinical environments, providing valuable data to clinicians and caregivers. The integration of DL methods such as CNNs and LSTM networks further enhances the analytical capacity of these systems. These models can learn complex, nonlinear patterns in time-series data, facilitating robust and accurate tremor classification and severity estimation.

In rehabilitation, wearable systems have evolved beyond passive monitoring to active components in therapy. Feedback-based systems, such as those providing real-time cues for movement correction, support personalized motor training and adaptive rehabilitation protocols. The deployment of such systems in clinical and home settings opens new avenues for continuous care and self-managed therapy, particularly valuable in resource-constrained environments or rural communities.

Despite significant advancements, several challenges persist. Data variability arising from individual differences, sensor placement, and activity context can affect model generalizability. Inter-device compatibility and standardization remain critical to ensure consistent, scalable solutions. Additionally, the ethical dimensions (such as data privacy, informed consent, and regulatory approval) must be carefully considered, especially as these systems transition from research to widespread clinical application.

REFERENCES

AlMahadin, G., Lotfi, A., Zysk, E., Siena, F. L., Mc Carthy, M., & Breedon, P. (2020). Parkinson's disease: Current assessment methods and wearable devices for evaluation of movement disorder motor symptoms-a patient and healthcare professional perspective. *BMC Neurology*, 20, 1–13.

Benba, A., Jilbab, A., & Hammouch, A. (2016). Discriminating between patients with Parkinson's and Neurological diseases using cepstral analysis. *IEEE Transactions on Neural Systems and Rehabilitation Engineering*, 24(10), 1100–1108.

Del Din, S., Godfrey, A., Mazzà, C., Lord, S., & Rochester, L. (2016). Free-living monitoring of Parkinson's disease: Lessons from the field. *Movement Disorders*, 31(9), 1293–1313. https://doi.org/10.1002/mds.26610

Dorsey, E. R., Vlaanderen, F. P., Engelen, L. J., Kieburtz, K., Zhu, W., Biglan, K. M., & Bloem, B. R. (2020). Moving Parkinson care to the home. *Movement Disorders*, 35(1), 11–20. https://doi.org/10.1002/mds.27868

Eskofier, B. M., Lee, S. I., Baron, M., Simon, A., Martindale, C. F., Gaßner, H., & Klucken, J. (2016). An overview of smart shoes in the internet of health things: Gait and mobility assessment in health promotion and disease monitoring. *Applied Sciences*, 6(11), 305. https://doi.org/10.3390/app6110305

Espay, A. J., Bonato, P., Nahab, F. B., Maetzler, W., Dean, J. M., Klucken, J., Eskofier, B. M., Merola, A., Horak, F., Lang, A. E., & Reilmann, R. (2016). Technology in Parkinson's disease: Challenges and opportunities. *Movement Disorders*, 31(9), 1272–1282.

Goetz, C. G., Tilley, B. C., Shaftman, S. R., & Stebbins, G. T. (2008). Movement disorder societ-sponsored revision of the unified Parkinson's disease rating scale (MDS-UPDRS): Scale presentation and clinimetric testing results, *Movement Disorders*, 23(15), 2129–2170.

Griffiths, R. I., Kotschet, K. E., Arfon, S., Xu, Z. M., Johnson, W., Drago, J., & Horne, M. K. (2020). Automated assessment of bradykinesia and dyskinesia in Parkinson's disease. *Journal of Parkinson's Disease*, 10(1), 233–245. https://doi.org/10.3233/JPD-191763

Hauser, R. A., McDermott, M. P., & Messing, S. (2006). Factors associated with the development of motor fluctuations and dyskinesias in Parkinson disease. *Archives Neurology*, 63, 1756–1760.

Izmailova, E. S., Wagner, J. A., & Perakslis, E. D. (2018). Wearable devices in clinical trials: Hype and hypothesis. *Clinical Pharmacology & Therapeutics*, 104(1), 42–52.

Kim, H. B., Lee, W. W., Kim, A., Lee, H. J., Park, H. Y., Jeon, H. S., ... & Park, K. S. (2018). Wrist sensor-based tremor severity quantification in Parkinson's disease using convolutional neural network. *Computers in Biology and Medicine*, 95, 140–146.

Kubota, K. J., Chen, J. A., & Little, M. A. (2016). Machine learning for large-scale wearable sensor data in Parkinson's disease: Concepts, promises, pitfalls, and futures. *MovDisord*, 31(9), 1314–1326.

Lang, A. E. (2011). A critical appraisal of the premotor symptoms of Parkinson's disease: Potential usefulness in early diagnosis and design of neuroprotective trials. *Movement Disorders*, 26(5), 775–783.

Lauraitis, A., Maskeliūnas, R., Damaševičius, R., & Krilavičius, T. (2020). A mobile application for smart computer-aided self-administered testing of cognition, speech, and motor impairment. *Sensors*, 20(11), 3236.

Lee, J. W., Lee, Y. J., Jeon, M., & Kim, J. W. (2019). A CNN-based EMG pattern classification approach for tremor detection in Parkinson's disease. *Biomedical Engineering Letters*, 9(1), 65–73. https://doi.org/10.1007/s13534-018-0074-9

López, C. D., Figueroa, M. C., Castro, A., & Tapia, A. (2020). Tele-rehabilitation in Parkinson's disease using wearable sensors: A systematic review. *Sensors*, 20(18), 5430. https://doi.org/10.3390/s20185430

Luis-Martínez, R., Monje, M. H. G., Antonini, A., Sánchez-Ferro, Á., & Mestre, T. A. (2020). Technology-enabled care: Integrating multidisciplinary care in Parkinson's disease through digital technology. *Frontiers in Neurology*, 11, 575975. 10.3389/fneur.2020.575975

Mahoney, D. F., Purtilo, R. B., Webbe, F. M., Alwan, M., Bharucha, A. J., Adlam, T. D., Jimison, H. B., Turner, B., & Becker, S. A. (2007). In-home monitoring of persons with dementia: Ethical guidelines for technology research and development. *Alzheimers Dement*, 3, 217–226.

Mazzetta, I., Zampogna, A., Suppa, A., Gumiero, A., Pessione, M., & Irrera, F. (2019). Wearable sensors system for an improved analysis of freezing of gait in Parkinson's disease using electromyography and inertial signals. *Sensors*, 19, 948.

Mei, J., Desrosiers, C., & Frasnelli, J. (2021). Machine learning for the diagnosis of Parkinson's disease: A review of literature. *Frontiers in Aging Neuroscience*, 13, 633752. https://doi.org/10.3389/fnagi.2021.633752

Miller, D. B., & O'Callaghan, J. P. (2015). Biomarkers of Parkinson's disease: Present and future. *Metabolism*, 64(3), S40–S46.

Mirelman, A., Rochester, L., Maidan, I., Del Din, S., Alcock, L., Nieuwhof, F., ... & Hausdorff, J. M. (2016). Addition of a non-immersive virtual reality component to treadmill training to reduce fall risk in older adults (V-TIME): A randomised controlled trial. *The Lancet*, 388(10050), 1170–1182. https://doi.org/10.1016/S0140-6736(16)31325-3

Murman, D. L. (2012). Early treatment of Parkinson's disease: Opportunities for managed care. *American Journal of Managed Care*, 18(7), S183.

Papadopoulos, A., Iakovakis, D., Klingelhoefer, L., Bostantjopoulou, S., Chaudhuri, K. R., Kyritsis, K., ... & Delopoulos, A. (2020). Unobtrusive detection of Parkinson's disease from multi-modal and in-the-wild sensor data using deep learning techniques. *Scientific Reports*, 10(1), 21370.

Papadopoulos, A., Kyritsis, K., Klingelhoefer, L., Bostanjopoulou, S., Chaudhuri, K. R., & Delopoulos, A. (2019). Detecting parkinsonian tremor from IMU data collected in-the-wild using deep multiple-instance learning. *IEEE Journal of Biomedical and Health Informatics*, 24(9), 2559–2569.

Patel, S., Lorincz, K., & Hughes, R. (Novemeber 2009). Monitoring motor fluctuations in patients with Parkinsons disease using wearable sensors. *IEEE Transactions on Information Technology in Biomedicine*, 13(6), 864–873.

Pham, M. H., Elshehabi, M., Haertner, L., Del Din, S., Dean, C. M., Maetzler, W., & Hobert, M. A. (2018). Validation of a wearable gait analysis system with multiple modalities for patients with Parkinson's disease. *Journal of NeuroEngineering and Rehabilitation*, 15(1), 77. https://doi.org/10.1186/s12984-018-0423-1

Phokaewvarangkul, O., Vateekul, P., Wichakam, I., Anan, C., & Bhidayasiri, R. (2021). Using machine learning for predicting the best outcomes with electrical muscle stimulation for tremors in Parkinson's disease. *Frontiers in Aging Neuroscience*, 13, 727654.

Prakash, K. M., Nadkarni, N. V., Lye, W. K., Yong, M. H., & Tan, E. K. (2016). The impact of non-motor symptoms on the quality of life of Parkinson's disease patients: A longitudinal study. *European Journal of Neurology*, 23(5), 854–860.

Rodríguez-Molinero, A., Samà, A., Pérez-Martínez, D. A., Pérez López, C., Romagosa, J., Bayés, A., ... & Català, A. (2015). A kinematic sensor and algorithm to detect motor fluctuations in Parkinson disease: Validation study under real conditions of use. *JMIR Rehabilitation and Assistive Technologies*, 2(1), e1. https://doi.org/10.2196/rehab.3982

Rodríguez-Martín, D., Cabestany, J., Pérez-López, C., Pie, M., Calvet, J., Samà, A., Capra, C., Català, A., & Rodríguez-Molinero, A. (2022). A new paradigm in Parkinson's disease evaluation with wearable medical devices: A review of STAT-ON™. *Frontiers in Neurology*, 13, 912343. https://doi.org/10.3389/fneur.2022.912343.

Sale, P., Franceschini, M., Waldner, A., & Hesse, S. (2021). Use of robotics in neurological rehabilitation: An update. *Current Physical Medicine and Rehabilitation Reports*, 9, 59–65. https://doi.org/10.1007/s40141-021-00288-y

Sama, A., Pérez-López, C., Rodríguez-Martín, D., Català, A., Cabestany, J., Moreno, J. M., & Bayés, À. (2017). Dyskinesia and motor state detection in Parkinson's disease patients with a single movement sensor. *Frontiers in Neurology*, 8, 457. https://doi.org/10.3389/fneur.2017.00457

San Segundo Hernández, R., Zhand, A., Cebulla, A., Panev, S., Tablor, G., Stebbins, K., ... & Hodgins, J. (2020). Parkinson's disease tremor detection in the wild using wearable accelerometers. *Parkinson's Disease Tremor Detection in the Wild Using Wearable Accelerometers*, 20(20), 5817.

Perumal, S. V. R. (2016). Gait and tremor assessment for patients with Parkinson's disease using wearable sensors. *Elsevier, ICT Express*, 2, 168–174.

Sigcha, L., Pavón, I., Costa, N., Costa, S., Gago, M., Arezes, P., ... & De Arcas, G. (2021). Automatic resting tremor assessment in Parkinson's disease using smartwatches and multitask convolutional neural networks. *Sensors*, 21(1), 291.

Silva de Lima, A. L., Smits, T., Darweesh, S. K., Valenti, G., Milosevic, M., Pijl, M., ... & Bloem, B. R. (2020). Home-based monitoring of falls using wearable sensors in Parkinson's disease. *Movement Disorders*, 35(1), 109–115.

Skinner, T. R., Scott, I. A., & Martin, J. H. (2016). Diagnostic errors in older patients: A systematic review of incidence and potential causes in seven prevalent diseases. *International Journal of General Medicine*, 9, 137–146.

Stamate, C., Donnelly, N., Smeaton, A. F., & McDonald, J. (2020). Multimodal deep learning for tremor assessment in Parkinson's disease. *IEEE Journal of Biomedical and Health Informatics*, 24(8), 2304–2315. https://doi.org/10.1109/JBHI.2020.2973712

Tanveer, M., Richhariya, B., Khan, R. U., Rashid, A. H., Khanna, P., Prasad, M., & Lin, C.-T. (2022). Parkinson's disease diagnosis using neural networks: Survey and comprehensive evaluation. *Information Processing & Management*, 59(3), 102909. https://doi.org/10.1016/j.ipm.2022.102909

Um, T. T., Pfister, F. M. J., Pichler, D., Endo, S., Lang, M., Hirche, S., & Kulić, D. (2017). Data augmentation of wearable sensor data for Parkinson's disease monitoring using convolutional neural networks. *Proceedings of the 19th ACM International Conference on Multimodal Interaction*, 216–220. New York, NY, USA: ACM. https://doi.org/10.1145/3136755.3136817

Van Den Eeden, S. K., Tanner, C. M., Bernstein, A. L., Fross, R. D., Leimpeter, A., Bloch, D. A., & Nelson, L. M. (2003). Incidence of Parkinson's disease: Variation by age, gender, and race/ethnicity. *American Journal of Epidemiology*, 157, 1015–1022.

Varghese, J., Alen, C. M. V., Fujarski, M., Schlake, G. S., Sucker, J., Warnecke, T., & Thomas, C. (2021). Sensor validation and diagnostic potential of smartwatches in movement disorders. *Sensors*, 21(9), 3139.

Vescio, B., Quattrone, A., Nistico, R., Crasa, M., & Quattrone, A. (2021). Wearable devices for assessment of tremor. *Frontiers in Neurology*, 12, 680011.

4 From Metrics to Meaning

An Embodied Cognition Framework for Conversational, Human-in-the-Loop Neurowearable Interfaces

Arun Sasidharan, Karthik Raghavendran, Vrinda M., Aditya Asopa, Soumya Bhattacharjee, Karthik Venkataraman, and Fayaz Pathan Khan

4.1 INTRODUCTION

The last decade has witnessed the rapid advancement and commercialization of neurotechnology, moving sophisticated brain monitoring from the lab environment to the consumer market (Centre for Future Generations (CFG), 2025). This "democratization of neurotechnology" has given rise to the concept of "The Quantified Mind," where consumer neurowearables – often in the form of headbands, earbuds, or other discreet form factors – offer users the promise of enhanced cognitive performance, deeper meditation, and improved sleep quality (Cinel et al., 2019; Girivirya et al., 2022; Simons et al., 2024). These devices leverage high-fidelity sensors and sophisticated signal-processing algorithms to provide unprecedented visibility into the brain's electrical activity, using electroencephalography (EEG) and corresponding states (Muvvala et al., 2025; Yang et al., 2025).

However, despite this technological progress, the industry faces a fundamental challenge: user retention. Many users adopt these devices with initial enthusiasm but ultimately abandon them; this high attrition rate is primarily driven by a significant gap between the raw data collected and the actionable insights provided, a phenomenon documented in the literature (Attig & Franke, 2020; Lazar et al., 2015). This chapter posits that the current, purely data-driven interface paradigm is fundamentally limited.

Drawing on the philosophical and scientific principles of Embodied Cognition, which asserts that cognitive processes are deeply interwoven with the body's interaction with its environment (Varela et al., 1991; Wilson, 2002), we propose a necessary paradigm shift. We argue for a transition from passive, data-monitoring dashboards to active, conversational, human-in-the-loop systems (Agarwal et al., 2020), in which

DOI: 10.1201/9781003500445-4

continuous user interaction, contextual awareness, and expert knowledge are integral to system behavior and adaptation. We call this proposed framework a "Context-Aware Neuro-Agent" that aims to go beyond mere brain-state measurement to actively guide the user's actions, thereby providing the missing "expert human touch." The following sections will detail the shortcomings of the current approach and introduce a novel three-layered framework that could address the "*What should I do?*" problem in neuro-interaction design.

4.2 PROBLEMS TO BE SOLVED: THE DATA-RICH, INSIGHT-POOR PARADOX

The commercial neurowearables market is currently facing a critical retention crisis, which we define as the "Data-Rich, Insight-Poor" (DRIP) Paradox. This paradox is the central problem that must be overcome for the technology to achieve widespread, sustained adoption.

4.2.1 The Crisis of Abstract Metrics

Contemporary neurowearable interfaces suffer from a foundational design flaw: they prioritize raw data accuracy and the communication of normative, prescriptive understandings over user interpretability and actionable insights (Di Lodovico et al., 2025). This design results in a user experience characterized by data overload, presenting the individual with a deluge of abstract, unprocessed metrics that utterly fail to convey immediate, relatable meaning or utility (Tzimourta, 2025). The information is technically correct yet practically useless to the lay user.

Users are consistently confronted with highly specialized and complex data representations (see Figure 4.1):

- **Spectral Power Graphs (or Electroencephalogram (EEG) Frequency Bands):** These are intricate visualizations of brain activity broken down into distinct frequency components—such as Delta, Theta, Alpha, Beta, and Gamma. While these bands correlate with specific cognitive states (Buzsáki,

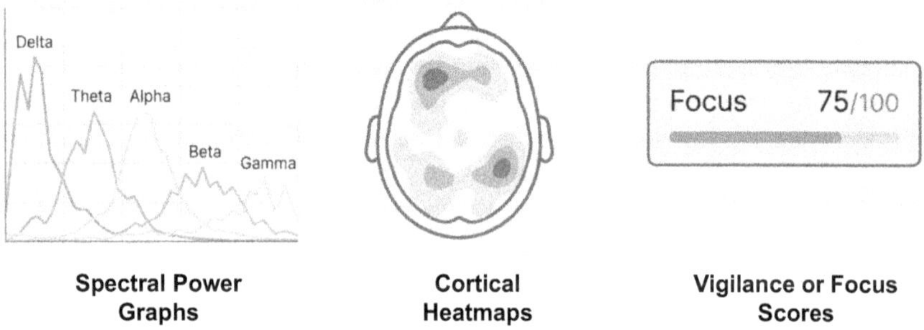

FIGURE 4.1 Highly Specialized and Complex Data Representations in Contemporary Neurowearable Interfaces.

2006) (e.g., Theta with deep relaxation or Beta with active thinking), their interpretation requires a strong foundation in neuroscience and signal processing. For the average user, they are merely complex, fluctuating lines on a graph, offering no direct instruction.

- **Abstract Cortical Heatmaps:** These are visually striking spatial representations that map the intensity of neural activity across different regions of the scalp. Although they appear engaging, showcasing the 'hotspots' of the brain, their functional meaning is deeply opaque. Without explicit knowledge of neuroanatomy and the functions of specific cortical areas (e.g., prefrontal cortex vs. parietal lobe), the heatmaps serve little more than as aesthetic novelty.
- **Raw Vigilance or Focus Scores:** These are often presented as simplistic, single-number metrics (e.g., a 'Focus Level' of 75/100) intended to summarize a complex internal state. While providing an instantaneous snapshot, they critically lack the necessary contextual scaffolding or prescriptive guidance. A user might know they are "unfocused," but the score itself offers zero insight into why this state is occurring or, more importantly, how to shift back into a desired state.

This pervasive reliance on technical presentation inevitably culminates in the most critical and unifying user complaint across the neurowearables sector: "*What am I supposed to do with all these metrics?*" The core functional disconnect is that the device, while highly sophisticated in its ability to monitor and accurately measure the brain's neurophysiological state, catastrophically fails at translation. The raw data remains locked in a technical domain, failing to serve as a meaningful, guiding principle for the user's immediate or long-term behavioral adjustment. The device effectively acts as a passive, high-fidelity observer—it monitors the current state, but it is fundamentally incapable of directing or prescribing actions to improve or maintain it. This gap between monitoring and meaningful action represents the central challenge that must be addressed for neurowearable technology to transition from a technical curiosity to a truly actionable, life-enhancing tool (Lotte et al., 2013).

4.2.2 The Missing "Expert Human Touch"

In therapeutic, clinical, or personalized coaching environments, the mere display of raw or minimally processed physiological data (e.g., heart rate variability (HRV), EEG frequency bands) is often insufficient for driving meaningful behavioral change. The true value is unlocked through a human-in-the-loop interpretation process provided by a trained professional, a clinician, therapist, or meditation coach. This professional integrates the objective biometric readings with the subjective reality of the patient or client through three crucial mechanisms:

- **Empathetic and Experiential Interpretation**
  The professional's role extends far beyond that of a data analyst. They serve as a bridge between the abstract numbers and the individual's inner world, providing:

    - **Linking Data to Lived Experience**: They contextualize the physiological changes within the patient's personal narrative. For example, instead of merely stating, "*Your alpha brainwaves decreased,*" they might say, "*The drop in your alpha activity during that session aligns with your report of feeling increasingly distracted and worrying about the upcoming meeting. The data confirms your subjective feeling of a shift from a relaxed focus to an anxious state.*"
    - **Validation and Trust Building:** By accurately reflecting the patient's internal state using external data, the coach validates the patient's experience, fostering a sense of being understood. This validation is foundational for building the therapeutic alliance and increasing engagement with the interface.
    - **Subjective-Objective Synthesis:** The coach actively seeks discrepancies or alignments between the quantitative metrics and the qualitative self-report, facilitating deeper insights into unconscious processes or habitual reactions.
- **Context-Aware and Adaptive Guidance**
  Effective guidance is never generic; it is deeply rooted in the user's current and historical situational context. This requires the professional to factor in a broad range of variables:
    - **Situational and Environmental Context:** They consider the external factors influencing the physiological state (e.g., time of day, noise level, whether the user had a conflict just before the session, or if they recently consumed caffeine). High HRV may be interpreted differently depending on whether it occurs during a high-stakes presentation or a quiet rest period.
    - **Goal and Baseline Alignment:** Guidance is tailored to the user's explicitly stated goals (e.g., reducing public speaking anxiety, improving sleep latency, deepening meditation practice). The data is interpreted relative to the individual's established baseline and trajectory toward their specific goals, not against a generalized population average.
    - **Activity-Specific Adaptation:** They adjust interpretations based on the user's current activity or task. For instance, increased sympathetic activity might be desirable during an exercise routine but detrimental during a focused meditation exercise. The coaching input is dynamically adjusted to the activity frame.
- **Translation into Actionable and Tangible Nudges**
  The final, critical step is to translate complex, often intimidating physiological states into simple, concrete, and immediately implementable actions. This transforms abstract data into practical wisdom:
    - **Simplification of Complexity:** Professionals filter out the noise and distill the physiological signal into a clear, single concept the user can grasp (e.g., translating "increased parasympathetic tone" into "*You have entered a state of deep rest, now gently sustain this breathing rhythm*").
    - **Tangible Steps and Behavioral Scripts:** The interpretation leads directly to a prescriptive intervention. Instead of merely informing the user

that they are stressed, the coach provides an "actionable nudge": "*When you notice your stress indicator rise, shift your focus to lengthening your exhale for a count of five.*" These nudges are small, specific behavioral modifications designed to regulate the observed physiological state.

- **Facilitating Self-Regulation:** Over time, the professional's guidance aims to internalize this process, equipping the user with the ability to self-interpret their own internal signals and initiate corrective actions without external prompting, effectively transitioning from human-in-the-loop guidance to autonomous self-regulation.

4.2.3 Missing "Time" from Interpretations

Current neurowearable systems rely on fixed, population-averaged interpretation models that do not account for users' evolving behavior over time. This temporal limitation compounds the DRIP paradox in several ways:

- **Static Interpretation Models:** Systems rely on fixed, universal population-averaged thresholds, which treat all users' brain signals identically. This critically ignores the fundamental principle of neuroplasticity and how neural signal patterns evolve with practice and learning trajectories. For example, expert practitioners exhibit fundamentally different neural signatures during meditation compared to novices (Davidson & Lutz, 2008). The inability to dynamically adjust to this evolution renders feedback instantly irrelevant to users who are showing progress.
- **Deteriorating Signal-to-Insight Ratio:** As a direct consequence of static models, the relevance and accuracy of the system's interpretations rapidly decline as the user's skill increases. This leads to high attrition rates (Attig & Franke, 2020). An app might flag "high beta activity" as problematic mind-wandering even when the user has progressed to a state of alert relaxation (Davidson & Lutz, 2008). Moreover, current systems fail to account for measurable changes in cortical representations that arise from motor skill consolidation over time, interpreting signs of learning as anomalies (Karni & Bertini, 1997).
- **Temporal Myopia (Lack of Longitudinal Narrative):** Each data point is treated in analytical isolation, preventing the interface from constructing a meaningful, longitudinal narrative of the user's journey. It fails to account for crucial factors such as baseline evolution, contextual learning history, and related lifestyle variables (e.g., last week's activities, yesterday's sleep) (Lazar et al., 2015). This absence of a temporal frame makes it impossible to distinguish between a negative state, such as maladaptive rumination, and a positive one, such as adaptive focused attention.
- **Ignoring Individualized Neurophysiology:** A related flaw is the reliance on standard, universal EEG frequency band definitions, which fail to capture individual peak frequencies that can vary significantly across healthy adults (Voytek et al., 2015). By missing these unique physiological signatures, the system consistently misinterprets a user's true state.

This combination of abstract metrics, a lack of expert guidance, and temporal blindness ultimately results in a heightened cognitive burden for the user, driving abandonment precisely when meaningful, long-term trends would be most informative.

4.3 SOLUTIONS: A CONTEXT-AWARE NEURO-AGENT FRAMEWORK

To address the DRIP Paradox and fundamentally shift the neurowearable paradigm, we outline a novel framework for a "Context-Aware Neuro-Agent" (see Figure 4.2). This agent should be designed to solve the "*What should I do?*" problem by integrating multiple critical layers of data ingestion and interpretation.

4.3.1 Multimodal Sensor Fusion: Understanding the Body

The first critical layer involves moving beyond isolated EEG data to establish a holistic view of the user's state. This view necessitates the simultaneous integration of situational context (e.g., calendar events, location, environmental data) alongside the user's physiological and subjective states.

Let's elaborate on the explanatory inadequacy of disembodied metrics by considering the context-dependency of neural signatures. Table 4.1 illustrates how identical brain signals yield divergent cognitive meanings when situated within different somatic and environmental contexts, demonstrating the inadequacy of brain-centric models. These patterns indicate that brain signals have no fixed meaning—their cognitive significance is constitutively dependent on the bodily and environmental contexts in which they are embedded.

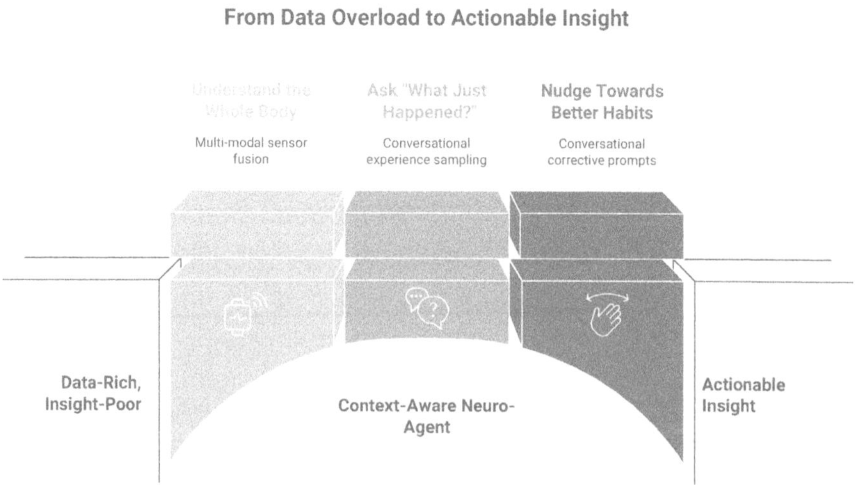

FIGURE 4.2 Outline of the Context-Aware Neuro-Agent Framework.

TABLE 4.1
Context-Dependency of Neural State Interpretation

Brain Signal	Body Context	Environmental Context	Interpreted State
High Frontal Alpha	Stable HRV, relaxed muscle tone	Meditation room, eyes closed	Deep relaxation, mindfulness (Cahn & Polich, 2006)
High Frontal Alpha	Postural collapse, declining HRV	Office desk, mid-afternoon	Mental fatigue, disengagement (Boksem et al., 2005)
High Frontal Beta	Low HRV, elevated GSR	Waiting outside the conference room	Pre-presentation anxiety (Miu et al., 2009)
High Frontal Beta	Stable HRV, normal GSR	Programming environment, flow cues	Sustained cognitive engagement (Harmony, 2013)
Parietal Alpha Asymmetry Spike	Jaw clenching (temporalis EMG (electromyography or electromyogram) artifact)	Office interruption detected	External distraction, context switch (Foxe & Snyder, 2011)
Parietal Alpha Asymmetry Spike	Relaxed facial muscles	No interruptions, prolonged task	Internal mind-wandering (Compton et al., 2019)

To understand the brain, the system must first understand the body. This is achieved through multimodal sensor fusion, integrating EEG with physiological data from the broader ecosystem of user wearables (e.g., smartwatches, rings).

- **Integration Methodology:** We discuss methodologies for correlating cortical activity (e.g., high Beta waves, often associated with cognitive activity) with autonomic biomarkers (e.g., decreased HRV or increased galvanic skin response (GSR)).
- **Validated Insights:** This fusion allows the system to differentiate between nuanced states. For example, high Beta activity correlated with increased GSR might signify physiological stress (fight-or-flight response). In contrast, the same high Beta activity with stable HRV might signify focused cognitive excitement. This moves the interface beyond generic feedback to offer biologically validated insights.

Beyond contextual disambiguation, multimodal fusion enables tracking of individual baseline evolution over time. Rather than applying static population thresholds, the system maintains rolling baselines for each physiological modality to detect systematic shifts that reflect learning and adaptation. For instance, a user's characteristic

HRV-beta coupling pattern during focused work may shift substantially over months of practice. By tracking these temporal trajectories across modalities simultaneously, the system distinguishes genuine skill development from day-to-day fluctuations, ensuring interpretations remain accurate as the user's psychophysiological profile evolves.

4.3.2 Conversational Experience Sampling : Subjective Context

The framework's second critical layer, which we term Conversational Experience Sampling (CES), moves beyond passive data collection. This novel approach actively captures the user's subjective psychological experience in real time, specifically during significant physiological shifts. CES integrates natural language processing (NLP) and large language models (LLMs), drawing on their proposed use to enhance telemedicine (Cunha Reis, 2025; T. Zhang et al., 2022).

CES fundamentally re-engineers the rigid, time-based structure of traditional Experience Sampling Method (ESM) surveys, transforming them into highly adaptable, context-aware, and naturalistic dialogues. By replacing impersonal, static forms with dynamic conversations, this approach directly addresses the pervasive issue of "survey fatigue." Crucially, it facilitates the capture of richer, qualitative nuance from unstructured responses, a depth inherently missed by the constraints of standard, quantifiable metrics alone.

Instead of relying on fixed, pre-scheduled questionnaires that often miss the moment of experience, the interface uses a sophisticated (artificial intelligence-driven) AI-driven conversational agent. This agent is designed to initiate a natural interaction immediately upon the system detecting a significant physiological or neurophysiological shift. This real-time, event-triggered methodology ensures maximum fidelity between the objective physiological state and the subjective psychological account.

The primary utility of this real-time interaction is the creation of a rich, labeled dataset. For instance, if the system detects a statistically significant spike in parietal alpha asymmetry, a neuro-physiological marker correlated with shifts in executive function or attentional focus, the agent would immediately query the user with a tailored, context-specific prompt, such as: "*I noticed a distinct shift in your focus just now. Could you tell me if a specific distraction just occurred, or if you intentionally shifted your attention to something new?*"

This immediate, targeted probing serves a triple function:

1. **Contextual Validation:** It instantly validates the raw physiological signal by connecting it directly to a verifiable behavioral or cognitive event in the user's conscious experience. This also makes it easy to improve the model iteratively and organically through regular supervised and reinforcement feedback from the user and their history.
2. **System Teaching:** Crucially, this iterative process builds a dense, highly labeled dataset that meticulously connects the raw, objective neurophysiological data (e.g., alpha asymmetry value) to the user's actual behavioral profile and internal experience (e.g., *"I was distracted by an email notification"*). This rich labeling effectively "teaches" the system the user's unique,

subjective language of their physiology, paving the way for truly personalized and actionable neuro-wearable interfaces.

3. **Coevolution of Model and User:** As mentioned above, this provides a continuous contextualized interaction between the model and the user, resulting in more accurate forecasting and interpretability.

Critically, CES enables the system to detect skill-stage transitions. As users progress from novice to intermediate to expert practitioners in domains like meditation or focus training, their physiological signatures and subjective interpretations shift systematically. The system uses these labeled transitions to adjust interpretive frameworks: what warrants intervention for a beginner (e.g., high beta as mind-wandering) becomes reframed for an advanced user (e.g., alert mindfulness). This developmental awareness prevents the deterioration of the signal-to-insight ratio that drives abandonment as users outgrow static interpretations (Attig & Franke, 2020).

4.3.3 Identifying Hidden, Non-Adaptive Habits

The third layer focuses on synthesizing the longitudinal neurophysiological data with the rich, labeled responses from CES to identify subconscious, adaptive, or maladaptive behavioral loops.

- **Synthesizing Maladaptive Loops:** The system could identify non-adaptive habits, such as subconscious jaw clenching (detectable via temporalis muscle artefact in EEG) during high-stress email processing, or shallow, rapid breathing patterns during deep work sessions. These are subconscious behaviors that drain cognitive resources.
- **Tracking Adaptive Patterns**: Conversely, the system identifies positive adaptations that reflect learning and skill acquisition. By comparing current patterns against the user's historical baseline, not population averages, the system detects improvements such as sustained increases in alpha power during meditation practice, reduced compensatory muscle tension during cognitive tasks, or faster autonomic recovery following stressors. These adaptive changes are highlighted conversationally. For instance, "Over the past month, your body has learned to maintain calm focus during email processing, your jaw tension has decreased by 40% while your attention metrics remained stable."
- **Conversational Nudges:** The interface would bring these subconscious behaviors to conscious awareness. This is done not through technical charts but through empathetic, conversational "nudges" that prompt the user to correct their behavior in real-time. The interface provides temporal context for both corrective and reinforcing feedback. Rather than treating each day's data as isolated, nudges reference relevant history: "I notice your stress pattern today mirrors what typically happens after reduced sleep. Last time this occurred, taking a ten-minute walk helped normalize your HRV." This longitudinal framing transforms the device from a moment-by-moment monitor into a

TABLE 4.2
Structural Overview of the Three Critical Layers and the Problems they are Designed to Solve

Framework Layer	Goal/Function	Key Inputs	Expected Output/ Action
Multimodal Sensor Fusion	Establish a holistic, physiological view of the user's state. Addresses "**The Crisis of Abstract Metrics**".	EEG, Autonomic Biomarkers (HRV, GSR), Situational Data (Calendar, Location)	Biologically Validated Insights (e.g., differentiating focused excitement from physiological stress).
Conversational Experience Sampling (CES)	Capture real-time subjective and psychological context from the user. Addresses "**The Missing Expert Human Touch**".	AI-Driven Probing, User Natural Language Responses	A rich, labeled dataset that connects raw neuro-physiological data to subjective experience.
Identifying Hidden, Non-Adaptive Habits	Synthesize longitudinal data to find and correct subconscious, maladaptive behaviors. Addresses "**Missing 'Time' from Interpretations**".	Fused Neuro-Physiological Data + Labeled Subjective Responses	Conversational Nudges that prompt real-time correction (e.g., correcting jaw clenching) or forecasts.

learning companion that understands the user's evolving patterns and can predict effective interventions based on personal history.

A condensed summary of the Context-Aware Neuro-Agent framework, detailing the goal, key inputs, and expected output for each layer, is provided in Table 4.2.

4.4 FUTURE DIRECTIONS: INTERACTIVE HYPER-PERSONALIZATION AND THE DIGITAL COACH

The Context-Aware Neuro-Agent framework's ultimate purpose is to move beyond mere feedback and achieve a **Virtualized Expert Presence**, culminating in the realization of the "Expert Human Touch." This section explores the future direction for deploying the system as a truly adaptive digital coach capable of facilitating Interactive Hyper-personalization and sustained behavioral change.

4.4.1 The Virtualized Expert and Dynamic Intervention

We argue that the human-in-the-loop must be the virtualized presence of an expert, a cognitive coach or clinician, rather than the user alone interpreting abstract neurophysiological data. With the widespread use of AI, conceptual frameworks for interactive personalization already exist (Khamaj & Ali, 2024; Mukti & Trisilia, 2025; Rane et al., 2023), and this needs to be optimized for the proposed Context-Aware Neuro-Agent framework. Accordingly, this virtual expert will need to operate on a continuous feedback loop driven by the two layers of the framework:

- **Curated and Dynamic Advice:** The system must transition from a static library of generic content to delivering advice dynamically. Developers would curate expert protocols, derived from clinical neuroscience, behavioral psychology, and meditation science, and give them based on the agent's real-time interpretation of the user's multimodal state (fusion), subjective labels (CES), and maladaptive habits.
- **Interactive Hyper-personalization:** This level of personalization is both biologically informed and immediately actionable. For example, if the system's fusion layer detects signs of fatigue coupled with high arousal (a "wired and tired" state), the interface would not suggest a generic "focus" exercise. Instead, it might offer a targeted intervention: "Your biology suggests you are over-stimulated. Let's try a three-minute physiological sigh protocol to reset your autonomic nervous system before we continue." The agent's next action would then be contingent on the user's response and the subsequent physiological change, creating a truly conversational and adaptive interaction.

4.4.2 Systemic and Ethical Design for Trust

For this Neuro-Agent to achieve sustained adoption, its design must explicitly address the user's fundamental concerns regarding trust, security, and the integration of deeply personal data. These elements are not features; they are foundational requirements for a system that aims to "know the user."

- **Design for Trust:** The interaction model must be transparent, with the agent providing clear, non-jargon explanations for its recommendations, grounded in the user's own data (e.g., "Based on the elevated GSR we detected..."). This transparency fosters a sense of collaborative agency, rather than a passive, obedience-based interaction with an opaque algorithm (Al-Othmani & De Vries, 2025). The agent's conversational tone should be empathetic and nonjudgmental, mirroring the supportive, motivational language of a human coach.
- **Security and Privacy-First Design:** Because neurophysiological data is sensitive, there are increasing privacy concerns (Szoszkiewicz & Yuste, 2025). Consequently, the framework must adopt a "security-by-design" approach, which is a required element. This approach includes:
  - **Edge Processing:** This is a vital architectural requirement for next-generation neurowearable interfaces, focusing on maximizing the local processing of raw physiological signals (like EEG) directly on the device rather than relying solely on the cloud (Nguyen et al., 2025). The key

benefits are: 1) enhanced privacy by minimizing the transmission of identifiable raw data, sending only aggregated or high-level semantic outputs instead; 2) low-latency responsiveness essential for real-time, human-in-the-loop conversational systems; 3) optimized power consumption by reducing the energy drain from extensive wireless data transmission; and 4) increased system robustness by allowing the interface to function reliably even with poor or intermittent network connectivity. Edge processing fundamentally transforms the neurowearable device into an intelligent, autonomous computing node, ensuring a private, responsive, and robust interface.

- **Strict Data Governance:** This is essential for the ethical integrity and trust of neurowearable interfaces. This comprehensive approach covers the entire data lifecycle through five key pillars (Davis III & Ruotsalo, 2025; Oh et al., 2024):
  1. **Mandatory Anonymization and Pseudonymization:** Sensitive neural data must be immediately processed to prevent re-identification.
  2. **Explicit, Granular, and Revocable Consent:** Users must give clear consent that specifies the data, purpose, and duration, and must be able to revoke it easily at any time.
  3. **Strict Purpose Limitation:** Data use is strictly limited to the consented purpose (e.g., user benefit/optimizing cognitive load) and prohibited for unapproved external uses like marketing or commercial aggregation.
  4. **Minimization and Retention Policies:** Only necessary data should be collected (minimization), and clear policies must govern storage duration and ensure secure, permanent deletion upon request or when the purpose is fulfilled.
  5. **Auditable Access Controls and Security:** Access to datasets must be secured through role-based controls, with all activities logged and auditable to ensure compliance and prevent breaches.

4.4.3 Long-Term Adaptation and Lifestyle Integration

The future direction also necessitates a shift from single-session optimization to long-term behavioral adaptation.

- **Integrate Lifestyle Factors for Better Actionable Insights:** The agent must learn to correlate neuro-states with longitudinal lifestyle data using an adaptive decision-making framework (C. Zhang et al., 2021). This involves factoring in sleep duration, nutrition, exercise, and social context (e.g., high-stress calendar days) to build a truly holistic, predictive model of the user's well-being. By integrating these factors, the agent can offer insights such as, "You tend to show non-adaptive jaw clenching during high-stress email processing after days with less than six hours of sleep. Prioritizing rest tonight may prevent this tomorrow." This predictive capability is key to preventative rather than purely reactive intervention.

- **Quantifying Behavioral Change:** Finally, the system needs to provide the user with clear, long-term metrics that demonstrate the tangible benefit of the intervention, moving past raw vigilance scores. Studies have shown that the technical and aesthetic elements of frameworks significantly influence users' psychological mechanisms and health promotion behaviors (Fu et al., 2025). Metrics should track reductions in non-adaptive habits and increases in self-reported positive states (e.g., "Reduction in clenching episodes by 30% this week," or "Subjective focus rating improved by 1.5 points"). This closes the loop on the DRIP Paradox by demonstrating that the data has led to meaningful, adaptive change.

4.5 CONCLUSION

The current limitations of neurowearable technology, encapsulated by the DRIP Paradox, stem from an interface design that treats brain data in isolation. By anchoring the user interface in the theory of Embodied Cognition, our proposed Context-Aware Neuro-Agent framework offers a robust roadmap for a fundamental paradigm shift.

By integrating multimodal sensor fusion, CES, longitudinal modeling, and the identification of non-adaptive habits, the system moves beyond mere measurement. It creates a bridge between raw physiological signals and the user's subjective, lived experience. This approach provides developers with a means to build neurowearables that do not merely display data, but:

- Understand context.
- Converse with empathy.
- Direct the user toward tangible, adaptive behavioral change.

The ultimate result of this transition is the evolution of the neurowearable from a passive device that merely measures the user to an active, deeply personalized system, fundamentally changing the human-technology relationship by holding the profound potential to truly and intimately *know* the user over time.

ACKNOWLEDGEMENTS

We thank all the other members of the Neurostellar Team for the discussions that made this chapter possible.

REFERENCES

Agarwal, M., Venkateswaran, S. K., & Sivakumar, R. (2020). Human-in-the-loop RL with an EEG wearable headset: On effective use of brainwaves to accelerate learning. In *Proceedings of the 6th ACM Workshop on Wearable Systems and Applications*, 25–30. Association for Computing Machinery (ACM). https://doi.org/10.1145/3396870.3400014

Al-Othmani, R., & De Vries, R. (2025). Trust in trust: A scoping review on trust and conversational agent design. In *Proceedings of the 16th Biannual Conference of the Italian*

SIGCHI Chapter, 1–6. Association for Computing Machinery (ACM). https://doi.org/10.1145/3750069.3750090

Attig, C., & Franke, T. (2020). Abandonment of personal quantification: A review and empirical study investigating reasons for wearable activity tracking attrition. *Computers in Human Behavior*, *102*, 223–237. https://doi.org/10.1016/j.chb.2019.08.025

Boksem, M. A. S., Meijman, T. F., & Lorist, M. M. (2005). Effects of mental fatigue on attention: An ERP study. *Cognitive Brain Research*, *25*(1), 107–116. https://doi.org/10.1016/j.cogbrainres.2005.04.011

Buzsáki, G. (2006). *Rhythms of the Brain* (pp. xv, 448). Oxford University Press. https://doi.org/10.1093/acprof:oso/9780195301069.001.0001

Cahn, B. R., & Polich, J. (2006). Meditation states and traits: EEG, ERP, and neuroimaging studies. *Psychological Bulletin*, *132*(2), 180–211. https://doi.org/10.1037/0033-2909.132.2.180

CFG. (2025, June 16). Neurotech consumer market atlas—How the sector is making moves into the mainstream. *Centre for Future Generations*. https://cfg.eu/neurotech-market-atlas/

Cinel, C., Valeriani, D., & Poli, R. (2019). Neurotechnologies for human cognitive augmentation: Current state of the art and future prospects. *Frontiers in Human Neuroscience*, *13*, 13. https://doi.org/10.3389/fnhum.2019.00013

Compton, R. J., Gearinger, D., & Wild, H. (2019). The wandering mind oscillates: EEG alpha power is enhanced during moments of mind-wandering. *Cognitive, Affective, & Behavioral Neuroscience*, *19*(5), 1184–1191. https://doi.org/10.3758/s13415-019-00745-9

Cunha Reis, T. (2025). Artificial intelligence and natural language processing for improved telemedicine: Before, during and after remote consultation. *Atención Primaria*, *57*(8), 103228. https://doi.org/10.1016/j.aprim.2025.103228

Davidson, R. J., & Lutz, A. (2008). Buddha's brain: Neuroplasticity and meditation [In the Spotlight]. *IEEE Signal Processing Magazine*, *25*(1), 174–175. https://doi.org/10.1109/MSP.2008.4431873

Davis III, K. M., & Ruotsalo, T. (2025). Physiological data: Challenges for privacy and ethics. *Computer*, *58*(1), 33–44. https://doi.org/10.1109/MC.2024.3404994

Di Lodovico, C., Houben, S., & Colombo, S. (2025). How to design with ambiguity: Insights from self-tracking wearables. In Proceedings of the 2025 CHI Conference on Human Factors in Computing Systems, 1–18. Association for Computing Machinery (ACM). https://doi.org/10.1145/3706598.3713267

Foxe, J. J., & Snyder, A. C. (2011). The role of alpha-band brain oscillations as a sensory suppression mechanism during selective attention. *Frontiers in Psychology*, *2*, 154. https://doi.org/10.3389/fpsyg.2011.00154

Fu, Y., Wu, C., & Li, P. (2025). The impact of smart wearable product influence elements on health promotion behaviors. *Humanities and Social Sciences Communications*, *12*(1), 1595. https://doi.org/10.1057/s41599-025-05903-8

Girivirya, S., Subekti, P., Indramayapanna, R., Marjoko, S., & Sutadi. (2022). Mind full or mindfulness! The effectiveness of mindfulness using brainwave entrainment portable EEG Muse™ S first generation. In *Proceedings of the 4th International Conference on Innovation in Education*, 96–102. SciTePress (Science and Technology Publications, LDA). https://doi.org/10.5220/0012197100003738

Harmony, T. (2013). The functional significance of delta oscillations in cognitive processing. *Frontiers in Integrative Neuroscience*, *7*, 83. https://doi.org/10.3389/fnint.2013.00083

Karni, A., & Bertini, G. (1997). Learning perceptual skills: Behavioral probes into adult cortical plasticity. *Current Opinion in Neurobiology*, *7*(4), 530–535. https://doi.org/10.1016/S0959-4388(97)80033-5

Khamaj, A., & Ali, A. M. (2024). Adapting user experience with reinforcement learning: Personalizing interfaces based on user behavior analysis in real-time. *Alexandria Engineering Journal*, *95*, 164–173. https://doi.org/10.1016/j.aej.2024.03.045

Lazar, A., Koehler, C., Tanenbaum, T. J., & Nguyen, D. H. (2015). Why we use and abandon smart devices. In *Proceedings of the 2015 ACM International Joint Conference on Pervasive and Ubiquitous Computing*, 635–646. Association for Computing Machinery (ACM). https://doi.org/10.1145/2750858.2804288

Lotte, F., Larrue, F., & Mühl, C. (2013). Flaws in current human training protocols for spontaneous brain-computer interfaces: Lessons learned from instructional design. *Frontiers in Human Neuroscience*, *7*, 568. https://doi.org/10.3389/fnhum.2013.00568

Miu, A. C., Heilman, R. M., & Miclea, M. (2009). Reduced heart rate variability and vagal tone in anxiety: Trait versus state, and the effects of autogenic training. *Autonomic Neuroscience*, *145*(1–2), 99–103. doi:10.1016/j.autneu.2008.11.010

Mukti, A. J., & Trisilia, M. (2025). AI-powered adaptive interface: Enhancing user experience through real-time personalization in digital platforms. *Procedia Computer Science*, *269*, 571–580. https://doi.org/10.1016/j.procs.2025.08.309

Muvvala, V. K., Kazen, A. B., Newton, T. J., Tosi, Z., Elwood, M., Lehmkuhle, M. J., Loddenkemper, T., Spitz, M. C., Strom, L., Friedman, D., & Frankel, M. A. (2025). Comparative analysis of signal quality and usability for a novel wireless, wearable EEG sensor. *Clinical Neurophysiology Practice*, *10*, 292–300. https://doi.org/10.1016/j.cnp.2025.05.004

Nguyen, M.-D., Do, T., Tran, X.-T., Nguyen, Q.-T., & Lin, C.-T. (2025). Edge AI-brain–computer interfaces system: A survey. *IEEE Transactions on Neural Systems and Rehabilitation Engineering*, *33*, 4051–4066. https://doi.org/10.1109/TNSRE.2025.3618688

Oh, J., Son, S., Kwon, D., Kim, M., Park, Y., & Park, Y. (2024). Design of secure and privacy-preserving data sharing scheme based on key aggregation and private set intersection in medical information system. *Mathematics*, *12*(11), 1717. https://doi.org/10.3390/math12111717

Rane, N., Choudhary, S., & Rane, J. (2023). Hyper-personalization for enhancing customer loyalty and satisfaction in Customer Relationship Management (CRM) systems. *SSRN Electronic Journal*. https://doi.org/10.2139/ssrn.4641044

Simons, S. B., Provo, M., Yanoschak, A., Schmidt, C., Gerrard, I., Weisend, M., Anderson, C., Shimizu, R., & Connolly, P. M. (2024). A randomized study on the effect of a wearable device using 0.75 Hz transcranial electrical stimulation on sleep onset insomnia. *Frontiers in Neuroscience*, *18*, 1427462. https://doi.org/10.3389/fnins.2024.1427462

Szoszkiewicz, Ł., & Yuste, R. (2025). Mental privacy: Navigating risks, rights and regulation: Advances in neuroscience challenge contemporary legal frameworks to protect mental privacy. *EMBO Reports*, *26*(14), 3469–3473. https://doi.org/10.1038/s44319-025-00505-6

Tzimourta, K. D. (2025). Human-centered design and development in digital health: Approaches, challenges, and emerging trends. *Cureus*. https://doi.org/10.7759/cureus.85897

Varela, F. J., Rosch, E., & Thompson, E. (1991). *The Embodied Mind: Cognitive Science and Human Experience*. The MIT Press. https://doi.org/10.7551/mitpress/6730.001.0001

Voytek, B., Kramer, M. A., Case, J., Lepage, K. Q., Tempesta, Z. R., Knight, R. T., & Gazzaley, A. (2015). Age-related changes in $1/f$ neural electrophysiological noise. *The Journal of Neuroscience*, *35*(38), 13257–13265. https://doi.org/10.1523/JNEUROSCI.2332-14.2015

Wilson, M. (2002). Six views of embodied cognition. *Psychonomic Bulletin & Review*, *9*(4), 625–636. https://doi.org/10.3758/BF03196322

Yang, R., Zhang, L., Yang, R., Hou, L., Zhu, D., & Zhong, B. (2025). Multiple entropy fusion predicts driver fatigue using forehead EEG. *Frontiers in Neuroscience*, *19*, 1567146. https://doi.org/10.3389/fnins.2025.1567146

Zhang, C., Lakens, D., & IJsselsteijn, W. A. (2021). Theory integration for lifestyle behavior change in the digital age: An adaptive decision-making framework. *Journal of Medical Internet Research*, *23*(4), e17127. https://doi.org/10.2196/17127

Zhang, T., Schoene, A. M., Ji, S., & Ananiadou, S. (2022). Natural language processing applied to mental illness detection: A narrative review. *Npj Digital Medicine*, *5*(1), 46. https://doi.org/10.1038/s41746-022-00589-7

5 Beyond Pristine Signals

A Paradigm Shift Towards Robust Multimodal Feature Analysis for Mental State Assessment with Consumer Neurowearables

Arun Sasidharan, Vrinda M., Varsha Vijayan, Fayaz Pathan Khan, and Karthik Raghavendran

5.1 INTRODUCTION

Consumer-grade neurowearables, which incorporate advanced neurophysiological and physiological sensing technologies such as electroencephalography (EEG) and photoplethysmography (PPG) for heart rate variability (HRV), have proliferated rapidly over the last decade. This increased sophistication and availability offer transformative potential: shifting mental-state assessment from restricted clinical laboratory settings to the dynamic, ecologically valid environment of daily life (Emish & Young, 2024). This shift promises scalable, longitudinal data collection, paving the way for accessible and personalized mental well-being support.

However, the enthusiasm for real-world application is tempered by a significant and pervasive challenge: signal quality (SQ). Data acquired from consumer neurowearables, which frequently employ dry electrodes and are inherently subject to movement artifacts, loose contact, and environmental interference, rarely achieve the "pristine" signal-to-noise ratio of gold-standard lab-based equipment (Hao et al., 2024). The traditional approach in biosignal analysis, rooted in lab settings, has been to treat noise and artifacts as contaminants to be meticulously filtered out (Islam et al., 2021). This approach, however, fundamentally limits the applicability and scalability of neurowearables.

This chapter argues that adhering to the pursuit of laboratory-standard signal purity in uncontrolled real-world environments is fundamentally impractical and misguided. We propose a critical paradigm shift in biosignal analysis. Instead of focusing on SQ, we advocate leveraging the rich, complex information embedded in the Gestalt of "noisy," multimodal data streams (Schmidt et al., 2019). The core hypothesis is that valuable psychophysiological information is not solely dependent on clean, isolated features from single channels, but is robustly preserved in the complex, dynamic

DOI: 10.1201/9781003500445-5

patterns and interactions that emerge across multiple physiological modalities, even in the persistent presence of real-world interference.

The following sections will detail the necessity and methodology of this new approach, outlining a robust framework for multimodal feature analysis essential for unlocking the true potential of consumer neurowearables.

5.2 THE REALITY OF REAL-WORLD BIOSIGNALS

Traditional biosignal analysis methodologies were developed for controlled laboratory settings, utilizing wet electrodes, shielded environments, and constrained subject movement. The application of these methods directly to data from consumer neurowearables (designed for convenience and everyday use) is deeply flawed, as the data profile is fundamentally different (Schmidt et al., 2019; Siddharth et al., 2019).

This section characterizes the specific noise and artifact profiles inherent to consumer-grade wearables:

- **Dry-Sensor EEG Artifacts:** Unlike wet electrodes, dry sensors are highly susceptible to changes in skin impedance due to movement, sweat, or minimal displacement (Taji et al., 2018). This often leads to high-amplitude, transient, or intermittent baseline drift and motion artifacts that severely corrupt the underlying neural signal. Traditional high-pass filtering, while useful, usually fails to fully suppress these artifacts without sacrificing low-frequency, physiologically relevant dynamics (Seok et al., 2021).
- **PPG Motion Artifacts:** PPG signals, crucial for estimating HRV, are particularly vulnerable to motion artifacts in active users. Slight device movement against the skin can introduce significant spectral energy that overlaps with the physiological signal of interest, rendering standard spectral filtering techniques ineffective at preserving the accurate pulse waveform needed for HRV calculations (Scardulla et al., 2023).
- **Environmental and Inter-Device Noise:** Data acquisition in real-world settings exposes the signals to ambient electromagnetic interference, radio frequency noise (Prekodravac Filipovic et al., 2025), and the inherent variability introduced by different device models and firmware versions (Canali et al., 2022).

These combined factors establish why conventional "denoising" techniques, designed for near-pristine lab data, frequently fail in real-world scenarios. By aggressively filtering, analysts risk eliminating genuine physiological dynamics that are intertwined with artifacts, thereby losing the very information they seek to measure. This reality underscores the need to change the analytical target from SQ to information quality (IQ).

5.3 THE CASE FOR A PARADIGM SHIFT

The core argument proposes shifting the analysis of consumer neurowearable data from prioritizing traditional SQ to focusing on IQ. Historically, lab-based analysis focused on achieving pristine SQ (clear, artifact-free single signals). However, in uncontrolled, "in-the-wild" scenarios typical of consumer devices, high SQ is difficult and often irrelevant due to motion artifacts and interference.

IQ operationalizes a new approach by shifting the analytical focus from the purity of a single signal to the robustness and discriminatory power of a multidimensional feature set. This means even a visually "noisy" signal (low SQ) can contribute to a high-IQ system if features extracted from multiple, imperfect signals collectively demonstrate: 1) Robustness to Noise and 2) Discriminatory Power (the ability to reliably separate target mental states) (Grosselin et al., 2019).

Consequently, "noise" is redefined not as an unwanted contaminant but as a complex artifact pattern that can be managed, modelled, and combined with other data (such as motion or heart rate) to enhance the overall IQ—the system's capacity to accurately assess mental states outside the lab.

Here is a breakdown of the contrast and the proposed metrics for operationalizing IQ.

5.3.1 Concept of Signal Quality vs. Information Quality

Table 5.1 provides a formal comparison between the traditional emphasis on SQ (i.e., signal quality) and the chapter's proposed focus on IQ (i.e., information quality),

TABLE 5.1
Comparison of Signal Quality and Information Quality

Concept	Goal (What is Sought)	Operationalization/ Measurement (How it is Measured)	Limitations in Real-World
Signal Quality (SQ)	**"Pristine" signal purity.** Achieving a clean, high signal-to-noise ratio (SNR) on individual channels.	**Signal-to-Noise Ratio (SNR):** The ratio of signal power to noise power. Success is measured by the efficacy of *filtering* and *denoising* techniques to suppress artifacts (e.g., dry-sensor EEG drift, PPG motion artifacts).	The pursuit of near-perfect SNR leads to aggressive filtering, risking the elimination of genuine physiological dynamics intertwined with artifacts, thereby losing **the very information sought.**
Information Quality (IQ)	**Resilient, complex patterns** that robustly represent the underlying psychophysiological state, even in the presence of noise.	**Classification Accuracy** and **Feature Pattern Stability** in a multi-dimensional space.	Requires computationally intensive advanced feature extraction and validation against established psychological benchmarks.

TABLE 5.2
Approaches for Measuring Information Quality

IQ Measurement Approach	Key Methodology	Operational Metric
Differentiation of Behavioral States	**Multimodal Fusion** (Feature-Level and Decision-Level Fusion of EEG and PPG)	**Superior Classification Accuracy:** The ability of the fused, multivariate features to correctly classify distinct mental states (e.g., focus and relaxation). The Case Study (Section 5.5) uses this as the primary evidence of success.
Stability of Patterns	**Cluster-Based Analysis of the Feature Gestalt** (Focusing on the sequence and stability of multi-dimensional feature clusters over time)	**Resilience to Artifact Load/Pattern Stability:** This is measured by the ability of the feature-cluster sequences to remain stable over a defined window of time, even when transient artifacts momentarily distort the raw signal. This is specifically highlighted as maintaining stable performance during periods of "high motion or environmental interference".

outlining the distinct goals, measurement approaches, and real-world limitations of each concept.

5.3.2 Operationalizing and Measuring Information Quality

The chapter defines IQ not by what is filtered out, but by what is retained and how reliably it can classify or represent a mental state. IQ is measured using two primary approaches: Differentiation of behavioral states and Stability of patterns (see Table 5.2).

5.3.3 Re-Interpreting Noise

Instead of viewing noise and artifacts solely as measurement errors, we must recognize that a compromise in individual channel SQ does not necessarily equate to a loss of psychophysiological information when multiple modalities are integrated. The core theory is based on the following principles:

- **Information Resilience through Modality Interaction:** The human mental state is not encapsulated by a single, isolated physiological channel, but by the complex, coordinated activity across multiple systems (e.g., neural, autonomic, somatic). Multimodal analysis, which examines the interaction, coherence, or phase relationships among different physiological signals (e.g., EEG-derived focus and HRV-derived stress from PPG), provides robust information. This information is superior to what can be gathered from unimodal sources alone (Mark et al., 2024). Furthermore, the correlated information across modalities enhances resilience, making the assessment less susceptible to the compromise of an individual sensor or channel (Vasilyev et al., 2019). Therefore, a momentary PPG artifact might obscure the HRV signal, but if the simultaneous EEG shows a strong, sustained pattern of focused attention, the overall assessment of the mental state remains robust.

- **Feature Complexity over Feature Fidelity:** The valuable information is not in the precise fidelity of a single data point (e.g., the exact voltage amplitude at a millisecond time point), but in the pattern and complexity of feature sets over time (Balasubramanian et al., 2025). A slight artifact-induced deviation in a raw signal may not corrupt a higher-order feature that describes the signal's complexity or its position relative to other features in a multidimensional space (Chen et al., 2025; Zhang et al., 2025).
- **Embracing Ecological Validity:** This shift embraces the inherent complexity and variability of the real world. By developing models that thrive on multimodal redundancy and statistical patterns rather than strict signal perfection (Pallapothula et al., 2025), we can build systems that are truly ecologically valid and relevant for continuous, personalized monitoring outside the confines of the lab.

This approach moves beyond simple univariate correlations, recognizing that the complex interplay of features provides a more robust signature of different mental states, such as focus and relaxation, than any single, artifact-prone channel could on its own.

5.4 METHODOLOGICAL FRAMEWORK – ADVANCED FEATURE EXTRACTION

This section details the technical core of the proposed framework (see Figure 5.1), focusing on advanced feature engineering and machine learning (ML) frameworks designed to operate effectively under real-world, noisy conditions. These are the wearable/nearable feature extractions that underpin the robust multimodal approach.

5.4.1 Multimodal Fusion of Electroencephalography and Photoplethysmography

Instead of treating EEG and PPG streams independently, this framework employs techniques to fuse the information at the feature or decision level.

- **Feature-Level Fusion:** Deriving a comprehensive feature vector that includes not only traditional power spectral densities from EEG and time/frequency domain features from HRV, but also cross-modal metrics such as

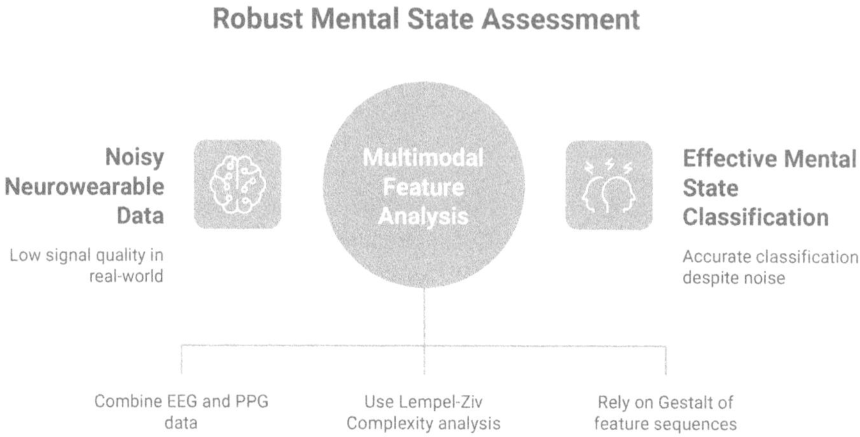

FIGURE 5.1 Proposed Framework for Robust Mental State Assessment.

the covariance, cross-correlation, or coherence between features from the two modalities (Suzuki et al., 2021; L. Wang et al., 2023).

- **Decision-Level Fusion:** Training separate classifiers for each modality and then using a meta-classifier (e.g., weighted voting, stacking) to combine their outputs (Hemakom et al., 2023; Kiejdo et al., 2025). The redundancy ensures that if one modality is temporarily compromised, the other can still contribute a reliable, weighted vote to the final classification of the mental state.

Large language models (LLMs) offer a more sophisticated approach to multimodal fusion of physiological signals, such as EEG and PPG, by converting them into a unified, tokenized vocabulary (C. Wang et al., 2025). This enables the LLM's self-attention mechanism to capture complex, nonlinear relationships. Benefits include dynamic, real-time cross-modal weighting and context-aware fusion through the integration of external metadata such as task descriptions. Furthermore, LLMs serve as powerful reasoning engines for decision-level fusion, enhancing interpretability in mental state classification by providing natural-language justifications that explain the synergy between neural and cardiovascular metrics.

5.4.2 Use of Nonlinear Dynamics

Moving beyond traditional linear time-series features, this framework heavily relies on nonlinear dynamics, which are often more resistant to additive white noise and motion artifacts.

- **Lempel-Ziv Complexity (LZC):** A robust measure of the complexity and randomness of a time series. LZC quantifies the number of distinct patterns or sub-sequences encountered as the data stream is parsed. It is a reliable marker of cognitive load and attention, exhibiting stability even when raw amplitude measurements are distorted.

- **Sample Entropy/Approximate Entropy:** These features quantify the predictability and regularity of the signal, providing an index of the underlying system's complexity that can be less sensitive to high frequency artifacts compared to simple band power.

5.4.3 Cluster-Based Analysis and the Feature Gestalt

The most critical aspect is the focus on the "Gestalt" of feature sequences rather than precise voltage amplitudes.

- **Multifeature Cluster Sequences:** This involves taking the comprehensive feature vector (including linear, nonlinear, and cross-modal features) and performing dimensionality reduction (e.g., principal components analysis (PCA) or uniform manifold approximation and projection (UMAP)), followed by a dynamic clustering algorithm (e.g., k-means, hierarchical density-based spatial clustering of applications with noise (HDBSCAN)) in the reduced feature space. The mental state is not classified based on the instantaneous feature vector, but on the sequence of cluster IDs that the subject's features occupy over a defined time window. The robust classification is achieved by analyzing the transition rate, dwell time, and typical sequence of these feature clusters, which are highly resistant to transient data anomalies that only momentarily push the feature vector away from its central cluster.

By employing these advanced frameworks, the analysis shifts from filtering out noise to robustly extracting psychophysiological information that survives, often leveraging the complexity of real-world data. These advanced, multimodal techniques collectively form a robust framework for achieving high IQ, which we validate in the following case study.

5.5 CASE STUDY AND VALIDATION

To ground this theory in practice, this section presents a validation summary comparing the proposed robust feature engineering approach against traditional, raw-signal-correlation methods.

The validation study, such as the recent Neurostellar study referenced, involves subjects using consumer-grade neurowearables in a representative, uncontrolled environment (e.g., working at a home office, engaging in light activity) (Marigowda et al., 2025). The study aimed to classify distinct mental states, such as focus and relaxation (key targets for mental well-being support), using a multimodal and multivariate approach (see Figure 5.2).

Key findings from the validation (Marigowda et al., 2025):

- **Moderate-to-Strong Correlations With Lab Measurements:** The analysis of device correlation ($r > 0.5$ & $p < 0.05$) showed significant agreement for a majority of features under both eyes closed and eyes open conditions. Specifically, under the eyes-closed condition, significant correlations were

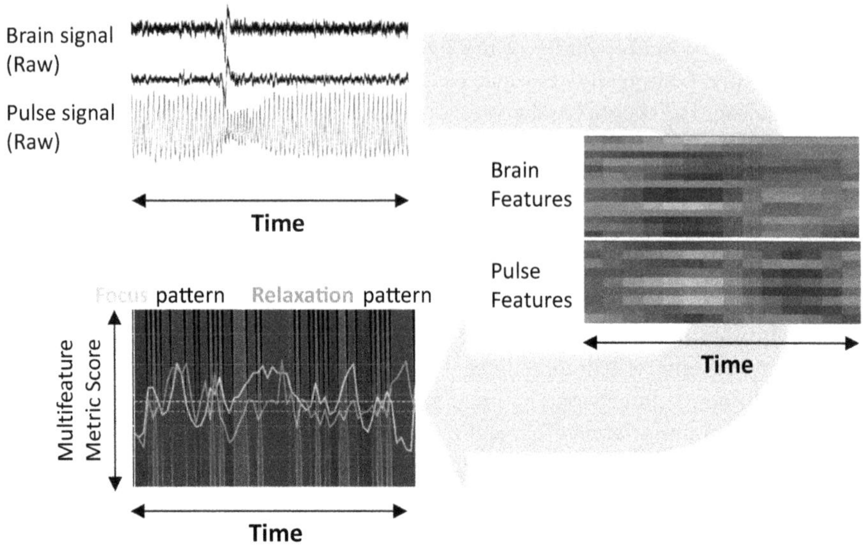

FIGURE 5.2 Multimodal and Multivariate Mapping Between Raw Signals and Mental States.

observed in at least 50% of recordings for 12 of 18 EEG features and 9 of 12 HRV features. Under the eyes open condition, the trend was similar, with 14 of 18 EEG features and 6 of 12 HRV features showing significant correlations in at least half of the recordings. The wearable reliably captured a wide range of standard psychophysiological features, including highly concordant HRV, despite hardware differences. Variation in feature and condition (eyes-open/closed) correlation strength is expected due to differing signal-to-noise ratios and artifact susceptibility, aligning with prior studies showing variable correlations, such as higher correlations in the EEG frequency domain (Jackson et al., 2013), and condition-dependent variation with dry electrodes (Pazuelo et al., 2024). The fact that over half the recordings showed significant correlations is encouraging for a consumer device prioritizing ease of use over strict lab standards.

- **Superior Classification Accuracy:** The study found that the advanced multimodal features were highly effective in classifying distinct mental states, as demonstrated by the significant results for both random forest (RF) ($z=13.08$-13.11, $p<0.001$) and Gradient Boosting ($z=13.00$-13.16, $p<0.001$) models when compared to chance. Furthermore, these features successfully predicted subjective ratings of relaxation and focus above chance levels, with RF achieving $z=2.37$ ($p<0.05$) and Gradient Boosting achieving $z=1.79$ ($p<0.05$). This finding aligns with previous research indicating that the combination of EEG and HRV features provides a clearer definition of psychophysiological states, such as stress (Attar et al., 2021). Furthermore, the inclusion of higher-order EEG complexity features has been shown to result in distinct predictions for focus and relaxation (Richer et al., 2018).

The empirical evidence from the case study demonstrates that, even with a moderate correlation to lab-grade recordings, a sophisticated, multifeatured analysis approach can effectively and reliably assess mental states outside of a controlled laboratory setting. This shift toward accommodating the complexity of real-world data, a necessity already recognized in the use of wearable accelerometer data for physical activity (Troiano et al., 2014) and wearable HRV data for mental state assessment (Tiwari & Falk, 2021), is essential. It is a core requirement for realizing the full potential of consumer neurowearables for accessible, personalized monitoring.

5.6 FUTURE CHALLENGES AND ETHICAL CONSIDERATIONS

While the paradigm shift towards robust multimodal analysis addresses the technical bottleneck of SQ, its implementation introduces new challenges and ethical responsibilities that must be addressed for widespread adoption.

5.6.1 Computational Trade-Offs and Battery Life

Advanced feature extraction techniques (e.g., nonlinear dynamics, cluster sequence analysis) are computationally intensive compared to simple time-domain or spectral-power calculations.

- **Challenge:** Implementing these advanced algorithms on resource-constrained consumer devices requires balancing the computational load of the robust extraction with the necessity of preserving device battery life.
- **Implication:** Future research must focus on optimizing these algorithms for energy efficiency, potentially through on-device edge computing or highly efficient feature selection to ensure the system is practical for continuous, long-term monitoring.

5.6.2 Standardization Challenges and Regulatory Approval

The departure from raw signal correlation creates a challenge for standardization and regulatory approval (Santra et al., 2024).

- **Challenge:** Medical devices and wellness regulators typically rely on established, traceable metrics derived directly from raw signals. Moving to complex, high-dimensional feature spaces and clustering sequences makes the underlying decision process less transparent (a "black-box problem").
- **Implication:** A new framework for validation and standardization is required. This may involve establishing a clear, validated link between the Gestalt feature space and established psychological/physiological benchmarks, ensuring that the model's output remains clinically and scientifically interpretable even if the intermediate features are abstract.

5.6.3 Ethical Considerations for Personalized Data

The detailed, longitudinal tracking of mental states raises significant ethical questions regarding data privacy and user autonomy (Pham, 2025).

- **Challenge:** Advanced algorithms can infer sensitive mental states with high accuracy. The data collected is highly personal and potentially vulnerable to misuse.
- **Implication:** Robust data security protocols, transparent user control over data usage, and ethical guidelines for the deployment of mental state assessment algorithms are paramount to maintaining user trust and ensuring this powerful technology is used responsibly for societal benefit.

5.7 CONCLUSION

The pursuit of "pristine" SQ from consumer neurowearables in real-world settings is an aspiration that must be abandoned. This chapter has argued for and outlined a necessary paradigm shift: Beyond Pristine Signals.

By embracing robust multimodal feature analysis (integrating signals such as EEG and PPG, employing nonlinear dynamics, and focusing on the complex, dynamic patterns (the Gestalt) of feature sets) we can move beyond the limitations of univariate, artifact-prone data. This new orientation is essential for developing the next generation of algorithms that can meaningfully and reliably track and support mental well-being in the diverse and dynamic conditions of daily life. The challenges of computational cost and regulatory standardization remain, but by addressing them directly, we can unlock the true, scalable potential of consumer neurowearables.

ACKNOWLEDGEMENTS

We thank all the other members of the Neurostellar Team for the discussions that made this chapter possible.

REFERENCES

Attar, E. T., Balasubramanian, V., Subasi, E., & Kaya, M. (2021). Stress Analysis Based on Simultaneous Heart Rate Variability and EEG Monitoring. *IEEE Journal of Translational Engineering in Health and Medicine*, *9*, 1–7. https://doi.org/10.1109/JTEHM.2021.3106803

Balasubramanian, K., Ranjani Rajendran, S., & Pati, S. (2025). Complexity Measures in Biomedical Signal Analysis: A Clinically-Grounded Survey Across EEG, ECG, Intracranial Pressure, and Photoplethysmogram Modalities. *IEEE Access*, *13*, 155285–155304. https://doi.org/10.1109/ACCESS.2025.3603848

Canali, S., Schiaffonati, V., & Aliverti, A. (2022). Challenges and Recommendations for Wearable Devices in Digital Health: Data Quality, Interoperability, Health Equity, Fairness. *PLOS Digital Health*, *1*(10), e0000104. https://doi.org/10.1371/journal.pdig.0000104

Chen, C.-S., Chang, S.-H., Liu, C.-W., & Pan, T.-M. (2025). Exploring the Potential of Electroencephalography Signal–Based Image Generation Using Diffusion Models: Integrative Framework Combining Mixed Methods and Multimodal Analysis. *JMIR Medical Informatics*, *13*, e72027. https://doi.org/10.2196/72027

Emish, M., & Young, S. D. (2024). Remote Wearable Neuroimaging Devices for Health Monitoring and Neurophenotyping: A Scoping Review. *Biomimetics*, *9*(4), 237. https://doi.org/10.3390/biomimetics9040237

Grosselin, F., Navarro-Sune, X., Vozzi, A., Pandremmenou, K., De Vico Fallani, F., Attal, Y., & Chavez, M. (2019). Quality Assessment of Single-Channel EEG for Wearable Devices. *Sensors*, *19*(3), 601. https://doi.org/10.3390/s19030601

Hao, S., Xin, Q., Xiandeng, H., Jian, W., Hongbin, C., Xiaoqin, W., Lifei, X., Jiaxin, J., Ruiying, X., Siping, F., Lu, L., Yuqi, S., Yuhang, Z., & Yuxi, Z. (2024). *Field Experiment on Wearable EEG/PPG-based Monitoring of Mental Fatigue in Drillers: Impact of Prolonged Working Hours and Night Shifts* (SSRN Scholarly Paper No. 4915905). Social Science Research Network. https://doi.org/10.2139/ssrn.4915905

Hemakom, A., Atiwiwat, D., & Israsena, P. (2023). ECG and EEG based Detection and Multilevel Classification of Stress using Machine Learning for Specified Genders: A Preliminary Study. *PLOS ONE*, *18*(9), e0291070. https://doi.org/10.1371/journal.pone.0291070

Islam, Md. K., Rastegarnia, A., & Sanei, S. (2021). Signal Artifacts and Techniques for Artifacts and Noise Removal. In M. A. R. Ahad & M. U. Ahmed (Eds.), *Signal Processing Techniques for Computational Health Informatics* (Vol. 192, pp. 23–79). Springer International Publishing. https://doi.org/10.1007/978-3-030-54932-9_2

Jackson, G., Radhu, N., Yinming, S., Tallevi, K., Ritvo, P., Daskalakis, Z. J., Grundlehner, B., Penders, J., & Cafazzo, J. A. (2013). Comparative Evaluation of an Ambulatory EEG Platform vs. Clinical Gold Standard. In *2013 35th Annual International Conference of the IEEE Engineering in Medicine and Biology Society (EMBC)*, 1222–1225. IEEE (Institute of Electrical and Electronics Engineers). https://doi.org/10.1109/EMBC.2013.6609727

Kiejdo, D., Depka Prądzinska, M., & Zawadzka, T. (2025). Late Fusion Model for Emotion Recognition from Facial Expressions and Biosignals in a Dataset of Children with Autism Spectrum Disorder. *Sensors*, *25*(24), 7485. https://doi.org/10.3390/s25247485

Marigowda, V., Sasidharan, A., Vijayan, V., Pathan, F. K., G, A., Raghavendran, K., Sree, D., Venkatesan, A., & Venkataraman, K. (2025). Evaluating Neurostellar's Wearable Device Along with Its Robust Multimodal Approach for Real-Time Mental State Assessment: A Validation Study. *Qeios*. Unique Article ID: HDMEQ5, Version 1. https://doi.org/10.32388/HDMEQ5

Mark, J. A., Curtin, A., Kraft, A. E., Ziegler, M. D., & Ayaz, H. (2024). Mental Workload Assessment by Monitoring Brain, Heart, and Eye with Six Biomedical Modalities During Six Cognitive Tasks. *Frontiers in Neuroergonomics*, *5*, 1345507. https://doi.org/10.3389/fnrgo.2024.1345507

Pallapothula, V. K. N., Anand, S., Das Bhattacharjee, S., & Yuan, J. (2025). Generalized Multisensor Wearable Signal Fusion for Emotion Recognition from Noisy and Incomplete Data. *Smart Health*, *36*, 100571. https://doi.org/10.1016/j.smhl.2025.100571

Pazuelo, J., Juez, J. Y., Moumane, H., Pyrzowski, J., Mayor, L., Segura-Quijano, F. E., Valderrama, M., & Le Van Quyen, M. (2024). Evaluating the Electroencephalographic Signal Quality of an In-Ear Wearable Device. *Sensors*, *24*(12), 3973. https://doi.org/10.3390/s24123973

Pham, T. (2025). Ethical and Legal Considerations in Healthcare AI: Innovation and Policy for Safe and Fair use. *Royal Society Open Science*, *12*(5), 241873. https://doi.org/10.1098/rsos.241873

Prekodravac Filipovic, J., Milenkovic, M., Kepic, D., Dorontic, S., Yasir, M., Nardin, B., & Jovanovic, S. (2025). Electromagnetic Interference in the Modern Era: Concerns, Trends, and Nanomaterial-Based Solutions. *Nanomaterials, 15*(20), 1558. https://doi.org/10.3390/nano15201558

Richer, R., Zhao, N., Amores, J., Eskofier, B. M., & Paradiso, J. A. (2018). Real-time Mental State Recognition using a Wearable EEG. In *2018 40th Annual International Conference of the IEEE Engineering in Medicine and Biology Society (EMBC)*, 5495–5498. IEEE (Institute of Electrical and Electronics Engineers). https://doi.org/10.1109/EMBC.2018.8513653

Santra, S., Kukreja, P., Saxena, K., Gandhi, S., & Singh, O. V. (2024). Navigating Regulatory and Policy Challenges for AI Enabled Combination Devices. *Frontiers in Medical Technology, 6*, 1473350. https://doi.org/10.3389/fmedt.2024.1473350

Scardulla, F., Cosoli, G., Spinsante, S., Poli, A., Iadarola, G., Pernice, R., Busacca, A., Pasta, S., Scalise, L., & D'Acquisto, L. (2023). Photoplethysmograhic Sensors, Potential and Limitations: Is it Time for Regulation? A Comprehensive Review. *Measurement, 218*, 113150. https://doi.org/10.1016/j.measurement.2023.113150

Schmidt, P., Reiss, A., Dürichen, R., & Van Laerhoven, K. (2019). Wearable-Based Affect Recognition—A Review. *Sensors (Basel, Switzerland), 19*(19), 4079. https://doi.org/10.3390/s19194079

Seok, D., Lee, S., Kim, M., Cho, J., & Kim, C. (2021). Motion Artifact Removal Techniques for Wearable EEG and PPG Sensor Systems. *Frontiers in Electronics, 2*, 685513. https://doi.org/10.3389/felec.2021.685513

Siddharth, N., Patel, A. N., Jung, T.-P., & Sejnowski, T. J. (2019). A Wearable Multi-Modal Bio-Sensing System Towards Real-World Applications. *IEEE Transactions on Bio-Medical Engineering, 66*(4), 1137–1147. https://doi.org/10.1109/TBME.2018.2868759

Suzuki, K., Laohakangvalvit, T., Matsubara, R., & Sugaya, M. (2021). Constructing an Emotion Estimation Model Based on EEG/HRV Indexes Using Feature Extraction and Feature Selection Algorithms. *Sensors, 21*(9), 2910. https://doi.org/10.3390/s21092910

Taji, B., Chan, A. D. C., & Shirmohammadi, S. (2018). Effect of Pressure on Skin-Electrode Impedance in Wearable Biomedical Measurement Devices. *IEEE Transactions on Instrumentation and Measurement, 67*(8), 1900–1912. https://doi.org/10.1109/TIM.2018.2806950

Tiwari, A., & Falk, T. H. (2021). New Measures of Heart Rate Variability Based on Subband Tachogram Complexity and Spectral Characteristics for Improved Stress and Anxiety Monitoring in Highly Ecological Settings. *Frontiers in Signal Processing, 1*, 737881. https://doi.org/10.3389/frsip.2021.737881

Troiano, R. P., McClain, J. J., Brychta, R. J., & Chen, K. Y. (2014). Evolution of Accelerometer Methods for Physical Activity Research. *British Journal of Sports Medicine, 48*(13), 1019–1023. https://doi.org/10.1136/bjsports-2014-093546

Vasilyev, V., Borisov, V., Syskov, A., & Kublanov, V. (2019). Case Study of Interrelation between Brain-Computer Interface based Multimodal Metric and Heart Rate Variability. In *Proceedings of the 12th International Joint Conference on Biomedical Engineering Systems and Technologies*, 532–538. https://doi.org/10.5220/0007694505320538

Wang, C., Li, M., He, J., Wang, Z., Darzi, E., Chen, Z., Ye, J., Li, T., Su, Y., Ke, J., Qu, K., Li, S., Yu, Y., Liò, P., Wang, T., Wang, Y. G., & Shen, Y. (2025). A Survey for Large Language

Models in Biomedicine. *Artificial Intelligence in Medicine*, *170*, 103268. https://doi.org/10.1016/j.artmed.2025.103268

Wang, L., Hao, J., & Zhou, T. H. (2023). ECG Multi-Emotion Recognition Based on Heart Rate Variability Signal Features Mining. *Sensors*, *23*(20), 8636. https://doi.org/10.3390/s23208636

Zhang, X., Liu, H., Sun, M., & Feng, S. (2025). Multimodal Approach to Public Health Interventions using EGG and Mobile Health Technologies. *Frontiers in Public Health*, *12*, 1520343. https://doi.org/10.3389/fpubh.2024.1520343

6 A Wearable Threshold-Based System for COVID-19 Severity Assessment

*Maria Inês Barbosa, Pedro Ribeiro,
Patrícia Batista, Ganesh R. Naik,
João Alexandre Lobo Marques, and
Pedro Miguel Rodrigues*

6.1 INTRODUCTION

Wearable technologies are increasingly being explored in healthcare for their simplicity, portability, and ability to provide real-time health monitoring (Khondakar and Kaushik 2023; Marques et al. 2021; Caldas et al. 2023; Cavalcante et al. 2023). In recent years, wearable devices have gained significant traction in the healthcare sector, offering a practical, noninvasive means to continuously monitor physiological parameters and are useful in both clinical and remote settings. Their ability to collect objective data and integrate with wireless systems enables real-time monitoring and clinical feedback, making them a promising solution for supporting early detection, continuous patient assessment, and personalized care delivery (Channa et al. 2021; Ding et al. 2020; Verde, De Pietro, and Sannino 2023; De Sario Velasquez et al. 2024). An example of this is the variety of wearable devices that have been developed to provide valuable insights into respiratory function and health, such as smartwatches (Trimpop et al. 2017), chest bands (De Fazio, De Vittorio, and Visconti 2022), smart bandages (Escobedo et al. 2020), electrical impedance tomography belts (Wu et al. 2019), smart patches (Lo Presti et al. 2022), proving their applicability in monitoring and managing pulmonary conditions, including COVID-19 (Aliverti 2017).

COVID-19, caused by the severe acute respiratory syndrome coronavirus 2 (SARS-CoV-2), is an infectious disease that significantly impacts the respiratory system. Symptoms reported by the World Health Organization (WHO) and the Centers for Disease Control and Prevention (CDC) include fever, dry cough, nasal congestion, difficulty breathing, weakness, chest pain, sore throat, dyspnea, diarrhea, vomiting, fatigue, headache, loss of taste and smell, and, in severe cases, pneumonia and breathing difficulties. The challenges posed by the pandemic have accelerated the adoption of wearable and intelligent healthcare technologies, underscoring the urgent

DOI: 10.1201/9781003500445-6

need for scalable, noninvasive, and data-driven solutions that support early detection, continuous monitoring, and clinical decision-making beyond traditional healthcare settings (Marques et al. 2021; Marques and Fong 2022). The convergence of wearable sensing, artificial intelligence (AI), and patient-centric data analytics has enabled the real-time acquisition and interpretation of physiological signals, facilitating proactive and personalized health management during both acute infection and post-acute recovery phases (Marques and Fong 2023; Luo et al. 2020). AI and deep learning (DL) methods have become central to processing the large volumes of heterogeneous data generated by wearable devices, transforming raw biosignals into clinically actionable insights for diagnosis, prognosis, and severity assessment (Marques, Bernardo Gois, et al. 2022; Marques, Gois, et al. 2022; Barbosa, Silva et al. 2025; Ribeiro, Barbosa et al. 2025). Within this context, advanced machine learning (ML) techniques have been successfully applied to wearable-compatible biosignals such as electrocardiogram (ECG) and electroencephalogram (EEG), enabling risk stratification, outcome prediction, and disease progression modeling through nonlinear analysis, recurrent neural networks (RNNs), and automated learning pipelines (Do Vale Madeiro et al. 2019; Fernandes et al. 2024; Guilherme Cunha Santos et al. 2023; Marques et al. 2019; Marques et al. 2020; Zacarias et al. 2024; Zhao et al. 2025). Furthermore, multimodal and decision-support frameworks that integrate physiological, behavioral, and contextual data have demonstrated particular relevance during the COVID-19 crisis, enhancing remote clinical oversight and public health intelligence while reducing the burden on healthcare infrastructure (Nguyen Van et al. 2021; Rodrigues et al. 2023; Yan et al. 2023). Complementary advances in medical information extraction, electronic health record summarization, and digital well-being analytics further support the deployment of wearable-based COVID-19 monitoring ecosystems capable of delivering timely, interpretable, and scalable responses to current and future pandemics (Singh et al. 2023).

More specifically, in the case of patients with respiratory symptoms, COVID-19 can also affect voice production, as the disease impacts the lungs, as well as the vocal and nasal tracts (Bartl-Pokorny et al. 2021; Despotovic et al. 2021; Bhattacharya et al. 2023; Tahir et al. 2023; Pancaldi et al. 2022; Pordeus, Ribeiro, Zacarias, de Oliveira, et al. 2023; Pordeus, Ribeiro, Zacarias, Paulo Madeiro, et al. 2023; Ribeiro et al. 2024; Ribeiro, Marques, and Rodrigues 2023).

Several studies have reported that the acoustic characteristics of voice, cough, speech, and breathing have changed in patients with COVID-19 compared with standard patterns, with even subtle changes observed in early cases (Despotovic et al. 2021; Shimon et al. 2021; Han et al. 2021). As a result, these studies can help to accelerate the development of quick, low-cost, noninvasive approaches for screening and monitoring the disease with high accuracy and ease of use (Despotovic et al. 2021; Shimon et al. 2021). The widespread disease has increased research into developing promising diagnostic solutions (Despotovic et al. 2021). Real-time Reverse Transcription-Polymerase Chain Reaction (RT-PCR) is the gold standard for COVID-19 diagnosis, but it is limited by false negatives, slow turnaround times, and specialized requirements. Antigen tests are faster but less sensitive, and computed tomography is limited by low specificity and radiation exposure (Al-Momani 2024; Hayden et al. 2023). These limitations have led to interest in new approaches, such as biochemical markers and voice-, cough-, or speech-based analysis (Despotovic et al. 2021; Chen et al. 2022; Silva, Batista, and Rodrigues 2022; Erdoğan and Narin 2021; Soltanian and Borna 2022). Acoustic features, such as fundamental frequency (F0), variation in the frequency of vocal fold vibration (e.g., F0SD), and the harmonics (Formants – F1, F2, F3, and F4), as well as the harmonic-to-noise ratio (HNR), the amplitude of the first and second harmonics (H1-H2), maximum phonation time (MPT), cepstral peak prominence (CPP), and perturbation measures of pitch (Jitter) and amplitude (Shimmer), have been systematically evaluated and utilized in the diagnosis of various diseases associated with the respiratory system (Sondhi et al. 2021; Bartl-Pokorny et al. 2020).

Recent advances in digital technology, such as automated signal-processing tools, have enabled continuous remote capture and analysis of bodily sounds. When integrated into commodity devices or wearable sensors, audio-based monitoring could unobtrusively track individuals throughout daily life, offering an affordable and widely deployable complement to traditional clinical assessments (Brown et al. 2020; Rodrigues, Freitas et al. 2014; Spachos, Gregori, and Deen 2022; Rodrigues, Madeiro et al. 2023). Such approaches are already being explored for applications like wheeze detection in asthma and for identifying vocal markers of diseases, including Parkinson's disease, cardiovascular diseases, depression, and various psychiatric conditions (Brown et al. 2020; Fischer et al. 2022; Islam, Abdel-Raheem, and Tarique 2022). For COVID-19, wearable and smartphone-based systems have been investigated for screening, early detection, and clinical management (Cheong et al. 2022). Commonly monitored parameters include heart rate, respiratory rate, body temperature, and blood oxygen saturation (SpO_2), along with clinical manifestations such as coughing, fever, and respiratory distress (Santos et al. 2021; Ding et al. 2020). Most existing approaches focus on heart rate-related metrics. In contrast, indicators such as body temperature and cough signals are less commonly utilized (Cheong et al. 2022). Different works have focused on physiological-signal-based detection: (Borhani et al. 2025) used data from Garmin watches and Oura rings to detect early physiological signs of infection, and similar investigations can be found in (Mishra et al. 2020), (Natarajan, Su, and Heneghan 2020), (Pho et al. 2023), (Quer et al. 2021), (Abdel-Ghani et al. 2024), and (Mason et al. 2022). Complementary efforts include smartwatch-based alerting systems capable of identifying pre-symptomatic and asymptomatic cases (Alavi et al. 2022), or wrist-worn devices integrating ML models to detect COVID-19 through combined vital-sign and cough-sound analysis (Abdel-Ghani et al. 2024). With regard to acoustics, sound inputs are usually captured using audio or mechanical sensors, including wearable or nearby microphones, as well as piezoelectric transducers and high-sensitivity accelerometers (Ding et al. 2020). Researchers have developed novel acoustic and respiratory wearables, such as a soft collar equipped with thermal and acoustic sensors for distinguishing mild from severe COVID-19-related respiratory dysfunction (Ishac et al. 2022), as well as voice-analysis frameworks using smartphone-based neural networks to detect respiratory changes linked to COVID-19 and asthma (Islam, Abdel-Raheem, and Tarique 2022). A similar work is also presented in (Maghded et al. 2020), where a smartphone-based framework was proposed to capture cough sounds, movement patterns, and temperature using built-in sensors, for COVID-19 detection and monitoring. More advanced multimodal AI-driven systems have also emerged, including CovidDeep, which integrates wearable signals with compact deep neural networks (DNNs) optimized for smartphone deployment, enabling daily noninvasive detection (Hassantabar et al. 2021). Finally, smartphone-based cough-analysis tools such as AI4COVID-19 have demonstrated the feasibility of rapid, scalable preliminary screening, distinguishing COVID-19 coughs from other cough types despite limited condition-specific data (Imran et al. 2020). Short-duration "snapshot" wearable sensing has also been explored, using a soft throat-mounted device with a high-resolution accelerometer to capture mechano-acoustic signals related to cardio-respiratory activity, motion, and cough sounds during brief activity sequences (Lonini et al. 2021). Nevertheless, most systems are still in the developmental stage, and evidence regarding the real-world performance and implementation of these technologies remains limited (Cheong et al. 2022).

The present study aims to develop a wearable application that runs an optimized speech analysis algorithm, supported by statistical methods, to distinguish between different COVID-19 severity levels across frequency bands and recording types. To enable efficient deployment in a wearable environment and facilitate rapid monitoring of disease progression, the study seeks to identify a single, robust metric that effectively quantifies and discriminates COVID-19 severity.

6.2 METHODOLOGY

The proposed approach comprises two components: (1) a back-end analytics pipeline – covering data ingestion, preprocessing, signal processing, feature extraction, and statistical analysis – and (2) a wearable front-end for on-device execution and user interaction.

The pipeline of back-end analytics was implemented entirely in Python (version 3.9.12; Python Software Foundation, Wilmington, Delaware, the United States of American), covering data ingestion, preprocessing, speech-band decomposition via discrete wavelet transforms (DWT), nonlinear feature extraction, data organization, and all statistical analyses (modeling, estimation, hypothesis testing). The wearable front-end was deployed on embedded, low-power devices and prototyped on Wear OS (user interface (UI) and app logic in Kotlin) and watchOS (UI and app logic in Swift). To satisfy real-time constraints, the DWT and the selected metric were implemented in a shared C/C++ library: on Android/Wear OS, it is compiled with the Native Development Kit (NDK) and invoked from Kotlin via Java Native Interface (JNI); on iOS/watchOS, it is linked and called from Swift through an Objective-C++ wrapper. The on-device pipeline includes: (i) audio acquisition with pre-emphasis and framing; (ii) real-time DWT for multiresolution decomposition of each frame; (iii) metric computation from the resulting wavelet coefficients/features; (iv) locally executed decision logic (e.g., thresholding or model scoring); and (v) user feedback/logging, with sliding-window buffering to meet latency and energy constraints. Figure 6.1 summarizes this two-layer architecture.

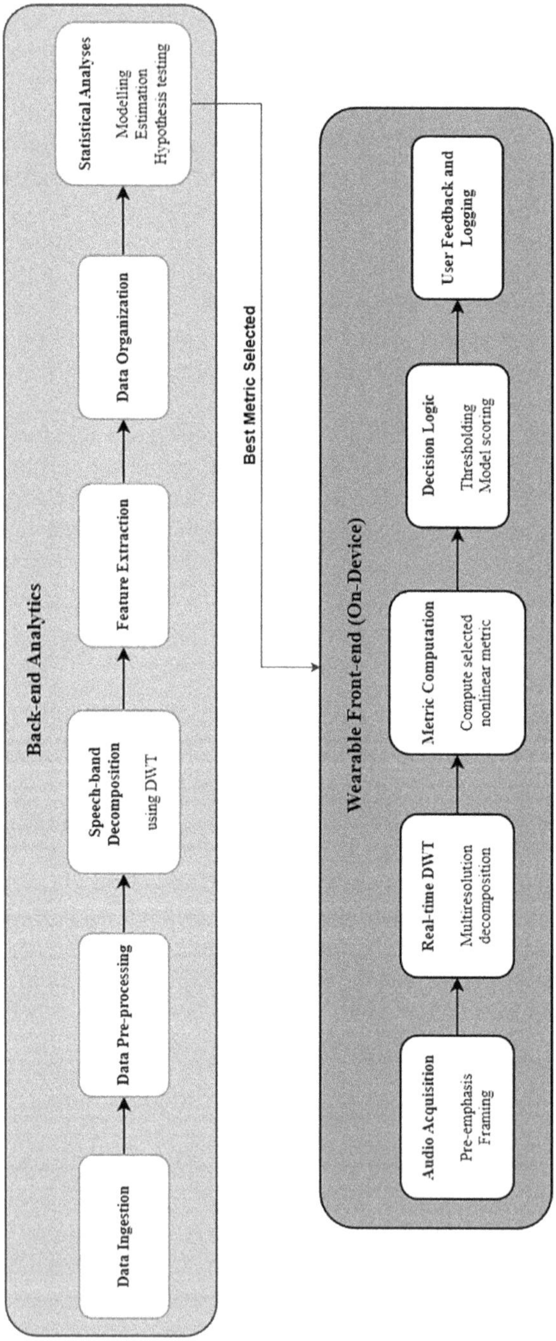

FIGURE 6.1 Methodology Workflow.

6.2.1 Database

This study used the Coswara public database, released on April 11, 2022, as detailed in (Bhattacharya et al. 2023). The database comprises sound samples collected via global crowdsourcing using the internet and is publicly accessible on the web. The samples are tagged with six COVID-19 statuses (no respiratory illness exposed (nRE), positive-asymptomatic (PA), positive-moderate (PMo), positive-mild (PM), recovered full (RF), and respiratory illness not identified (RIn)) and one group of control (healthy controls – HC).

Each participant in the dataset has nine different sound types, including breathing-deep, breathing-shallow, cough-heavy, cough-shallow, counting-fast, counting-normal, and vowel sounds /a/, /e/, and /o/, with a sampling frequency of 44100 Hz. After selecting 78.6 % of the samples marked as excellent by the expert human annotators of the original dataset, removing samples with missing audio files or demographic data, and removing all the participants with an age below ten, 1993 participants were identified, with ages ranging from ten to 87 years old, and more male participants (70.4 %). Find more details in Table 6.1.

The participants were from various locations, most from India (92.3%) and the United States (3.1%). However, the study also included participants from other countries, such as Argentina, Australia, Bahrain, Bangladesh, Belgium, Brazil, Canada, China, Finland, France, Germany, Greece, Hungary, Indonesia, Italy, Japan, Korea South, Malaysia, Netherlands, Oman, Pakistan, Philippines, Portugal, Romania, Russia, Saudi Arabia, Singapore, South Africa, Spain, Sri Lanka, Sweden, Switzerland, Syria, Thailand, Turkey, United Arab Emirates, United Kingdom. Upon analyzing the data, it was observed that a significant portion of the participants (50%) belonged to the healthy controls group. Furthermore, 28.4% of the participants were identified as infected with the virus, presenting with diverse symptoms or asymptomatic (3.2%).

6.2.2 The Algorithm

6.2.2.1 Preprocessing

All signals follow the guidelines described in (Coleman 1993). For each participant, it was ensured that all nine types of sound recordings were stable, at least 2.2-s in duration, and free of artifacts. To eliminate the effect of speaker–microphone distance, all signal amplitudes were normalized to the range [−1, 1]. Using a hamming window, the signals were then divided into nonoverlapping 20-ms segments for subsequent analysis.

6.2.2.2 Signal Processing and Feature Extraction

This section describes the set of features extracted from each voice-type sound recording.

6.2.2.2.1 Multiband Decomposition via Wavelet Transform

The DWT dissects a discrete signal of finite energy into a set of base functions composed of a limited number of prototype sequences and their time-shifted variations. This process, as described in Guido's research in 2022 (Guido 2022), is

TABLE 6.1
Socio-Demographic and Clinical Characteristics of the Participants

	Continuous Measure	Min	Max	Mean			SD
Age (Years)		10	87	36.29			14.06
	Categorical Measure				**N**	**%**	
	Gender						
	Female				616	30.9	
	Male				1377	69.1	
	Country						
	India				1832	91.9	
	United States of America				65	3.3	
	Germany				10	0.5	
	Other				86	4.3	
	Clinical Information						
	Healthy Controls				998	50	
	No respiratory illness exposed				181	9.1	
	Positive – asymptomatic				77	3.8	
	Positive– mild				370	18.7	
	Positive – moderate				120	5.9	
	Recovered full				127	6.4	
	Respiratory illness not identified				120	6.1	

advantageous for analyzing signals in the time-frequency domain because it enables switching between the time and frequency domains, helping to localize the sources of frequency components in time (Rodrigues, Freitas et al. 2018).

To perform the expansion and subsequent reconstruction, an octave-band critically decimated filter bank is employed, as outlined in works by Malvar in 1992 and Vetterli in 1995 (Malvar 1992; Vetterli and Kovacevic 1995). Considering only the positive frequencies, the mth sub-band is confined to:

$$W_k = \begin{cases} \left[0,\ \pi/2^S\right], & m = 0 \\ \left[\pi/2^{S-m+1}, \pi/2^{S-m}\right], & m = 1, 2, \ldots, S \end{cases} \tag{1}$$

where S is the number of levels, $S+1$ is the number of sub-bands, and π is the normalized angular frequency equivalent to half the sampling rate. The DWT utilizes an analysis scale function $\tilde{\phi}_1(n)$ and an analysis wavelet function $\tilde{\psi}_1(n)$, which are defined as follows:

$$\tilde{\phi}_1(n) = h_{\text{LP}}(n) \tag{2}$$

and

$$\tilde{\psi}_1(n) = h_{\text{HP}}(n) \tag{3}$$

in this context, $h_{LP}(n)$ and $h_{HP}(n)$ refer to the impulse responses of the half-band low-pass and high-pass analysis filters, respectively.

Defining the following recursion formulas:

$$\widetilde{\phi}_{i+1}(n) = \widetilde{\phi}_i\left(n/2\right) * \widetilde{\phi}_1(n) \tag{4}$$

$$\widetilde{\psi}_{i+1}(n) = \widetilde{\phi}_i(n) * \widetilde{\psi}_1\left(n/2^i\right) \tag{5}$$

where the symbol $*$ represents the convolution operator, and the analysis filter for the mth sub-band can be expressed as follows:

$$h_m(n) = \begin{cases} \widetilde{\phi}_S(n), & m = 0, \\ \widetilde{\psi}_{S+1-m}(n), & m = 1, 2, \ldots, S \end{cases} \tag{6}$$

The mth sub-band signal is given by:

$$x_m(n) = \begin{cases} \sum_{k=-\infty}^{\infty} x(k) h_m\left(2^S n - k\right), & m = 0 \\ \sum_{k=-\infty}^{\infty} x(k) h_m\left(2^{S-m+1} n - k\right), & m = 1,\ 2,\ \ldots,\ S \end{cases} \tag{7}$$

The present study applied the DWT to individual voice segments, decomposing them into sub-bands up to the third level, denoted as $S = 3$. The sub-band signals, represented by $x_m(n)$ with m ranging from zero to three, underwent resampling to match the original sampling rate using the wavelet interpolation method (Rioul and Vetterli 1991; Rodrigues, Freitas et al. 2012, Rodrigues, Freitas et al. 2018). The frequency ranges for each component are as follows:

- x_3: 11,050 Hz to 22,100 Hz
- x_2: 5,525 Hz to 11,050 Hz
- x_1: 2,762.5 Hz to 5,525 Hz
- x_0: 0 Hz to 2,762.5 Hz

6.2.2.2.2 *Nonlinear Analysis*

Nonlinear analysis of a signal refers to methods for extracting information from signals that exhibit nonlinear behavior, characterized by irregular, unpredictable patterns that change nonlinearly over time. Speech signals are ideally suited for nonlinear analysis due to their inherently complex production mechanisms, which involve nonlinear interactions among the vocal folds, airflow, and articulators. Additionally, the dynamic and non-stationary nature of speech – where pitch, tone, and speed continuously vary – demands analysis methods capable of capturing these fluctuations. Nonlinear features excel in this regard, effectively capturing the rich, nuanced information in speech, such as intonation, emotion, and stress, which linear methods may miss. This combination of factors makes nonlinear analysis particularly effective for comprehensively characterizing the intricate and variable nature of speech signals (Esposito and Marinaro 2005; Birgmeier, Bernhard, and Kubin 1997; Abreu Araujo et al. 2020; Kumar and Mullick 1996).

Nonlinear features are associated with entropy, exponents, and fractal-dimension parameters.

- Energy (EN)

The energy concept can be understood within a system framework as its potential to do work. More precisely, when considering a speech signal, energy pertains to the quantity of exertion employed by the speaker's respiratory system and vocal tract in generating sound across time. Thus, energy holds substantial importance since it offers crucial insights into the mechanisms of the vocal system during speech production (Guido 2016; Akbari and Arjmandi 2014).

The energy of $x(n)$ is defined as:

$$EN = \sum n = 1^{N} \left| x(n) \right|^{2} \tag{8}$$

- Entropy

Entropy is a measure of the level of information hidden or obscured within a signal. For speech signals affected by pathological conditions, entropy can be used to build a model and quantify abnormalities in the signal within a specific frequency range with maximal accuracy. This method allows a more detailed speech signal analysis, leading to a deeper understanding of the pathology affecting the signal's production (Akbari and Arjmandi 2014). The Shannon (SE), logarithmic (LE), and approximate $(AnEp)$ entropies are three commonly utilized estimates of entropy and can be estimated as (Hu and Zhang 2019; Sanei and Chambers 2013; Sairamya et al. 2021):

$$SE = -\sum_{n=1}^{N} \left| x(n) \right|^{2} log \left[\left| x(n) \right|^{2} \right] \tag{9}$$

$$LE = \sum_{n=1}^{N} log \left[\left| x(n) \right|^{2} \right] \tag{10}$$

$$AnEp(m, r, N) = H^{m}(r) - H^{m+1}(r) \tag{11}$$

where N is the data length, r is the similar tolerance (0.2 in the present work), and m represents the embedding dimension (2.5 in this study). The variable H denotes the Heaviside function derived during intermediate calculations (Faust and Bairy 2012).

- Chaos Theory

Chaos theory concerns dynamic systems and their unpredictable behavior arising from the absence of equilibrium properties.

Two primary exponents provide a comprehensive framework for understanding chaos (Sanei and Chambers 2013; Albertovich and Aleksandrovna 2017). At any given time, the state of a dynamic system, described by m variables can be visualized as points in an m-dimensional space.

As time progresses, a state sequence is generated, producing curves known as trajectories within the state or phase space. This space illustrates the system's states. When these trajectories are observed over a significant period, they can converge to a specific geometric form, known as an attractor, regardless of the system's initial parameters.

– Correlation Dimension (CD): It characterizes the distribution of attractor points, offering valuable information about the complexity of a dynamic system. It can be estimated using the following approach:

$$CD = \lim_{r \to 0} \frac{\log\left(C(r,M)\right)}{\log(r)} \tag{12}$$

where

$$C(r,M) = \frac{2}{M(M-1)} \sum_{i=1}^{M} \sum_{\substack{j=1 \\ j \neq i}}^{M} \Theta\left(r - |\boldsymbol{x}_i - \boldsymbol{x}_j|\right) \tag{13}$$

is the probability of the pair of points $\{x_i, x_j\}$ on the attractor is separated by a distance less than or equal to r and Θ is the Heaviside function (Rodriguez-Bermudez and Garcia-Laencina 2015; Faust and Bairy 2012).

– Lyapunov Exponent (L): It is related to the analysis of the trajectories over time that affect the stability dynamics of a system. This information, as highlighted in Faust's study in 2012 (Faust and Bairy 2012), offers insight into the evolution of trajectories and the behavior of the underlying system.

$$L\left(x_0\right) = \lim_{n \to \infty} \frac{1}{n} \sum_{k=1}^{n} \ln \left| f'\left(x_k - 1\right) \right| \tag{14}$$

where f' is the iterator function f derivative (Sanei and Chambers 2013).

– Detrended Fluctuation Analysis: It is a method that provides a parameter for quantifying long-range correlations (self-similarity) of a non-stationary time series (Gifani et al. 2007). From $x(n)$ the cumulative deviation series can be computed as follows,

$$y(k) = \sum_{i=1}^{k} \left[x(i) - \bar{x}\right] \tag{15}$$

Then, an estimation is made for each segment of $y(k)$ with length of m, resulting in a linear approximation denoted as $y_m(k)$. The average fluctuation of the signal, as a function of m, is then defined as follows:

$$F(m) = \sqrt{\frac{1}{N} \sum_{k=1}^{N} \left[y(k) - y_m(k)\right]^2} \tag{16}$$

The slope of the best linear approximation of $log\left|F(m)\right|$ as a function of $log(m)$ is the scaling exponent α that represents the correlation properties of the signal $x(n)$ (Lee et al. 2002).

- Fractal Dimension

The self-similar properties of fractal structures make them suitable for characterizing irregular structures and processes. Fractal geometry has been demonstrated as an effective method for identifying anomalies caused by various biomedical disorders in signals such as the voice, as evidenced in previous studies (Ali et al. 2015). Monitoring speech self-similarity enables evaluation of a patient's clinical condition. Extracting fractal dimension (FD) features, such as the Higuchi fractal dimension, are considered a valuable approach to classifying voice signals (Albertovich and Aleksandrovna 2017). Using such techniques can enhance the classification of voice signals, thus improving the detection of voice-related disorders.
– Higuchi Exponent (D):

$$L(k)\alpha k^{-D} \tag{17}$$

where the variable k indicates the time interval under consideration. Within each time interval, the length of the curve is denoted as $L(k)$, while the Higuchi Exponent, cited as reference (Wijayanto, Hartanto, and Nugroho 2019), is represented by D.
– Katz Algorithm: According to Katz (Katz 1988), the FD of a waveform $x(n)$ can be defined as:

$$FDk = \frac{log\left(L/a\right)}{log\left(d/a\right)} \tag{18}$$

where L represents the cumulative distance between adjacent points in the sequence $x(n)$. a denotes the average distance between consecutive points, while d represents the maximum distance between $x(1)$ and the remaining points in $x(n)$.

6.2.2.2.3 Feature extraction process

Per each voice recording of all study participants, nine nonlinear features (EN, SE, LE, AE, CD, L, α, D, FDk) have been extracted from every 20-ms-long signal segment and their respective sub-bands. DWT decomposed the 20-ms-long segments into sub-bands up to decomposition level three using biorthogonal 3.1 as the selected wavelet. In previous works (Alves et al. 2023; Alves et al. 2020; Silva, Batista, and Rodrigues 2022)wavelet biorthogonal 3.1 emerges as an excellent option for analyzing speech signals. To reduce the problem's dimensionality and maintain equal metrics per subject for statistical analysis, the nine extracted features from all segments were treated as time-series distributions. The mean statistic was employed to compress the data within each sub-band and across the broadband over time. This reduced the number of metrics while ensuring equal representation for each subject.

6.2.2.3 Statistical Analysis

In this study, statistical differences were assessed for each pair of study groups in each voice recording. The normality and homoscedasticity of the time-series feature vector distributions have been assessed with the Kolmogorov-Smirnov and Levene tests, respectively. The hypothesis of parametric tests was met. Therefore, the parametric test, the independent-samples t-test, has been applied. It is a statistical hypothesis test used to determine whether a significant difference exists between the means of two data groups (Zar 2010).

The total number of statistical tests done was 8910, resulting from the 22 binary comparisons individually applied on the nine compressed time-series nonlinear feature distributions for each signal's band (five bands – one broadband & four subbands reached by signal's DWT decomposition) for the nine different types of voice recordings.

In every 22 binary comparisons, all data subsets were equally balanced for statistical analysis. For that, subgroups were randomly selected from the main database previously defined in Table 6.1, based on the lower maximum number of samples per group within each study group pair. Using voice analysis and binary comparison, the data have been normalized by the z-score algorithm (Rodrigues et al. 2021) and then subjected to a t-test to evaluate the significance of the parameter distribution. The application step of the z-score method helps standardize the data, detect outliers, assess normality assumptions, and enable comparability and interpretation.

6.2.3 Wearable Implementation

The wearable front-end was implemented as a real-time, on-device pipeline that captures incoming speech, processes it in short frames, and produces local decisions that are surfaced to the user interface. The application layer was developed in Kotlin on Wear OS (i.e., operating system) and Swift on watchOS to manage permissions, lifecycle, and UI/notifications, while the compute-intensive digital signal processing – the DWT and the computation of the selected metric (*AnEp*) – was implemented in a shared C/C++ library to guarantee predictable latency and portability across platforms. The application layer was developed in Kotlin on Wear OS and Swift on watchOS to manage permissions, lifecycle, and UI/notifications, while the compute-intensive digital signal processing – the DWT and the computation of the selected metric (*AnEp*) – was implemented in a shared C/C++ library to guarantee predictable latency and portability across platforms. On Android/Wear OS, the library is compiled with the NDK and called from Kotlin via JNI; on iOS/watchOS, it is linked and invoked from Swift through an Objective-C++ wrapper. Once the microphone permission is granted, the application (App) configures an audio session at the target sample rate and begins frame-based acquisition. Each frame is first pre-emphasized to compensate for high-frequency roll-off and then windowed (e.g., Hann) to reduce spectral leakage. Frames are pushed into a circular buffer that supports sliding-window processing with controlled overlap, so that feature computation remains both responsive and statistically stable. The resulting *AnEp* features (selected as the most robust and informative acoustic marker for this work – for more information, check the results at Section 6.3 and their discussion at subsection 6.4). fed into a decision module that applies calibrated thresholds for multiclass severity classification. Threshold calibration follows a systematic process: first, the mean *AnEp* value (μ) is calculated for each severity class (e.g., μ_{HC} for healthy controls, μ_{nRE} for No respiratory illness exposed, μ_{PA} for Positive – asymptomatic, etc. …) using training data; next, pairwise midpoint thresholds are computed between adjacent class means ($T_{HC,\ \ nRE} = \left(\mathrm{HC} + \mathrm{nRE}\right)/2$, $T_{nRE,\ \ PA} = \left(\mu_{\mathrm{nRE}} + \mu_{\mathrm{PA}}\right)/2$, etc.); these pairwise thresholds are then ordered into a monotonic threshold ladder ($T < T < \ldots < T$, where k equals to seven – the number of classes – minus one); finally, test samples are classified based on where their *AnEp* value falls within this threshold ladder, enabling group-level distinctions between severity classes in the wearable processing pipeline. At runtime, the device calculates the selected metric (*AnEp*) for the incoming signal and applies these precomputed, ordered thresholds to assign the sample to the appropriate class via a simple cascading comparison (e.g., if selected metric (*AnEp*) $< T \rightarrow$ class HC; else if selected metric (*AnEp*) $< T \rightarrow$ class nRE; else if selected metric (*AnEp*) $< (T_3 \rightarrow$ class PA; and so on). This threshold-based, multiclass decision logic is lightweight and predictable, avoids heavy classifiers, and supports real-time severity differentiation entirely on-device while maintaining stable execution time and minimal resource usage – making it suitable for continuous operation on consumer wearable devices. All decisions are executed locally to avoid network dependence, and the results are immediately reflected in the UI (e.g., a glanceable indicator, haptic feedback, and concise logs). Only minimal summaries persisted to conserve storage and protected privacy. The runtime is engineered for real-time: buffers and workspaces are pre-allocated to avoid heap churn, CPU-intensive (i.e., central processing unit-intensive) loops are vectorization-friendly, and (where appropriate) fixed-point arithmetic is available to reduce floating-point pressure on lower-power SoCs (i.e., system-on-chips). The app also adapts to OS policies by utilizing user-initiated sessions or foreground modes when continuous processing is required, and it gracefully throttles or suspends the pipeline when the device enters low-power states.

Deploying this class of algorithms on a wearable imposes several limitations that shape design choices. Energy and thermal budgets are tight: continuous audio capture and DWT + *AnEp* computation can drain the battery and, under sustained load, trigger thermal throttling that increases latency and jitter. To mitigate this, the pipeline uses conservative frame sizes and overlap, opportunistic duty-cycling (e.g., voice-activity-triggered processing), and adaptive load shedding (such as reducing DWT levels) as thermal headroom shrinks. Compute and memory constraints limit the sub-band count, feature breadth, and model complexity; hence, the digital signal processor (DSP) core is carefully optimized using a lifting-scheme DWT, and numerical formats are chosen to balance precision and speed. Audio path variability – microphone characteristics, built-in AGC/AEC/noise (i.e., automatic gain control/acoustic echo cancellation) suppression, sampling-rate drift, and environmental noise – can perturb wavelet coefficients and, consequently, *AnEp*; the front end therefore standardizes preprocessing parameters, performs basic input validation, and, where feasible, includes device-specific calibration to stabilize metric ranges. OS background-execution policies are another constraint: watchOS restricts long-running background audio work, and Wear OS requires foreground services and strict resource management. The app aligns with these policies by using short, user-visible sessions or explicit foreground processing with clear affordances. Privacy and permissions are central: microphone access is sensitive, and strong raw audio increases risk. The system processes audio on devices, avoids persisting raw waveforms, retains only derived summaries or event markers, and provides transparent consent and revocation paths. Finally, portability and numerical reproducibility are nontrivial: differences in CPU architecture, compiler flags, and floating- vs. fixed-point math can shift *AnEp* scores subtly across devices; to address this, the C/C++ implementation is deterministic, unit-tested against a Python ground truth, and shipped with tight tolerances and continuous checks during integration testing. Together, these measures enable a practical, responsive wearable front end that executes DWT and *AnEp* in real-time while acknowledging and managing the inherent constraints of battery-powered, sensor-rich devices.

6.3 RESULTS

To improve the organization of the results, we divided this section into two parts: the backend results and algorithm optimization for the wearable application, and the wearable application itself.

6.3.1 The Algorithm Results

The number of significant features per voice recording type and binary comparison is shown in the heatmap of Figure 6.2.

The number of significant features for each band of voice recording type for all binary comparisons is illustrated in the heatmap of Figure 6.3.

The total number of occasions on which a feature was found to be statistically significant across all sub-band analyses is shown in Figure 6.4.

The feature's ability to distinguish intra-binary binary groups (binary comparisons) is illustrated in Figure 6.5.

6.3.2 The Wearable Results

After selecting the optimal feature from the back-end analyses (*AnEp*), the real-time version of the algorithm was deployed to the wearable platform (iOS/watchOS). Figure 6.6 shows the model operating on the wearable device.

The results confirm that the real-time wearable implementation showed predictable latency, strong numerical agreement with the offline reference, and stable behavior across realistic operating conditions. Each audio frame was processed within real-time, with no noticeable delays. Because buffers were pre-allocated and the main loops were optimized, there were no pauses from memory allocation and no circular-buffer overruns. The three-level biorthogonal 3.1 DWT ran smoothly on all tested smartwatch chips. *AnEp* values produced on the watches closely matched the reference values used during testing. Differences were small and never large enough to change the model decisions. The behavior remained consistent across devices and processors. Continuous audio capture and processing

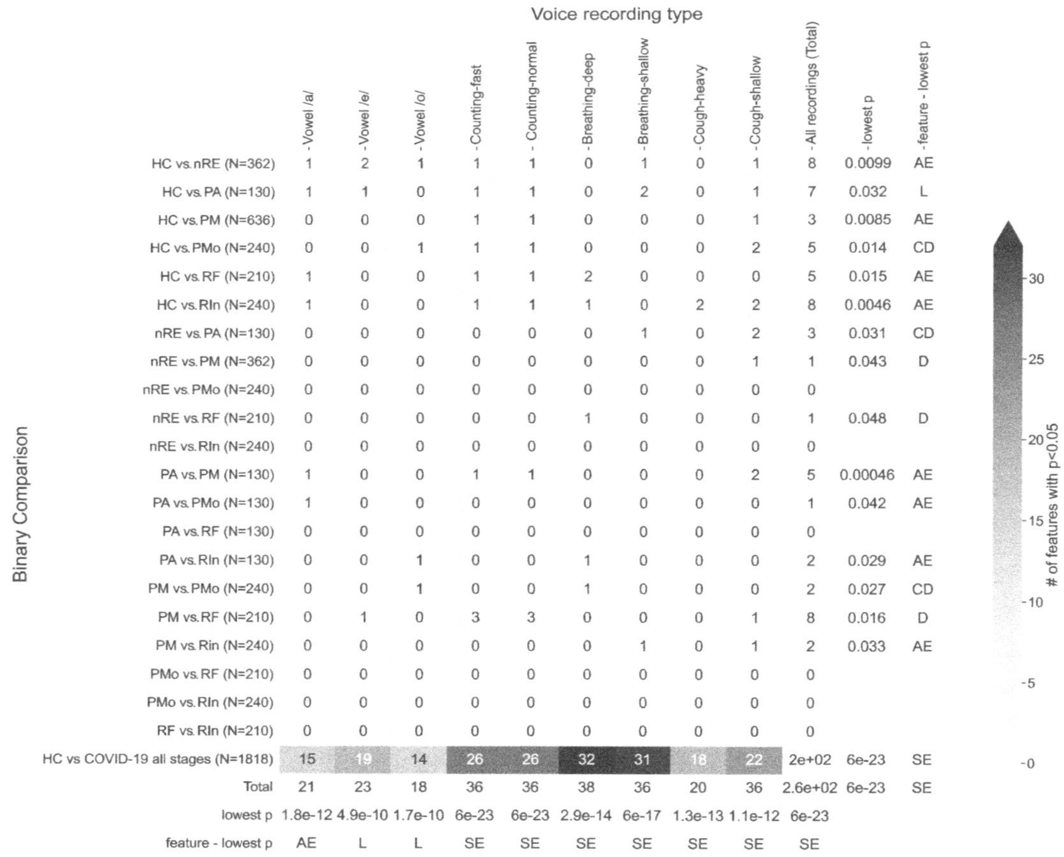

FIGURE 6.2 Heatmap – Analysis Per Voice Type Recording, a Global Results Overview (here, *AE* = *ApEn*).

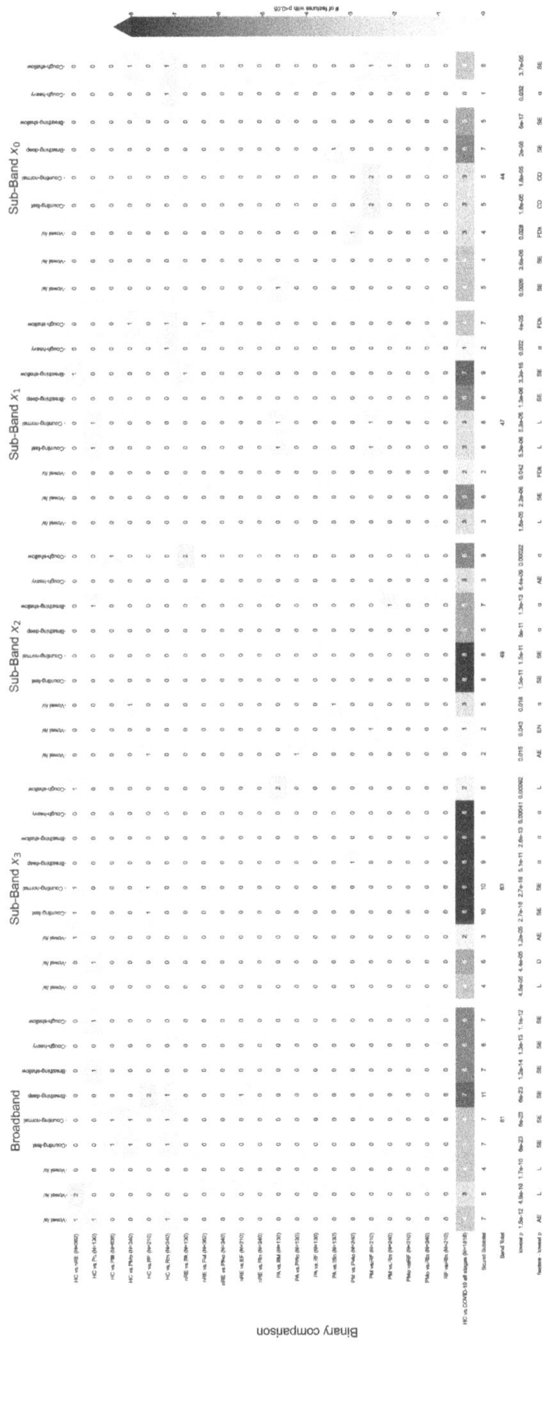

FIGURE 6.3 Heatmap – Signals Bands Analysis Results (here, $AE = ApEn$).

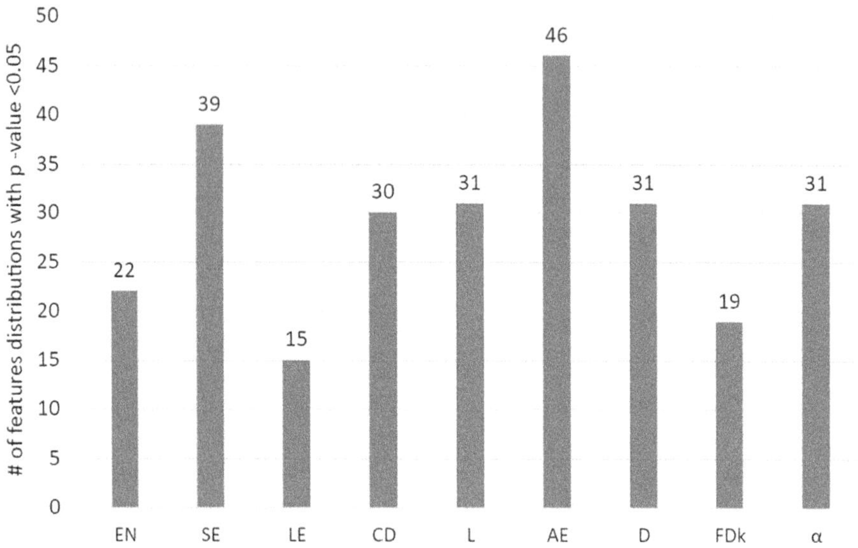

FIGURE 6.4 The Total Number of Occasions a Feature Demonstrated to be Statistically Significant Across All Sub-Band Analyses (here, *AE* = *ApEn*).

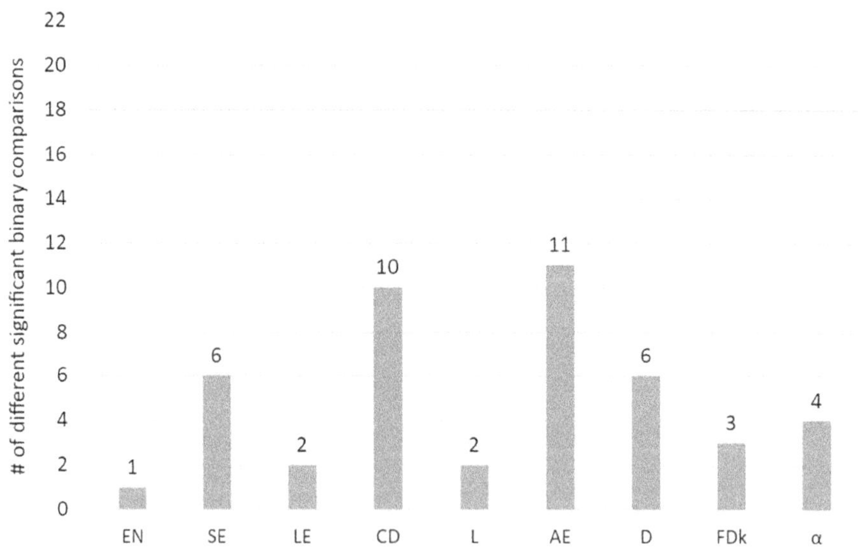

FIGURE 6.5 Features' Discriminant Capability to Distinguish Intra-Binary Groups (here, *AE* = *ApEn*).

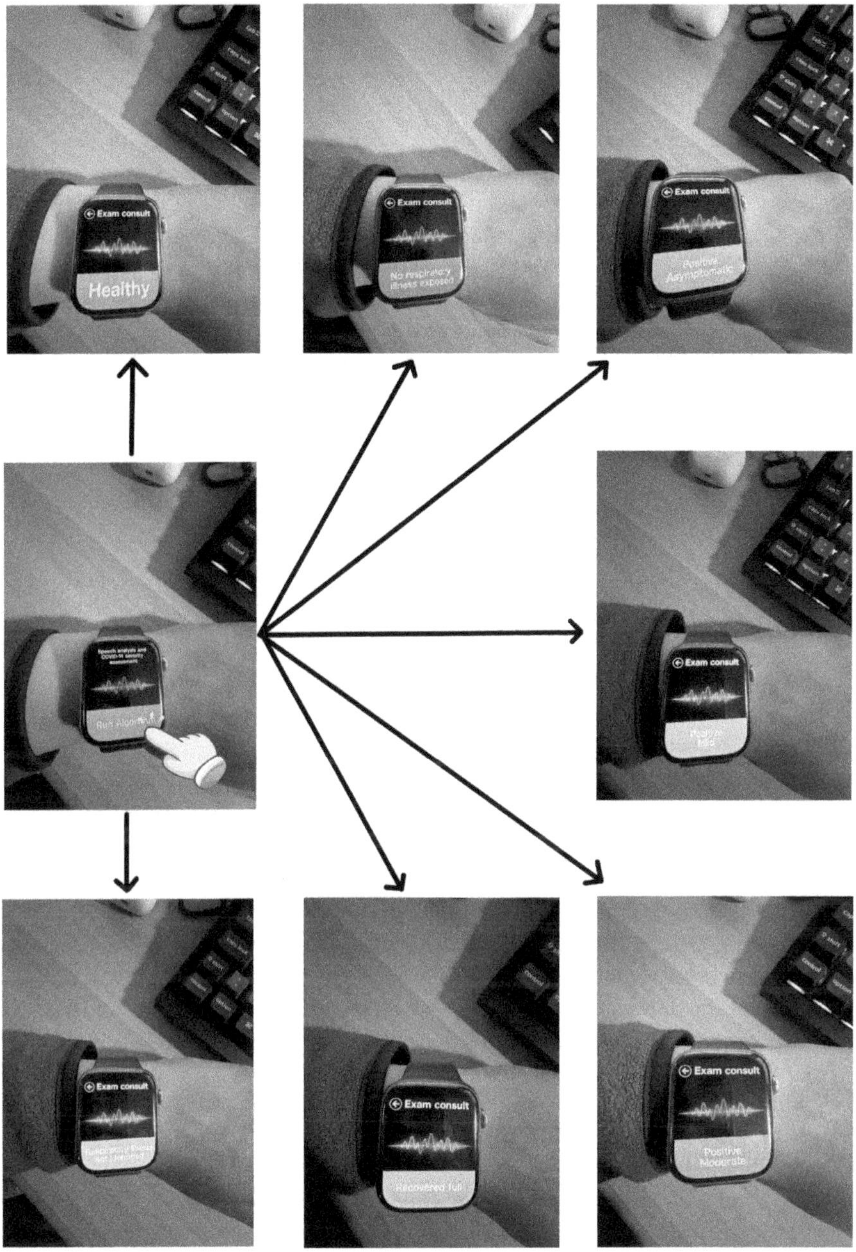

FIGURE 6.6 Wearable Application Front-End Operability.

increased power use, but the optimized DSP pipeline kept battery impact reasonable for short-term use. Standard preprocessing steps helped stabilize the audio prior to DWT, and simple input checks prevented corrupted frames from affecting *AnEp*. Optional device-specific calibration reduced differences between wearable models. Because all decisions were made locally, results appeared on the screen immediately. Foreground modes on Wear OS and user-started sessions on watchOS provided the app with continuous microphone access without violating OS rules. Over long tests, the app remained stable with no crashes, memory leaks, or buffer issues. Memory stayed within fixed limits, CPU load behaved as expected, and real-time performance held up even with normal background activity. Storage use stayed low because only summary data was saved.

After selecting the optimal feature from the back-end analyses (*AnEp*), the real-time version of the algorithm was deployed to the wearable platform (iOS/watchOS). The results confirm that the core digital signal processing engine achieves predictable latency, numerical consistency with the offline reference implementation, and stable on-device behavior across realistic operating conditions.

6.4 DISCUSSION

6.4.1 The Algorithm Results

Scrutiny of the heatmap illustrated in Figure 6.2 reveals that the nature of the studied sounds significantly influences the results. The entropy-based features, such as *SE* and *AnEp*, yielded the greatest number of lowest *p*-values, accounting for 78% of the lowest *p*-values across the different recording types and 53% across the different binary comparisons. This analysis is supported by Figure 6.4, which shows that *SE* and *AnEp* distributions were not only the ones with the lowest *p*-values, but they could also find more differences between groups over all the sub-band investigations. However, examining Figure 6.5, which demonstrates the statistical significance of the distribution of a particular feature by showing the number of distinct binary combinations observed, we can see that, despite *SE* remaining a good pattern in this analysis, it has been surpassed by the *CD* feature. Nevertheless, *AnEp* remains the most reliable and comprehensive feature for identifying the different severity statuses of COVID-19.

Among the analyzed sounds shown in Figure 6.2, breathing sounds had the highest number of statistically significant features, with 28 for deep breathing and 36 for shallow breathing. On the other hand, both counting sound analyses provided the lowest *p*-values of all the sounds (6×10^{-23}) for both sorts. As the two counting sound analyses yielded the same number of statistically significant features in the exact binary comparisons, with approximately identical *p*-values, we conclude that counting speed does not affect the results.

The other two types of sounds, namely the vowels and cough sounds, also show variability within the group. Although the vowel /e/ analysis provided the most significant features, the analysis of vowel /a/ provided the lowest *p*-value, and an entropy-based feature (*AnEp*) successfully achieved this outcome. Lastly, the shallow cough speech analysis provided much more significant features than the one applied for the heavy cough. These results show that breathing sounds adjust pathological activity better than other types of sounds. We can also see that shallow breathing and coughing produce better discrimination performance than their heavier counterparts. This indicates that the extracted features can be employed for early diagnosis of mild symptoms, when the disease is most likely to be misdiagnosed as a cold or seasonal flu. In the binary comparison analyses, the pairs in which HC was matched yielded the best overall results, with at least three significant features. The comparison of HC vs. all COVID-19 stages provided the maximum number of significant features (200) and the lowest overall p-value (6×10^{-23}) through an entropy-based feature, namely SE. Entropy often measures the degree of complexity or irregularity of the signal. This could be interpreted as the human body adapting to different conditions or situations; if it's high, it might indicate a healthy state. Conversely, low entropy often suggests regular, predictable, or repetitive signal patterns, which could indicate a disease state. In the context of this study, changes in entropy could be related to the physiological changes induced by COVID-19, such as inflammation or damage in the respiratory tract (Schwartz et al. 2020).

The results showed that it's possible to distinguish severe cases of disease from healthy controls, asymptomatic patients, and recovered patients, suggesting that COVID-19 may affect the voice from the outset and that changes can persist after recovery. On the other hand, six pairs of comparisons showed no statistical differences (nRE vs. PMo, nRE vs. RIn, PA vs. RF, PMo vs. RF, PMo vs. RIn, and RF vs. RIn).

Figure 6.3 allows us to conduct a more comprehensive impact assessment of the statistical significance of the DWT frequency-band decomposition employed for each voice recording type. This heatmap is composed of five bands: the first is the signal's broadband, and the others are the sub-bands resulting from the DWT decomposition of the signal's broadband (x_0, x_1, x_2, and x_3). Firstly, we can see that broadband and sub-band x3 yielded the most statistically significant features, as well as the lowest p-values of 6×10^{-23} and 2.7×10^{-16}, respectively. Once again, the concepts of the amount and quality of the features do not quite match, and even though x_3 has more significant features, and the lowest p-value originates in the broadband analysis. As the subband x_3 is the frequency domain, the band with the highest analyzed frequency may yield the highest number of significant features across all band analyses, because most of the time pathological patterns are related to small, rapid changes in the full-band signal, captured at higher frequencies.

The features extracted from higher frequency bands effectively distinguished HC from the other groups. However, when examining lower frequency bands, such as sub-band x_0. The number of features that can differentiate HC from others diminishes. Instead, these lower-frequency bands reveal a growing number of significant features that are more indicative of different phases of disease severity. The sound observations do not differ significantly from the global overview analysis illustrated in Figure 6.3, as breathing, counting, and coughing sounds outperform vowels in both quantity and quality of the significant features.

When we compare the results of the present study with those of other studies, we see that, first and foremost, the studied nonlinear features constitute a novel strategy for achieving the same goals. When distinguishing COVID-19-infected patients from healthy patients, nonlinear measures yield the best results (Sondhi et al. 2021; Asiaee et al. 2022). In addition to this general distinction, the studied metrics, compared to healthy controls vs. recovered patients, outperform almost all the literature metrics except one. However, the study that achieved this outcome performed a statistical analysis by gender (male and female), and the best result was achieved only for the male participants using the Formant F3 metric. Although our study yields lower p-values than the best reported in the literature, a careful comparison should be made, as different databases were used, and most studies do not accurately identify the severity status of COVID-19 patients or provide separate results for male and female patients. Furthermore, our study offers novel insights that advance the state of the art by addressing gaps not previously covered in the literature. By applying this approach of evaluating all the different recording sources per different ranges of frequencies via DWT, contrary to the state-of-the-art that used all broadband analysis, we make future research easier by 1) identifying the best recording types for distinguishing COVID-19 severity levels and 2) specifying the most effective and higher significant parameters and frequency bands for efficient triage of COVID-19 severity. Based on this analysis, *AnEp* was found to be the most effective feature for distinguishing among different COVID-19 severity levels. Thus, it was selected as the primary discriminative feature for the wearable implementation. In the wearable processing pipeline, group-level distinctions were derived by comparing the average *AnEp* distributions associated with each severity class, enabling a simple but efficient and reliable decision mechanism for severity differentiation in real-time that can be executed entirely on-device, while maintaining predictable execution time and minimal resource usage, making it suitable for continuous operation on consumer wearable devices.

6.4.2 The Wearable Solution Results

The results show that the proposed pipeline can be reliably deployed on consumer smartwatches, enabling real-time monitoring directly on the device. The system runs continuously on the wearable, processing voice input as the user speaks, with no need for external hardware or network connectivity. This demonstrates that real-time, on-device speech analysis is both technically feasible and practical in everyday use.

The optimized DSP implementation, along with pre-allocated buffers and vectorization-friendly loops, allowed the pipeline to meet strict real-time requirements without memory pauses or circular-buffer overruns. The three-level DWT and *AnEp* computation ran smoothly on all tested watch platforms. Energy and thermal control strategies, such as conservative frame sizes and optional duty cycling, kept power consumption and device heating within safe limits, enabling short-term monitoring.

Preprocessing steps, input validation, and optional device-specific calibration helped stabilize output across different microphones and acoustic conditions, demonstrating the system's robustness to everyday variability. Because decisions are produced locally, feedback appears instantly on the watch, and OS-compliant session management ensures uninterrupted access to the microphone.

Overall, the findings show that the wearable implementation performs accurately, efficiently, and responsively, enabling real-time monitoring through simple voice interaction. This supports the broader potential of this pipeline for on-device applications such as speech monitoring, health assessment, and other real-time audio-sensing tasks. By enabling these multimodal signals to be analyzed directly on a wearable device, the system enables continuous, natural data collection without specialized clinical equipment. This creates an opportunity for monitoring subtle, short-term changes in a person's speech, breathing, or vocal behavior in everyday environments. Such is particularly valuable in real-world scenarios where frequent screening or symptom tracking is needed, as occurred during the COVID-19 pandemic. Beyond COVID-19, the same framework can be applied to other respiratory or vocal health applications, offering a scalable way to investigate multimodal biomarkers.

6.5 LIMITATIONS

Data for the training threshold-based approach algorithm were collected across multiple countries using different measurement systems, which included variations in microphones, amplifiers, frequency response, signal-to-noise ratio, and dynamic range, which might have impacted the results. Additionally, the dataset used to develop the threshold-based approach algorithm is geographically imbalanced, with most samples originating from India, which may limit the model's generalizability to other populations due to differences in language patterns, acoustic environments, respiratory pathophysiology prevalence, or demographic characteristics. Besides that, features were extracted from relatively short 20-ms signal windows. The influence of longer analysis intervals on feature quality and model performance remains unclear. Understanding these effects could enhance the reliability and generalizability of the findings.

All wearable tests were conducted under controlled and typical conditions. Real-world deployments with different users and acoustic environments may affect wearable performance and should be considered in future analyses. Very noisy or unusual acoustic environments could still perturb *AnEp* computation, potentially affecting decision accuracy.

6.6 CONCLUSION

In conclusion, this work demonstrates that accurate differentiation of COVID-19 severity can be achieved fully on-device with consumer wearables, eliminating reliance on external hardware, cloud connectivity, or offline post-processing. By prioritizing a lightweight, energy-efficient implementation tailored to the memory and timing constraints of smartwatches and similar devices, the system enables stable, continuous operation in everyday environments. The decision logic is driven by statistically derived thresholds applied to DWT-based *AnEp*, thereby keeping the model interpretable and predictable while avoiding heavy ML classifiers. This threshold-based approach supports consistent execution time, prevents buffer overruns, and fits within the limited power and memory budgets typical of wearable platforms. The low cost, hands-free use, and portability make the voice-based wearable pipeline especially valuable for real-world screening and short-term monitoring. Beyond COVID-19, the same wearable framework – and its threshold-driven decision strategy – can be extended to other respiratory and vocal health applications, enabling scalable, continuous data collection and biomarker investigation without specialized clinical infrastructure.

ACKNOWLEDGMENTS

This work was supported by the FCT – Fundação para a Ciência e a Tecnologia under project UID/50016/2025.

REFERENCES

Abdel-Ghani, Ayah, Amira Abdalla, Zaineh Abughazzah, Mahnoor Akhund, Khalid Abualsaud, and Elias Yaacoub. 2024. Wearable bracelet and machine learning for remote diagnosis and pandemic infection detection. *Discover Applied Sciences* 6 (9):451.

Abreu Araujo, F., M. Riou, J. Torrejon, S. Tsunegi, D. Querlioz, K. Yakushiji, A. Fukushima, H. Kubota, S. Yuasa, M. D. Stiles and J. Grollier. 2020. Role of non-linear data processing on speech recognition task in the framework of reservoir computing. *Scientific Reports* 10 (1):328.

Akbari, Ali, and Meisam Khalil Arjmandi. 2014. An efficient voice pathology classification scheme based on applying multi-layer linear discriminant analysis to wavelet packet-based features. *Biomedical Signal Processing and Control* 10:209–223.

Alavi, A., G. K. Bogu, M. Wang, E. S. Rangan, A. W. Brooks, Q. Wang, E. Higgs, A. Celli, T. Mishra, A. A. Metwally, and K. Cha. 2022. Real-time alerting system for COVID-19 and other stress events using wearable data. *Nature Medicine* 28(1):175–184.

Albertovich, Tayurskii Dmitrii, and Rusanova Inna Aleksandrovna. 2017. The fractal analysis of the images and signals in medical diagnostics. *Fractal Analysis-Applications in Health Sciences and Social Sciences*:57.

Ali, Zulfiqar, Irraivan Elamvazuthi, Mansour Alsulaiman, and Ghulam Muhammad. 2015. Detection of voice pathology using fractal dimension in a multiresolution analysis of normal and disordered speech signals. *Journal of Medical Systems* 40 (1):20.

Aliverti, A. 2017. Wearable technology: Role in respiratory health and disease. *Breathe (Sheff)* 13 (2):e27–e36.

Al-Momani, Hafez. 2024. A literature review on the relative diagnostic accuracy of chest CT scans versus RT-PCR testing for COVID-19 diagnosis. *Tomography* 10 (6):935–948.

Alves, Marco A. R., Gabriel A. R. Silva, Bruno C. Bispo, María E. Dajer, and Pedro M. Rodrigues. 2020. Detecção de distúrbios vocais através de parâmetros cepstrais multibanda de vogal sustentada. In *Paper read at XXXVIII Simpósio Brasileiro de Telecomunicações e Processamento de Sinais.*

Alves, Marco, Gabriel Silva, Bruno C. Bispo, María E. Dajer, and Pedro M. Rodrigues. 2023. Voice disorders detection through multiband cepstral features of sustained vowel. *Journal of Voice* 37 (3):322–331.

Asiaee, Maral, Amir Vahedian-Azimi, Seyed Shahab Atashi, Abdalsamad Keramatfar, and Mandana Nourbakhsh. 2022. Voice quality evaluation in patients with COVID-19: An acoustic analysis. *Journal of Voice* 36 (6):879. e13–879. e19.

Barbosa, M. I., G. Silva, P. Ribeiro, E. Vieira, A. Perrotta, P. Moreira, and P. M. Rodrigues. 2025. Unraveling the microbiome–environmental change nexus to contribute to a more sustainable world: A comprehensive review of artificial intelligence approaches. *Sustainability* 17 (16):7209.

Bartl-Pokorny, K. D., F. B. Pokorny, A. Batliner, S. Amiriparian, A. Semertzidou, F. Eyben, E. Kramer, F. Schmidt, R. Schönweiler, M. Wehler, and B. W. Schuller. 2020. The voice of COVID-19: Acoustic correlates of infection. *arXiv preprint arXiv:2012.09478.*

Bartl-Pokorny, K. D., F. B. Pokorny, A., Batliner, S. Amiriparian, A. Semertzidou, F. Eyben, E. Kramer, F. Schmidt, R. Schönweiler, M. Wehler, and B. W. Schuller. 2021. The voice of COVID-19: Acoustic correlates of infection in sustained vowels. *Journal of the Acoustical Society of America* 149 (6):4377–4383.

Bhattacharya, D., N. K. Sharma, D. Dutta, S. R. Chetupalli, P. Mote, S. Ganapathy, C. Chandrakiran, S. Nori, K. K. Suhail, S. Gonuguntla, and M. Alagesan. 2023. Coswara: A respiratory sounds and symptoms dataset for remote screening of SARS-CoV-2 infection. *Scientific Data* 10 (1):397.

Birgmeier, Martin, H-P. Bernhard, and Gernot Kubin. 1997. Nonlinear long-term prediction of speech signals. In *Paper read at 1997 IEEE International Conference on Acoustics, Speech, and Signal Processing.*

Borhani, S., I. Silva, R. J. Damiano, T. Feng, C. Wang, L. Liu, E. Salvati, S. Mariani, and B. Conroy. 2025. Automatic detection of persistent physiological changes after COVID infection via wearable devices with potential for long COVID management. *Scientific Reports* 15 (1):29443.

Brown, C., J. Chauhan, A. Grammenos, J. Han, A. Hasthanasombat, D. Spathis, T. Xia, P. Cicuta, and C. Mascolo. 2020, August. Exploring automatic diagnosis of COVID-19 from crowdsourced respiratory sound data. In *Proceedings of the 26th ACM SIGKDD International Conference On Knowledge Discovery & Data Mining* (pp. 3474–3484).

Caldas, W. L., J. P. do Vale Madeiro, R. C. Pedrosa, J. P. P. Gomes, W. Du, and J. A. L. Marques. 2023. "Noise Detection and Classification in Chagasic ECG Signals Based on One-Dimensional Convolutional Neural Networks." In R. Lee (Ed.), *Computer and Information Science* (pp. 117–129). Springer International Publishing.

Cavalcante, A. F., V. H. D. L. Kunst, T. D. M. Chaves, J. D. de Souza, I. M. Ribeiro, J. P. Quintino, and A. E. F. da Gama. 2023. Deep learning in the recognition of activities of daily living using smartwatch data. *Sensors* 23 (17):7493.

Channa, Asma, Nirvana Popescu, Justyna Skibinska, and Radim Burget. 2021. The rise of wearable devices during the COVID-19 pandemic: A systematic review. *Sensors* 21 (17):5787.

Chen, Z., M. Li, R. Wang, W. Sun, J. Liu, H. Li, T. Wang, Y. Lian, J. Zhang, and X. Wang. 2022. Diagnosis of COVID-19 via acoustic analysis and artificial intelligence by monitoring breath sounds on smartphones. *Journal of Biomedical Informatics* 130:104078.

Cheong, Shing Hui Reina, Yu Jie Xavia Ng, Ying Lau, and Siew Tiang Lau. 2022. Wearable technology for early detection of COVID-19: A systematic scoping review. *Preventive Medicine* 162:107170.

Coleman, Robert F. 1993. Sources of variation in phonetograms. *Journal of Voice* 7 (1):1–14.

De Fazio, Roberto, Massimo De Vittorio, and Paolo Visconti. 2022. A BLE-connected piezoresistive and inertial chest band for remote monitoring of the respiratory activity by an android application: Hardware design and software optimization. *Future Internet* 14 (6):183.

Despotovic, Vladimir, Muhannad Ismael, Maël Cornil, Roderick Mc Call, and Guy Fagherazzi. 2021. Detection of COVID-19 from voice, cough and breathing patterns: Dataset and preliminary results. *Computers in Biology and Medicine* 138:104944.

Ding, X., D. Clifton, N. Ji, N. H. Lovell, P. Bonato, W. Chen, X. Yu, Z. Xue, T. Xiang, X. Long, and K. Xu. 2020. Wearable sensing and telehealth technology with potential applications in the coronavirus pandemic. *IEEE Reviews in Biomedical Engineering* 14:48–70.

Do Vale Madeiro, J. P., Barreto, D., Marques, J. A. L., and Salinet, J. L. 2019. Evaluating mathematical models for morphological classification of the QRS complex. *Computing in Cardiology*. https://doi.org/10.23919/CinC49843.2019.9005790

Erdoğan, Yunus Emre, and Ali Narin. 2021. COVID-19 detection with traditional and deep features on cough acoustic signals. *Computers in Biology and Medicine* 136:104765.

Escobedo, Pablo, Mitradip Bhattacharjee, Fatemeh Nikbakhtnasrabadi, and Ravinder Dahiya. 2020. Smart bandage with wireless strain and temperature sensors and batteryless NFC tag. *IEEE Internet of Things Journal* 8 (6):5093–5100.

Esposito, Anna, and Maria Marinaro. 2005. Some notes on nonlinearities of speech. In *Paper read at Nonlinear Speech Modeling and Applications, 2005, Berlin, Heidelberg*.

Faust, Oliver, and Muralidhar G. Bairy. 2012. Nonlinear analysis of physiological signals: A review. *Journal of Mechanics in Medicine and Biology* 12 (4):1240015.

Fernandes, J. V. M. R., A. R. D. Alexandria, J. A. L. Marques, D. F. D. Assis, P. C. Motta, and B. R. D. S. Silva.2024. Emotion detection from EEG signals using machine deep learning models. *Bioengineering* 11 (8):782.

Fischer, Aurelie, Abir Elbeji, Gloria Aguayo, and Guy Fagherazzi. 2022. Recommendations for successful implementation of the use of vocal biomarkers for remote monitoring of COVID-19 and long COVID in clinical practice and research. *Interactive Journal of Medical Research* 11 (2):e40655.

Gifani, Peyman, Hamid R. Rabiee, M. H. Hashemi, P. Taslimi, and Mohammed Ghanbari. 2007. Optimal fractal-scaling analysis of human EEG dynamic for depth of anesthesia quantification. *Journal of the Franklin Institute* 344 (3-4):212–229.

Guido, Rodrigo Capobianco. 2016. A tutorial on signal energy and its applications. *Neurocomputing* 179:264–282.

Guido, Rodrigo Capobianco. 2022. Wavelets behind the scenes: Practical aspects, insights, and perspectives. *Physics Reports* 985:1–23.

Han, J., C. Brown, J. Chauhan, A. Grammenos, A. Hasthanasombat, D. Spathis, T. Xia, P. Cicuta, and C. Mascolo. 2021. June. Exploring automatic COVID-19 diagnosis via voice and symptoms from crowdsourced data. In *ICASSP 2021-2021 IEEE International Conference on Acoustics, Speech and Signal Processing (ICASSP)* (pp. 8328–8332). IEEE.

Hassantabar, S., N. Stefano, V. Ghanakota, A. Ferrari, G. N. Nicola, R, Bruno, I. R. Marino, K. Hamidouche, and N. K. Jha. 2021. CovidDeep: SARS-CoV-2/COVID-19 test based on wearable medical sensors and efficient neural networks. *IEEE Transactions on Consumer Electronics* 67 (4):244–256.

Hayden, M. K., K. E. Hanson, J. A. Englund, F. Lee, M. J. Lee, M. Loeb, D. J. Morgan, R. Patel, A. El Alayli, I. K. El Mikati, and S. Sultan. 2024. The Infectious Diseases Society of America guidelines on the diagnosis of COVID-19: antigen testing (January 2023). *Clinical Infectious Diseases* 78 (7):e350–e384.

Hu, Li, and Zhiguo Zhang. 2019. *EEG Signal Processing and Feature Extraction*. Springer.

Imran, A., I. Posokhova, H. N. Qureshi, U. Masood, M. S. Riaz, K. Ali, C. N. John, M. I. Hussain, and M. Nabeel. 2020. AI4COVID-19: AI enabled preliminary diagnosis for COVID-19 from cough samples via an app. *Informatics in Medicine Unlocked* 20:100378.

Ishac, D., S. Matta, S. Bin, H. Aziz, E. Karam, A. Abche, and G. Nassar. 2022. Objective assessment of Covid-19 severity affecting the vocal and respiratory system using a wearable, autonomous sound collar. *Cellular and Molecular Bioengineering* 15 (1):67–86.

Islam, Rumana, Esam Abdel-Raheem, and Mohammed Tarique. 2022. A study of using cough sounds and deep neural networks for the early detection of Covid-19. *Biomedical Engineering Advances* 3:100025.

Katz, Michael J. 1988. Fractals and the analysis of waveforms. *Computers in Biology and Medicine* 18 (3):145–156.

Khondakar, Kamil Reza, and Ajeet Kaushik. 2023. Role of wearable sensing technology to manage long COVID. *Biosensors* 13 (1):62.

Kumar, Arun, and S. K. Mullick. 1996. Nonlinear dynamical analysis of speech. *Journal of the Acoustical Society of America* 100 (1):615–629.

Lee, Jong-Min, Dae-Jin Kim, In-Young Kim, Kwang-Suk Park, and Sun I Kim. 2002. Detrended fluctuation analysis of EEG in sleep apnea using MIT/BIH polysomnography data. *Computers in Biology and Medicine* 32 (1):37–47.

Lo Presti, Daniela, Daniele Bianchi, Carlo Massaroni, Alessio Gizzi, and Emiliano Schena. 2022. A soft and skin-interfaced smart patch based on fiber optics for cardiorespiratory monitoring. *Biosensors* 12 (6):363.

Lonini, L., N. Shawen, O. Botonis, M. Fanton, C. Jayaraman, C. K. Mummidisetty, S. Y. Shin, C. Rushin, S. Jenz, S. Xu, and J. A. Rogers. 2021. Rapid screening of physiological changes associated with COVID-19 using soft-wearables and structured activities: a pilot study. *IEEE Journal of Translational Engineering in Health and Medicine*, 9:1–11.

Luo, R., J. A. L. Marques, K.-L. Ong, and, S. Fong. 2020. Crowdsensing-based gamification for collective assistance for post-era of coronavirus epidemic in community living. *International Journal of Extreme Automation and Connectivity in Healthcare (IJEACH)* 2 (2):54–64. https://doi.org/10.4018/IJEACH.2020070106

Maghded, Halgurd S., Kayhan Zrar Ghafoor, Ali Safaa Sadiq, Kevin Curran, Danda B Rawat, and Khaled Rabie. 2020. A novel AI-enabled framework to diagnose coronavirus COVID-19 using smartphone embedded sensors: design study. In *Paper read at 2020 IEEE 21st international conference on information reuse and integration for data science (IRI).*

Malvar, Henrique S. 1992. *Signal Processing with Lapped Transforms*. Artech House, Inc.

Marques, J. A. L., and S. Fong. (Eds.). 2022. *Epidemic Analytics for Decision Supports in COVID19 Crisis*. Springer.

Marques, J. A. L., and S. J. Fong (Eds.). 2023. *Computerized Systems for Diagnosis and Treatment of COVID-19*. Springer.https://doi.org/10.1007/978-3-031-30788-1

Marques, J. A. L., F. N. B. Gois, J. P. do V. Madeiro, T. Li, and S. J. Fong. 2022. Artificial neural network-based approaches for computer-aided disease diagnosis and treatment. In A. K. Bhoi, V. H. C. de Albuquerque, P. N. Srinivasu, and G. Marques (Eds.), *Cognitive and Soft Computing Techniques for the Analysis of Healthcare Data* (pp. 79–99). Academic Press. https://doi.org/10.1016/B978-0-323-85751-2.00008-6

Marques, J. A. L., F. N. B. Gois, J. Xavier-Neto, and S. J. Fong. 2021. *Predictive Models for Decision Support in the COVID-19 Crisis*. Springer.

Marques, J. A. L., F. N. Bernardo Gois, J. A. Nunes da Silveira, T. Li, and S. J. Fong. 2022. AI and deep learning for processing the huge amount of patient-centric data that assist in clinical decisions. In A. K. Bhoi, V. H. C. de Albuquerque, P. N. Srinivasu, and G. Marques (Eds.), *Cognitive and Soft Computing Techniques for the Analysis of Healthcare Data* (pp. 101–121). Academic Press. https://doi.org/10.1016/B978-0-323-85751-2.00001-3

Marques, J. A. L., P. C. Cortez, J. P. D. V. Madeiro, S. J. Fong, F. S. Schlindwein, and V. H. C. D. Albuquerque. 2019. Automatic cardiotocography diagnostic system based on hilbert transform and adaptive threshold technique. *IEEE Access* 7:73085–73094. https://doi.org/10.1109/ACCESS.2018.2877933

Marques, J. A. L., P. C. Cortez, J. P. V. Madeiro, V. H. C. Albuquerque, S. J. Fong, and F. S. Schlindwein. 2020. Nonlinear characterization and complexity analysis of cardiotocographic examinations using entropy measures. *Journal of Supercomputing* 76 (2):1305–1320. https://doi.org/10.1007/s11227-018-2570-8

Mason, A. E., F. M. Hecht, S. K. Davis, J. L. Natale, W. Hartogensis, N. Damaso, K. T. Claypool, S. Dilchert, S. Dasgupta, S. Purawat, and V. K. Viswanath. 2022. Detection of COVID-19 using multimodal data from a wearable device: results from the first TemPredict Study. *Scientific Reports* 12 (1):3463.

Mishra, T., M. Wang, A. A. Metwally, G. K. Bogu, A. W. Brooks, A. Bahmani, A. Alavi, A. Celli, E. Higgs, O. Dagan-Rosenfeld, and B. Fay. 2020. Pre-symptomatic detection of COVID-19 from smartwatch data. *Nature Biomedical Engineering* 4 (12):1208–1220.

Natarajan, Aravind, Hao-Wei Su, and Conor Heneghan. 2020. Assessment of physiological signs associated with COVID-19 measured using wearable devices. *npj Digital Medicine* 3 (1):156.

Pancaldi, F., G. S. Pezzuto, G. Cassone, M. Morelli, A. Manfredi, M. D'Arienzo, C. Vacchi, F. Savorani, G. Vinci, F. Barsotti, and M. T. Mascia. 2022. VECTOR: An algorithm for the detection of COVID-19 pneumonia from velcro-like lung sounds. *Computers in Biology and Medicine*, 142:105220.

Pho, Gerald Norman, Nina Thigpen, Shyamal Patel, and Hal Tily. 2023. Feasibility of measuring physiological responses to breakthrough infections and COVID-19 vaccine using a Wearable Ring Sensor. *Digital Biomarkers* 7 (1):1–6.

Pordeus, D., P. Ribeiro, L. Zacarias, J. Paulo Madeiro, J. A. Lobo Marques, P. Miguel Rodrigues, C. Leite, M. Alves Neto, A. Aires Peixoto Jr, and A. de Oliveira. 2023. Classification of severity of COVID-19 patients based on the heart rate variability. In *Computerized Systems for Diagnosis and Treatment of COVID-19* (pp. 155–177). Cham: Springer International Publishing.

Pordeus, D., Ribeiro, P., Zacarias, L., de Oliveira, A., Marques, J.A.L., Rodrigues, P.M., Leite, C., Neto, M.A., Peixoto Jr, A.A. and do Vale Madeiro, J.P., 2023, June. Training Strategies for Covid-19 Severity Classification. In *International Work-Conference on Bioinformatics and Biomedical Engineering* (pp. 514–527). Cham: Springer Nature Switzerland.

Quer, G., J. M. Radin, M. Gadaleta, K. Baca-Motes, L. Ariniello, E. Ramos, V. Kheterpal, E. J. Topol, and S. R. Steinhubl. 2021. Wearable sensor data and self-reported symptoms for COVID-19 detection. *Nature Medicine* 27(1):73–77.

Ribeiro, Pedro, João Alexandre Lobo Marques, and Pedro Miguel Rodrigues. 2023. COVID-19 detection by means of ECG, voice, and X-ray computerized systems: A review. *Bioengineering* 10 (2):198.

Ribeiro, P., J. A. L. Marques, D. Pordeus, L. Zacarias, C. F. Leite, M. A. Sobreira-Neto, A. A. Peixoto Jr, A. de Oliveira, J. P. do Vale Madeiro, and P. M. Rodrigues. 2024. Machine learning-based cardiac activity non-linear analysis for discriminating COVID-19 patients with different degrees of severity. *Biomedical Signal Processing and Control* 87:105558.

Rioul, O., and M. Vetterli. 1991. Wavelets and signal processing. *IEEE Signal Processing Magazine* 8 (4):14–38.

Rodrigues, P. M., D. Freitas, and J. P. Teixeir. 2012. Alzheimer electroencephalogram temporal events detection by K-means. *Procedia Technology* 5:859–864.

Rodrigues, P. M., D. Freitas, J. P. Teixeira, B. Bispo, D. Alves, and C. Garrett. 2018. Electroencephalogram hybrid method for Alzheimer early detection. *Procedia Computer Science* 138:209–214.

Rodrigues, P. M., J. P. Madeiro, and J. A. L. Marques. 2023. Enhancing health and public health through machine learning: Decision support for smarter choices. *Bioengineering* 10 (7):792.

Rodrigues, Pedro M., Bruno C. Bispo, Carolina Garrett, Dílio Alves, Joao P Teixeira, and Diamantino Freitas. 2021. Lacsogram: A new EEG tool to diagnose Alzheimer's disease. *IEEE Journal of Biomedical and Health Informatics* 25 (9):3384–3395.

Rodriguez-Bermudez, German, and Pedro J. Garcia-Laencina. 2015. Analysis of EEG signals using nonlinear dynamics and chaos: A review. *Applied Mathematics & Information Sciences* 9 (5):2309.

Sairamya, N. J., M. S. P. Subathra, Easter S. Suviseshamuthu, and S. Thomas George. 2021. A new approach for automatic detection of focal EEG signals using wavelet packet decomposition and quad binary pattern method. *Biomedical Signal Processing and Control* 63:102096.

Sanei, Saeid, and Jonathon A Chambers. 2013. *EEG Signal Processing*. Wiley.

Santos, A. G., J. A. Marques, L. O. Rigo, and J. P. Madeiro. 2023. October. Exploring EEG signal features for predicting post cardiac arrest prognosis. In *2023 Computing in Cardiology (CinC)* (Vol. 50, pp. 1–4). IEEE. https://doi.org/10.22489/CinC.2023.312

Santos, M. D., C. Roman, and M. A. F. Pimentel. 2021. A real-time wearable system for monitoring vital signs of COVID-19 patients in a hospital setting. *Front Digit Heal* 3:1–16 [online].

Schwartz, Laurent, Anne Devin, Frédéric Bouillaud, and Marc Henry. 2020. Entropy as the driving force of pathogenesis: An attempt of diseases classification based on the laws of physics. *Substantia* 4 (2):1–154.

Shimon, Carmi, Gabi Shafat, Inbal Dangoor, and Asher Ben-Shitrit. 2021. Artificial intelligence enabled preliminary diagnosis for COVID-19 from voice cues and questionnairesa). *Journal of the Acoustical Society of America* 149 (2):1120–1124.

Silva, G., Batista, P. and Rodrigues, P.M., 2025. COVID-19 activity screening by a smart-data-driven multi-band voice analysis. *Journal of Voice* 39(3): 602–611.

Singh, P., G. Chaudhary, and J. A. L. Marques. 2023. Medical information extraction of clinical notes and pictorial visualisation of electronic medical records summary interface. In Preeti Nagrath, Jafar A. Alzubi, Bhawna Singla, Joel J. P. C. Rodrigues, and A. K. Verma (Eds.), *Smart Distributed Embedded Systems for Healthcare Applications* (pp. 29–40). CRC Press.

Soltanian, Mohammad, and Keivan Borna. 2022. Covid-19 recognition from cough sounds using lightweight separable-quadratic convolutional network. *Biomedical Signal Processing and Control* 72:103333.

Sondhi, S., A. Salhan, C. A. Santoso, M. Doucoure, D. M. Dharmawan, A. Sureka, B. N. Natasha, A. D. Danusaputro, N. S. Dowson, M. S. L. Yap, and M. A. Hadiwidjaja. 2021. Voice processing for COVID-19 scanning and prognostic indicator. *Heliyon 7*(10).

Spachos, P., S. Gregori, and M. J. Deen. 2022. Voice activated IoT devices for healthcare: Design challenges and emerging applications. *IEEE Transactions on Circuits and Systems II: Express Briefs* 69 (7):3101–3107.

Tahir, Emel, Esra Kavaz, Senem Çengel Kurnaz, Fatih Temoçin, and Aynur Atilla. 2023. Patient reported voice handicap and auditory-perceptual voice assessment outcomes in patients with COVID-19. *Logopedics Phoniatrics Vocology* 48 (2):88–97.

Trimpop, John, Hannes Schenk, Gerald Bieber, Friedrich Lämmel, and Paul Burggraf. 2017. Smartwatch based respiratory rate and breathing pattern recognition in an end-consumer environment. In *Proceedings of the 4th International Workshop on Sensor-based Activity Recognition and Interaction*. Association for Computing Machinery.

Van, S. N., J. L. Marques, T. A. Biala, and Y. Li. 2021. Identification of latent risk clinical attributes for children born under IUGR condition using machine learning techniques. *Computer Methods and Programs in Biomedicine* 200:105842. https://doi.org/10.1016/j.cmpb.2020.105842

Velasquez, G.D.D.S., S. Borna, M. J. Maniaci, J. D. Coffey, C. R. Haider, B. M. Demaerschalk, and A. J. Forte. 2024. Economic perspective of the use of wearables in health care: a systematic review. *Mayo Clinic Proceedings: Digital Health* 2 (3):299–317.

Verde, Laura, Giuseppe De Pietro, and Giovanna Sannino. 2023. Artificial intelligence techniques for the non-invasive detection of COVID-19 through the analysis of voice signals. *Arabian Journal for Science and Engineering* 48 (8):11143–11153.

Vetterli, Martin, and Jelena Kovacevic. 1995. *Wavelets and Subband Coding*. Vol. 87. Prentice Hall PTR Englewood Cliffs, NJ.

Wijayanto, I., R. Hartanto, and H. A. Nugroho. 2019. October. Higuchi and katz fractal dimension for detecting interictal and ictal state in electroencephalogram signal. In *2019 11th International Conference on Information Technology and Electrical Engineering (ICITEE)* (pp. 1–6). IEEE.

Wu, Yu, Dai Jiang, Andy Bardill, Richard Bayford, and Andreas Demosthenous. 2019. A 122 fps, 1 MHz bandwidth multi-frequency wearable EIT belt featuring novel active electrode architecture for neonatal thorax vital sign monitoring. *IEEE Transactions on Biomedical Circuits and Systems* 3:927–937.

Yan, K., T. Li, J. A. L. Marques, J. Gao, S. J. Fong, K. Yan, T. Li, J. A. L. Marques, J. Gao, and S. J. Fong. 2023. A review on multimodal machine learning in medical diagnostics. *Mathematical Biosciences and Engineering* 20 (5):8708–8726. https://doi.org/10.3934/mbe.2023382

Zacarias, H., J. A. L. Marques, V. Felizardo, M. Pourvahab, and N. M. Garcia. 2024. ECG forecasting system based on long short-term memory. *Bioengineering* 11 (1):89.

Zar, J. H. 2010. *Biostatistical Analysis*. Prentice Hall.

Zhao, T., F. N. B. Gois, J. A. L. Marques, B. R. dos Santos Silva, P. Cortez, S. K. Jagatheesaperumal, and V.H.C. de Albuquerque. 2025. AutoML-based EEG signal analysis in neuro-marketing classification using biclustering method. *Applied Soft Computing* 181:113412.

7 Wearable-Cloud Based System for COVID-19 Severity Discrimination Through Multiband Nonlinear Modeling

Pedro Ribeiro, João Alexandre Lobo Marques, Daniel Pordeus, Maria Inês Barbosa, Laíla Zacarias, Manoel Alves Sobreira-Neto, Arnaldo Aires Peixoto Jr., Bruno Catarino Bispo, Adriel de Oliveira, Victor Hugo C. de Albuquerque, Ganesh R. Naik, Camila Ferreira Leite, João Paulo Madeiro, and Pedro Miguel Rodrigues

7.1 INTRODUCTION

The COVID-19 pandemic, declared by the World Health Organization (WHO) in March 2020, exposed persistent gaps in rapid, scalable tools for early severity assessment—particularly in critical care and resource-limited settings (Yesudhas, Srivastava, and Gromiha. 2020; Hosseini et al. 2020; Ciotti et al. 2020). The development of digital technologies was strongly encouraged in both computational (Marques et al. 2021; Marques and Fong 2022) and artificial intelligence (AI) and computational solutions for diagnostic and treatment (Marques and Fong 2023). The issues and limitations of the clinic support during the outbreak have underscored the critical role of wearable technologies as scalable, noninvasive tools for diagnostics, risk stratification, and continuous monitoring, which are reliable and widely used tools (Marques et al. 2021; Caldas et al. 2023; Cavalcante et al. 2023) and can be applied in both acute and post-acute phases of the disease. The rapid deployment of wearable electrocardiogram (ECG) devices, combined with advances in AI, has enabled continuous acquisition and real-time interpretation of cardiac and autonomic biomarkers reflecting systemic inflammation, hypoxia, and cardiovascular stress associated with *severe* acute respiratory syndrome coronavirus 2 (SARS-CoV-2) infection. AI and deep

DOI: 10.1201/9781003500445-7

learning (DL) techniques have proven fundamental for processing the large volumes of patient-centric ECG data generated by wearables, supporting computer-aided diagnosis, severity assessment, and clinical decision-making in resource-constrained and remote settings (Marques, Bernardo Gois, et al. 2022; Marques, Gois, et al. 2022). Recent studies demonstrate that machine learning (ML) models—ranging from nonlinear dynamical analysis to recurrent neural networks and automated learning pipelines—can extract diagnostically relevant patterns from ECG signals, enabling early detection, prognosis, and forecasting of disease progression in wearable-compatible scenarios (Do Vale Madeiro et al. 2019; Fernandes et al. 2024; Guilherme Cunha Santos et al. 2023; Marques et al. 2019; Marques et al. 2020; Zacarias et al. 2024; Zhao et al. 2025). In parallel, multimodal decision-support systems integrating ECG-derived biomarkers with complementary clinical and contextual data have shown strong potential to enhance remote COVID-19 diagnostics and public health surveillance while reducing dependence on centralized testing infrastructure (Nguyen Van et al. 2021; Rodrigues et al. 2023; Yan et al. 2023). These developments are further reinforced by advances in medical information extraction, electronic health record summarization, and digital health analytics, which collectively support the integration of wearable ECG diagnostics into resilient, interpretable, and scalable healthcare ecosystems for pandemic response (Singh et al. 2023).

Clinical management of SARS-CoV-2 infection spans a broad severity spectrum—from *low* (mild/no pneumonia) to *moderate* (pneumonia with fever/respiratory symptoms), *severe* (e.g., respiratory distress >30 breaths/min; SpO_2 <93%; PaO_2/FiO_2 <300 mmHg; rapid radiologic progression), and critical (e.g., respiratory failure requiring ventilation, shock, or other organ failure necessitating intensive care unit (ICU) care) (Yan et al. 2020). Timely stratification across these categories is essential for triage, care escalation, and optimal resource allocation.

While diagnostic confirmation relies primarily on RT-PCR (i.e., reverse transcription-polymerase chain reaction), ancillary tools such as rapid antigen/antibody assays and chest CT have been employed to gauge disease status and burden (Lai and Lam 2021; Pordeus, Ribeiro, Zacarias, de Oliveira, et al. 2023; Pordeus, Ribeiro, Zacarias, Paulo Madeiro, et al. 2023). However, the cost, logistics, and limited availability of advanced imaging can hinder frequent monitoring, especially outside tertiary centers. In parallel, cardiovascular involvement in COVID-19—manifesting as acute cardiac injury, cardiogenic shock, thromboembolic events, right ventricular dysfunction, tachyarrhythmias, and electrocardiographic changes—underscores the disease's systemic impact (Long et al. 2021; Farshidfar, Koleini, and Ardehali 2021; Ribeiro, Marques, and Rodrigues 2023). Notably, ECG abnormalities such as ST-segment elevation/depression and T-wave inversion have been associated with adverse outcomes, making ECG an attractive, low-cost modality for continuous risk assessment (Wang et al. 2020; Duca et al. 2022; da Silva et al. 2023).

Building on this premise, wearable devices equipped with single-lead ECG sensors offer a practical route to large-scale, near-continuous physiologic monitoring without chest electrodes—particularly valuable for bedridden patients and contexts where repeat computed tomography (CT) imaging is impractical or unavailable. Their affordability, portability, and broad availability position smartwatch ECG as a promising screening adjunct for early severity stratification (Klén et al. 2022; Kotnis et al.

2022; Rodrigues, Madeiro, and Marques 2023). Yet, effective clinical deployment requires robust signal processing, security, and architectural choices that minimize on-device compute while enabling reliable, interpretable predictions. While Cheong et al. (2022) noted that the use of wearables for early COVID-19 detection is still relatively new and often relies on untested technologies, these devices have already proven effective in other clinical areas. For example, Perez et al. (2019) demonstrated that wearables could detect atrial fibrillation using an irregular pulse algorithm. More recently, a systematic review and meta-analysis by Murray et al. (2025) concluded that wearables are a promising strategy for managing high-risk heart failure patients, effectively reducing both hospitalization and mortality. This study aims to:

1. Design a wearable-to-cloud architecture for early COVID-19 severity assessment using consumer smartwatches (Apple watchOS and Android Wear OS) that acquire single-lead ECG in WaveForm DataBase (WFDB) format.
2. Constrain on-device workload by limiting the wrist application to ECG acquisition, secure data upload, and results visualization, delegating all computational tasks to the cloud backend.
3. Establish secure, reliable data transmission with end-to-end encryption and integrity checks, ensuring robust handling of acquisition metadata (e.g., sampling rate, duration, device operating system (OS)).
4. Implement a cloud-hosted signal processing pipeline that applies a discrete wavelet transform (DWT) to decompose raw ECG into frequency subbands suitable for subsequent analysis.
5. Engineer feature representations by computing ten nonlinear dynamical features per subband and compressing them via statistical metrics into fixed-size descriptors for efficient modeling.
6. Train and evaluate supervised ML classifiers on the compact descriptors under an 80/20 hold-out protocol to enable automated severity stratification (*low, moderate, severe*).
7. Deploy and integrate the pretrained classification model within a secure, scalable cloud backend, exposing inference via REST/gRPC (i.e., representational state transfer/Google remote procedure call) application programming interfaces (APIs) and ensuring end-to-end encryption, audit logging, model versioning, CI/CD (i.e., continuous integration/continuous delivery or deployment), and real-time monitoring for reliability and compliance.
8. Deliver predictions and associated metadata back to the wrist application through secure APIs, enabling timely on-device visualization and facilitating clinical decision-support workflows.

7.2 METHODOLOGY

7.2.1 Machine Learning algorithm training stage

In this section, we describe each step of the experimental study and introduce the database.

Figure 7.1 illustrates the methodology diagram for the steps described below.

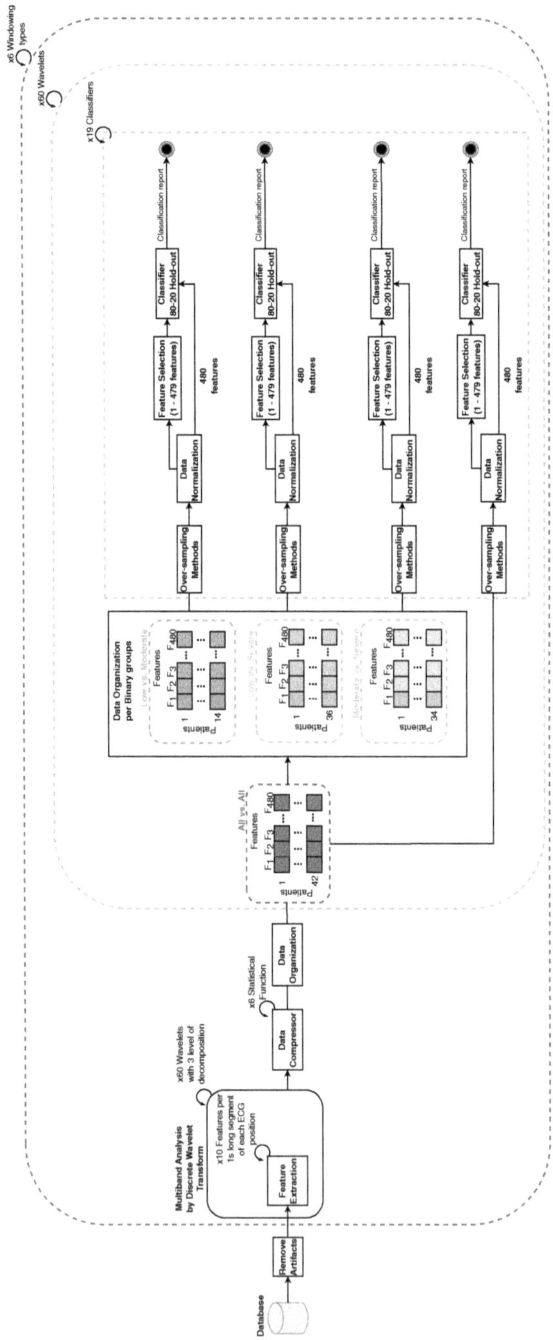

FIGURE 7.1 Methodology Workflow Diagram.

7.2.1.1 Experimental Setup

In accordance with the study objectives, the experimental workflow was implemented using matrix laboratory (MATLAB) (R2022a) for signal processing and feature engineering, and Python (3.9.12) for model design, training, and evaluation. Although the target runtime is a cloud-coupled architecture, all experiments reported here were executed locally to ensure reproducibility and controlled benchmarking; cloud deployment details are described in the implementation section of the manuscript.

All work was conducted using two MacBook laptops:

- 2019 MacBook Pro with a 2.6 GHz Intel Core i7 (six-core), advanced micro devices (AMD) Radeon Pro 5300M 4 GB graphics processing unit (GPU), and 16 GB RAM.
- MacBook Pro 14 with an M1 Pro (eight-core CPU, 14-core GPU) and 16 GB RAM.

7.2.1.2 The Database

The database is a cross-sectional, descriptive quantitative study conducted at Hospital Universitário Walter Cantídio (HUWC) and Hospital Estadual Leonardo da Vinci (HELV), Ceará, Brazil, from May 2021 to January 2022, corresponding to the first, second, and third waves of COVID-19 in Brazil.

The Ethics Committee approved the study for Research on Humans (CAAE – HELV: 47229221.9.3001.5684; CAAE – HUWC: 47229221.9.0000.5045).

The database includes eight patients with *low* severity, ten with *moderate* severity, and 33 with *severe* disease.

The youngest patient was 18 years old, and the oldest was 88, with an average age of 54.59 and a standard deviation of 17.23.

Table 7.1 provides an overview of the socio-demographic and clinical characteristics of the database. Additionally, it includes the results of the corresponding statistical analyses: the Mann-Whitney U test ($p<0.05$) for the Gender distribution and the Kruskal-Wallis test ($p<0.05$) for the Clinical Information.

TABLE 7.1
Socio-Demographic and Clinical Characteristics of the Database

		Age					
		Min	**Max**	**%**	**Avg.**	**Std**	***p*-value**
Full Database		18	88	-	54.59	17.23	-
Gender	Male	27	82	60	53.16	15.51	0.5455
	Female	18	88	40	56.80	19.85	
Clinical Information	Low	18	78	16	47.63	18.09	0.2313
	Moderate	30	80	18	49.89	19.65	
	Severe	27	88	66	57.64	16.37	

The ECG recordings were performed with the participants being placed in two different body positions, the supine (*Down*) position and the orthostasis (*Up*) position.

The signals were sampled at a frequency rate of 256Hz and an elliptic band-pass filter with the frequency cut-offs of 1Hz and 40Hz (Kalidas and Tamil 2017), a *steepness* of 0.85, and a *A StopBandAttenuation of 60 dB was applied to each* signal's lead. Participants were monitored during spontaneous breathing on the modified Lead II.

The database is registered with Mendeley Data under doi:10.17632/cy8b8kvfdf.2, and it can be accessed at: https://data.mendeley.com/datasets/cy8b8kvfdf/2. Inside the designated "COVID-19 Database" folder, it can be found:

- An Excel file (*.xlsx*) named "COVID-19 Patients Information", containing the following physiological data about patients:
  - Patient Information – Identifier number, age, and gender.
  - Clinical Data – COVID-19 severity level, comorbidities, symptoms, medication, oxygen therapy, invasive mechanical ventilation, noninvasive ventilation, prone positioning, shock, acute respiratory distress syndrome (ARDS), PCR, heart injury, kidney injury, and secondary injury.
  - Vital Signs – Heart rate, respiration rate, oxygen saturation ($SatO_2$ or SpO_2), systolic blood pressure, diastolic blood pressure and body mass index (BMI).
  - Laboratory Exams – Red cell count, hemoglobin, hematocrit, neutrophil count, leukocyte count, lymphocyte count, platelets, thrombin time, thromboplastin time, ferritin, troponin, PCR, urea, creatinine, D-dimer, aspartate aminotransferase, alanine aminotransferase, and creatine kinase.
- A folder named "ECG Signals" contains participants' raw ECGs in *.mat* extension files. After being loaded in Matlab, each ECG *.mat* file includes three variables:
  - DATA – The date that the ECG has been collected.
  - sinalf1 – ECG raw signal.
  - Timing of Pulsars (TEMPO1) – Duration of the raw signal in seconds.

It is worth noting that each patient signal alias file is assigned a unique identifier following the structure "Patient_{#patient}_{body position}". This identifier was designed to safeguard patient anonymity.

7.2.1.3 Artifacts Removal

At this stage, a medical doctor on our team analyzed the quality and integrity of the raw ECG collected signals by identifying artifacts. Figure 7.2 shows an example of an artifact present in the database. Subsequently, one of two actions was performed for each signal, as performed in other state-of-the-art studies (Jiang et al. 2007; Kumar and Singh 2015): (1) full signal deletion or (2) removal of the signal portions related to the artifacts if the rest of the signal is acceptable. Initially, 51 patients' signals were present. After artifact removal, the number of patients available for further analysis decreased to 42 (comprising data from eight patients with *low* severity, six with *moderate* severity, and 28 with a *severe* stage of the disease), as the ECG data from nine

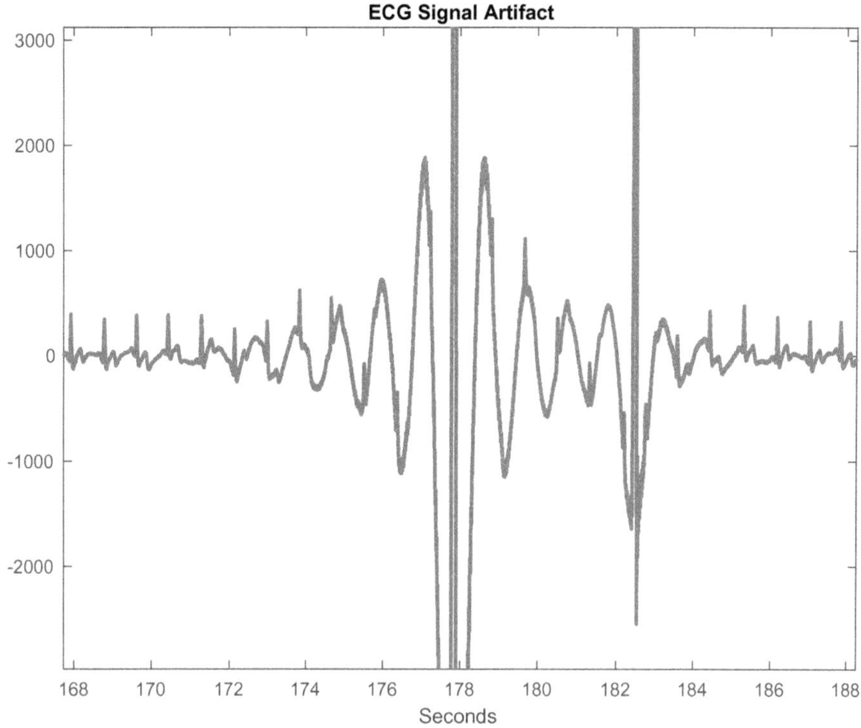

FIGURE 7.2 Example of an Electrocardiogram Artifact Present in the Database.

participants was full of artifacts related to contact, movement, and other equipment interference, rendering it unusable as it is too corrupted to yield any usable information. It is important to note that this data was collected under the challenging conditions of one of humanity's most complex pandemics.

7.2.1.4 Electrocardiogram Multiband Decomposition Via Wavelet Transform and Feature Extraction

The DWT is a multiresolution technique that represents a finite-energy discrete signal across multiple frequency bands, highlighting localized time-domain features at each frequency scale (Guido 2022; Rioul and Vetterli 1991). Unlike the Short-Time Fourier Transform (STFT), which uses a fixed-resolution window, the DWT employs an adaptive filter bank that divides the signal into low-frequency (approximation) and high-frequency (detail) subbands across several levels. The standard DWT implementation often relies on an octave-band critically decimated filter bank (Malvar 1992; Kovačević 1995). Let $h_0(n)$ be the low-pass filter (LP) and $h_1(n)$ be the high-pass filter (HP). Each subband occupies a distinct frequency band, for $m = 0, 1, \ldots, S$, as

$$W_m = \begin{cases} [0, \ /2^S], & m = 0, \\ [/2^{\{S-m+1\}}, \ /2^{\{S-m\}}], & m = 1, 2, \ldots, S, \end{cases} \tag{1}$$

where S is the total number of decomposition levels and π is the normalized angular frequency (half the sampling rate).

In a more standard notation, we define the scale function $\phi_0(n)$ and wavelet function $\psi_0(n)$ at the initial level:

$$_0(n) = h_0(n), \quad _0(n) = h_1(n). \tag{2}$$

Using the standard dyadic expansion, the scale and wavelet functions at level $j+1$ can be written as

$$\phi_{j+1}(n) = \phi_j\left(n/2\right) * \phi_0(n), \tag{3}$$

$$\psi_{j+1}(n) = \phi_j\left(n/2\right) * \psi_0(n), \tag{4}$$

where $*$ denotes convolution and j runs from zero to $S-1$.

For each level j, the low-pass and high-pass subbands correspond to coefficients obtained by filtering and downsampling. Equivalently, their filter impulse responses can be seen as

$$h_m(n) = \begin{cases} \phi_S(n), & m = 0, \\ \psi_{S-m}(n), & m = 1, 2, \ldots, S. \end{cases} \tag{5}$$

Here, $\phi_S(n)$ corresponds to the lowest subband (approximation coefficients) and $\psi_{S-m}(n)$ accounts for each higher-frequency subband (detail coefficients).

The subband signals $x_m(n)$ are computed by convolving $x(n)$ with the appropriate $h_m(n)$ filter and performing the downsampling (often expressed by 2^j):

$$x_m(n) = \begin{cases} \sum_{k=-\infty}^{\infty} x(k) h_m(2^S n - k), \&m = 0, \\ \sum_{k=-\infty}^{\infty} x(k) h_m(2^{S-m+1}\ n - k), \&\ m = 1,2,\ldots,S. \end{cases} \tag{6}$$

This process generates a set of subband signals suitable for multiresolution analysis.

In this study, a diverse set of 60 wavelet functions is applied to one-second ECG segments for a robust performance evaluation (Daamouche et al. 2012; Smital et al. 2013; Ribeiro, Sá, et al. 2024; Li, Zheng, and Tai 1995; Zhi, Faust, and Yu 2014; Sivannarayana and Reddy 1999; Mourad and Fethi 2016; Cui et al. 2021; Shen and Zayed 2014). These wavelets differ in frequency response, noise robustness, and capability to highlight distinct ECG features (e.g., normal vs. wide QRS complexes, biphasic vs. monophasic P and T waves), providing a comprehensive testing framework for analyzing physiological signals (Rodrigues, Freitas, and Teixeir 2012; Rodrigues, D.Freitas, et al. 2018).

- Haar (*haar*): The simplest wavelet function representing the Haar wavelet.
- Daubechies (*db1* to *db10*): A family of orthogonal wavelets designed by Ingrid Daubechies, with different orders denoted by numbers one to ten.

- Symlet (*sym2* to *sym8*): Symmetrical wavelets designed to balance regularity and localization.
- Coiflet (*coif1* to *coif5*): Coiflet wavelets designed to achieve smoother signal approximation.
- Biorthogonal (*bior1.1* to *bior6.8*): Biorthogonal wavelets offer distinct functions for decomposition and reconstruction.
- Reverse Biorthogonal (*rbio1.1* to *rbio6.8*): Reverse biorthogonal wavelets with reversed roles between analyzing and synthesizing wavelets.
- Farras-Kovacevic (*fk4* to *fk22*): Wavelets introduced by Farras and Kovacevic are known for favorable localization properties in time and frequency domains.
- Daubechies Meyer (*dmey*): A specific wavelet that balances regularity and localization.

The decomposition of ECG signals using the DWT is performed via six distinct sliding-window analyses. These analyses include rectangular nonoverlapping windowing (*Rect*), rectangular 0.5s overlapping windowing (*RecO*), Hamming nonoverlapping windowing (*Hm*), Hamming 0.5s overlapping windowing (*HmO*), Hanning nonoverlapping windowing (*Hn*), and Hanning 0.5s overlapping windowing (*HnO*). The choice of these windowing methods is driven by the need to evaluate a reliable set of sliding-window analyses to identify those that enhance the accuracy and reliability of ECG signal analysis, thereby contributing to better COVID-19 diagnostic outcomes. In each windowing signal cropping analysis, this process generates signal subbands denoted as $x_m(n)$, extending up to the third level of decomposition ($S = 3$). We choose level three of decomposition based on the reasonable number of data points (32 points per second) available for analysis during the DWT decimation process up to level three. Level four, with only 16 points per second, is insufficient for thorough ECG analysis. Additionally, this level of decomposition is commonly used in state-of-the-art works (Pal and Mitra 2010; Mohamed Suhail and Abdul Razak 2022). In Figure 7.3, we show ten seconds of the signal along with its corresponding decomposition levels. Notably, the DWT level one and two signal details ($x_3(n)$and $x_2(n)$, respectively) display a higher concentration of power at QRS (Q, R and S waves) complexes.

In Figure 7.4, we present two seconds of the raw signal from each class used in this study. Notably, there is a clear reduction in cardiac activity in the *severe* class.

To maintain consistency with the original sampling rate, the subband signals $x_m(n)$ underwent resampling using the wavelet interpolation method (Rioul and Vetterli 1991). Following this, for each windowing signal cropping analysis, ten non-linear features (refer to Table 7.2 for more information) were extracted from each signal subband. Subsequently, the resulting time series for each feature, windowing signal analysis, and subband were compressed over time using six distinct statistical functions: average (*Avg*), standard deviation (*Std*), 95th percentile (*P95*), variance (*Var*), median (*Med*), and Kurtosis (*Kur*) (Ribeiro, Marques, et al. 2024). In the final step, the data matrix per body position, consisting of all one-second time-series vectors of features extracted from all subbands over time for all patients, underwent normalization using the z-score method (Peck, Olsen, and Devore 2008).

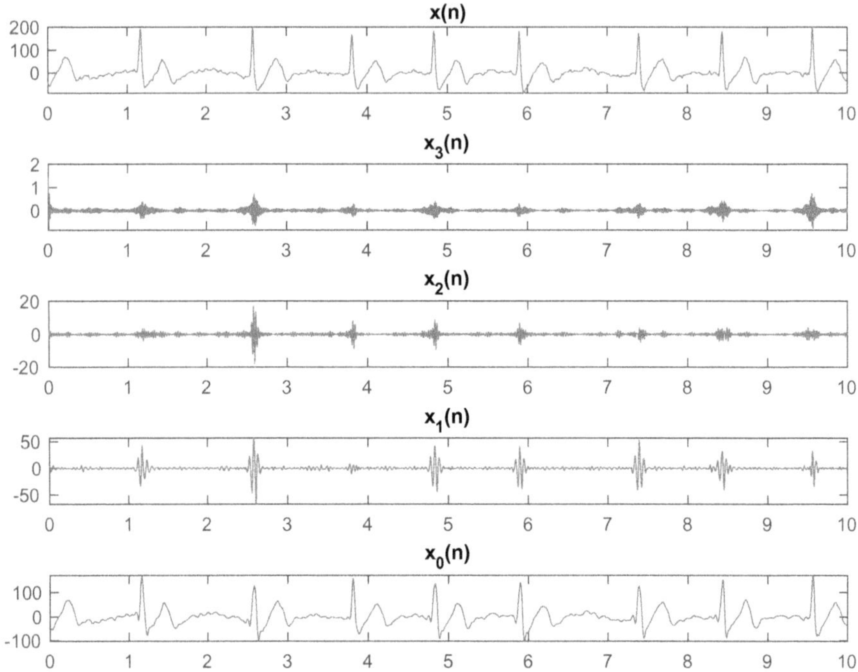

FIGURE 7.3 Ten Seconds of Raw Signal with the Decomposition Levels.

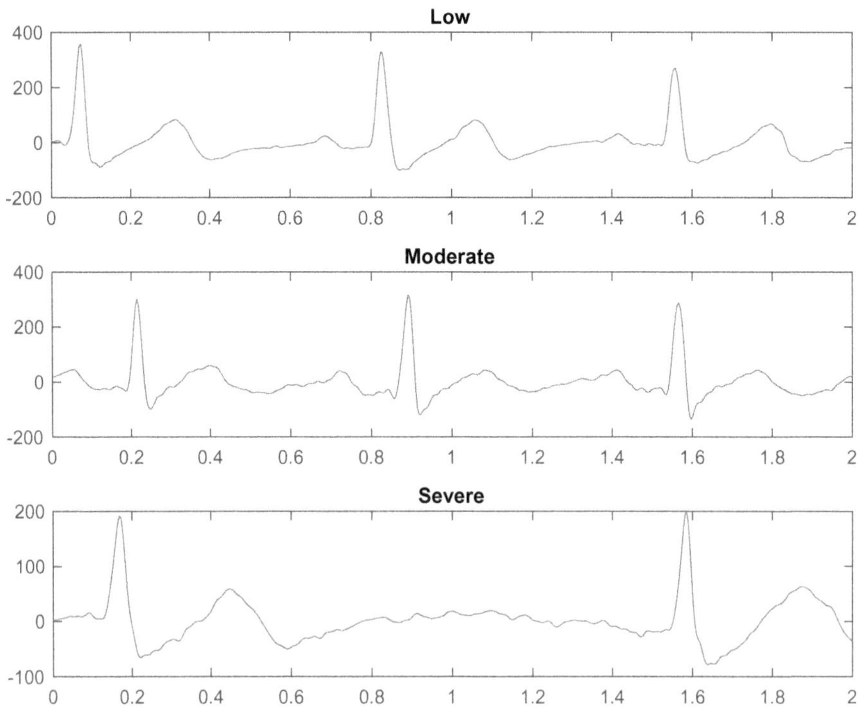

FIGURE 7.4 Two Seconds of Raw Signal for Each Severity Class.

TABLE 7.2
Extracted Features with Corresponding Equations and Definitions

Feature	Definition	Equation
Approximate Entropy (*AE*)	*AE* assesses the likelihood that similar patterns within the data remain consistent when additional data points are included. A lower *AE* suggests more regular or predictable data, while a higher *AE* indicates greater complexity or irregularity.	$AE(m,r) = \lim_{N\to\infty} \Theta^m(r) - \Theta^{m+1}(r)$, Θ is the Heaviside step function, and m is the dimension (Caesarendra et al. 2013).
Correlation Dimension (*CD*)	*CD* measures self-similarity, with higher values indicating greater complexity and less similarity.	$CD = \lim_{M\to\infty} \frac{2\sum_{i=1}^{M-k}\sum_{j=i+k}^{M}\Theta\left(l\lvert X_i - X_j\rvert\right)}{M^2}$, where $\Theta(x)$ is the Heaviside step function, X_i and X_j are position vectors on the attractor, l is the distance under consideration, k is the summation offset, and M is the number of reconstructed vectors from $x(n)$ (Caesarendra et al. 2013).
Detrended Fluctuation Analysis (*DFA*)	*DFA* measures power scaling observed through R/S analysis.	$DFA(n) = \sqrt{\frac{\sum_{k=1}^{N}\left[y(k) - y_n(k)\right]^2}{N}}$, where N is the length, $y_n(k)$ is the local trend, and $y(k)$ is defined as $y(k) = \sum_{i=1}^{k}\left[x(i) - \overline{x}\right]$, with $x(i)$ as the inter-beat interval and $\overline{x}$ as its average (Hardstone et al. 2012).
Energy (*En*)	*En* represents the system's capacity to perform work (Sundararajan 2015).	$En = \sum_{n=0}^{N-1} \lvert x(n) \rvert^2$
Higuchi Fractal Dimension (*H*)	*H* estimates the fractal dimension of a time series (M. Silva et al. 2023).	$H = \frac{ln(L(k))}{ln\left(\frac{1}{k}\right)}$, where k is the number of composed subseries, and $L(k)$ is the averaged curve size.
Hurst Exponent (*EH*)	*EH* quantifies the chaos or unpredictability of a time series.	$K_q(\tau) \sim \left(\frac{\tau}{\nu}\right)^{qEH(q)}$, with $K_q(\tau) = \frac{\left(\lvert X(t+\tau) - X(t)\rvert^q\right)}{\left(\lvert X(t)\rvert^q\right)}$, where q is the order moments of the distribution increments, ν is the time resolution, τ is the incorporation time delay of the attractor, and t is the period of a given time series signal $X(t)$ (Garcia et al. 2022).

TABLE 7.2 (Continued)
Extracted Features with Corresponding Equations and Definitions

Feature	Definition	Equation
Katz Fractal Dimension (K)	K estimates fractal dimensions using waveform analysis of a time series (Garcia et al. 2022).	$K = \frac{log(n)}{log(n)+log\left(\frac{max_n\left(\sqrt{(n-1)^2+(x(n)-x(1))^2}\right)}{\sum_{n=2}^{N}\sqrt{1+(x(n-1)-x(n))^2}}\right)}$,
Logarithmic Entropy or Boltzmann–Gibbs entropy (LE)	LE quantifies the average amount of information (in bits) needed to represent each event in the probability distribution. Higher logarithmic entropy values indicate greater unpredictability or randomness, while lower values suggest more certainty or order (Sundararajan 2015).	$LE = \sum_{n=1}^{N} log_2\left[\,\lvert x(n)\rvert^2\right]$
Lyapunov Exponent (ELy)	ELy evaluates the system's predictability and sensitivity to change.	$ELy\left(x_0\right) = \lim_{n\to\infty} \frac{\sum_{k=1}^{n} ln\lvert f'\left(x_k-1\right)\rvert}{n}$, where f' is the derivative of f (Silva, Batista, and Rodrigues 2025).
Shannon Entropy (SE)	SE is measured in bits when the base-two logarithm (log2) is used, quantifying the average number of bits required to represent each outcome in a probability distribution. Higher entropy values indicate greater uncertainty, unpredictability, or randomness, while lower values suggest more order or certainty (Sundararajan 2015).	$SE = -\sum_{n=1}^{N}\lvert x(n)\rvert^2 log_2\left[\,\lvert x(n)\rvert^2\right]$

7.2.1.5 Data Driven Framework Analysis

7.2.1.5.1 Combined Features Power Analysis to Discriminate between groups – Per each Wavelet Analysis

We evaluated the model's performance in discriminating between pairs of study groups and in the *All* vs. *All* scenario, using a comprehensive ML approach. The evaluation employed 19 selected scikit-learn ML models (presented in Table 7.3) (Pedregosa et al. 2011) within an 80/20 hold-out validation procedure (Barbosa et al. 2025).

TABLE 7.3
Nineteen Sci-Learn Machine Learning Classifiers Configurations

Classifier	Hyperparameters
AdaBoostClassifier (AdaBoost)	Default parameters
BaggingClassifier (BaggC)	Default parameters
DecisionTreeClassifier (DeTreeC)	max_depth: 5
ExtraTreesClassifier (ExTreeC)	n_estimators: 300
GaussianNB (GauNB)	Default parameters
GaussianProcessClassifier (GauPro)	1.0 x RBF(1.0)
GradientBoostingClassifier (GradBoost)	Default parameters
KNearestNeighborsClassifier (KNN)	Default parameters
LinearDiscriminantAnalysis (LinDis)	Default parameters
LinearSVC (LinSVC)	Default parameters
LogisticRegression (LogReg)	solver: "lbfgs"
LogisticRegressionCV (LogRegCV)	cv: 3
MLPClassifier (MLP)	α: 1, max_iter: 1000
OneVsRestClassifier (OvsR)	random_state: 0
RandomForestClassifier (RF)	c max_depth: 5, n_estimators: 300, max_features: 1
SGDClassifier (SGD)	max_iter: 100, tol: 0.001
SGDClassifierMod (SGDCMod)	Default parameters
Support Vector Machine (SVC)	γ: "auto"

TABLE 7.4
Six Over-Sampling Methods Configurations

Method	Parameters
RandomOverSampler	default parameters
SMOTE	k_neighbors: 4
SVMSMOTE	k_neighbors: 4
SMOTEN	k_neighbors: 4
ADASYN	default parameters
BorderlineSMOTE	k_neighbors: 4

We used a combined feature set of 480 features per participant to feed and test the ML models. These features were derived by extracting ten features from each of the four subbands, compressing them using six statistical measures, and collecting data from two different body positions. This comprehensive feature set was used for each group comparison analysis.

To mitigate class imbalance, six oversampling techniques were applied to balance class distributions in the training sets (Table 7.4 for more details): RandomOverSampler, Synthetic Minority Over-sampling TEchnique (SMOTE), Support Vector Machine

SMOTE (SVMSMOTE), SMOTE for Nominal features (SMOTEN), Adaptive Synthetic Sampling (ADASYN), and Borderline SMOTE (BorderlineSMOTE). The entire process was repeated using each of the 60 wavelets previously selected for the DWT signal analysis. This methodological variation for performing combined-feature discrimination assessment is illustrated in Figure 7.1.

7.2.1.5.2 Classification evaluation metrics

The models' performance has been evaluated within the testing stage:

- Accuracy (*Acc*): Proportion of correctly labeled cases out of all cases.

$$Acc = \frac{TP + TN}{TP + TN + FP + FN} \times 100\% \quad (7)$$

where *TP* (True Positives), *TN* (True Negatives), *FP* (False Positives), *FN* (False Negatives) (Ribeiro et al. 2025).

- Precision (*Prec*): Proportion of true positives among all positive predictions.

$$Prec = \frac{TP}{TP + FP} \times 100\% \quad (8)$$

- Recall (*Rec*): Proportion of true positives among all actual positives.

$$Rec = \frac{TP}{TP + FN} \times 100\% \quad (9)$$

- Specificity (*Spec*): Proportion of true negatives among all actual negatives.

$$Spec = \frac{TN}{TN + FP} \times 100\% \quad (10)$$

- $F1-Score$: Harmonic mean of *Prec* and *Rec*.

$$F1-Score = 2 \times \frac{Prec \times Rec}{Prec + Rec} \times 100\% \quad (11)$$

- The negative predictive value(*NPV*) shows the proportion of true negatives out of all cases predicted as negative (Safari et al. 2018). Formally, the *NPV* can be defined as,

$$NPV = \frac{TN}{TN + FN} \times 100\%, \quad (12)$$

The area under the curve (AUC) of the receiver operating characteristic (ROC) is a measure of how well a model distinguishes between positive and negative classes.

A perfect classifier gets an AUC of one, a random one gets 0.5, and a poor one gets less than 0.5. AUC helps compare models, especially when dealing with unbalanced classes.

7.2.2 Cloud-Coupled Architecture (Runtime Overview)

This section details the end-to-end execution path of the proposed system, from wearable ECG acquisition to cloud-hosted signal processing, model inference, and return of results to the wrist application. The architecture is designed to (i) minimize on-device computation, (ii) enforce a stable, versioned data contract between preprocessing and classification, and (iii) meet security, reliability, and scalability requirements expected for clinical research settings.

7.2.2.1 Acquisition and Secure Upload (WatchOS/Wear OS)

A single-lead ECG is acquired on the smartwatch in WFDB format, together with metadata (sampling rate, acquisition duration, device OS/firmware, and optional recording-quality indicators). The wrist app performs a secure upload over transport layer security (TLS) to the API gateway using background transfer (e.g., URLSession on watchOS, WorkManager on Wear OS), with certificate pinning, integrity checks (e.g., SHA-256 checksum), and idempotent request semantics keyed by a session_id. Personally identifiable information is avoided; a pseudonymized patient_id is used to support privacy-preserving analytics. The gateway validates the payload (format, size, metadata), persists the raw file in object storage, and enqueues the processing request.

Outcome: the upload endpoint acknowledges receipt with a unique session_id, which the client uses to poll for results or receive push notifications.

7.2.2.2 Cloud Signal Processing Service

A dedicated, containerized microservice retrieves the WFDB recording from storage and executes the signal-processing pipeline described between sections 7.2.1.2 and 7.2.1.4.

7.2.2.3 Model Serving and Inference

A separate model-serving API loads the pre-trained severity classifier and exposes inference via REST/gRPC. The API validates feature-vector compatibility with the current model version, performs prediction (severity class: *low, moderate,* or *severe*)

7.2.2.4 Result Delivery to the Wearable

Results are delivered to the wrist app through secure APIs. The client may poll by session_id or receive push notifications when processing completes. The on-device user interface (UI) renders the severity label and, when appropriate, displays signal-quality feedback or guidance for re-acquisition. Results and event traces are stored server-side to support reproducibility, clinical review, and performance monitoring.

7.2.2.5 Security, Compliance, and Operations

The system enforces end-to-end encryption (TLS in transit) and encryption at rest (e.g., advanced encryption standard-246 (AES-256) for databases and object storage). Authentication and authorization use Open Authorization 2.0/JSON Web Token (OAuth2/JWT) with scoped access and least-privilege policies. Audit logging captures access and processing events; data retention and erasure policies adhere to applicable privacy regulations (e.g., General Data Protection Regulation or GDPR). Production operations include observability (metrics, logs, traces), alerting on latency and error rates, data/model-drift monitoring, and resilience mechanisms (exponential retries, circuit breakers, asynchronous queues with dead-letter handling)(Rodrigues, Freitas, and Gabriel 2014).

7.3 RESULTS

7.3.1 Machine Learning training pipeline results

Tables 7.5, 7.6, 7.7, and 7.8 showcase the optimal outcomes obtained through feature selection across binary groups and *the All vs. All setting*.

Table 7.5 shows the best results for the *low* vs. *moderate* group when the wavelet-mother *coif1* and the window type *RO* were used.

Table 7.6 shows the best results for the *low* vs. *severe* group when wavelet-mother *sym7* and window type *RO* were used.

Table 7.7 shows the best results for the *moderate* vs. *severe* group when the wavelet-mother *db6* and the window type *Hm* were used.

Table 7.8 shows the best results for the *All* vs. *All* group when the wavelet-mother *rbio2.8* and the window type *Hm* were used.

Figure 7.5 shows the ROC curves for the best overall results.

The discrimination index reporting results regarding AUC, $F1-score$, and *Acc* achieved in the current study are compared to our previous results in the study (Ribeiro, Marques, et al. 2024) at Figure 7.6, for the combined feature power analysis.

7.3.2 Cloud-Coupled Architecture

Figure 7.7 shows the WatchOS application created in this study.

7.4 DISCUSSION

7.4.1 Machine Learning Training Pipeline Algorithm Discussion

Looking into Tables 7.5, 7.6, and 7.7, we can see that every over-sampling technique allowed to obtain the maximum possible performance, with the *Acc*, *Rec*, *Prec*, $F1-score$ Spec and NPV reached 100%, and the AUC was one.

In Table 7.8, which presents the *All* vs. *All* comparison results, three data synthesizers (RandomOverSampler, SVMSMOTE, and BorderlineSMOTE) were allowed to achieve optimal performance with perfect scores (100%) across all evaluation metrics (*Acc*, *Rec*, *Prec*, $F1-score$, *Spec*, and NPV) and an ideal AUC value

TABLE 7.5
Classification Outcomes for the *Low* vs. *Moderate* – best *Acc, Rec, Prec, F1–Score, Spec,* AUC, and NPV Results for Each Over-Sampling Technique

Over-sampling Methods	# of Features	Algorithm	Acc (%)	Rec (%)	Prec (%)	Spec (%)	F1–Score (%)	NPV (%)	AUC
RandomOverSampler	1	SVC	100	100	100	100	100	100	1
SMOTE	1	SVC	100	100	100	100	100	100	1
SVMSMOTE	1	SVC	100	100	100	100	100	100	1
SMOTEN	1	SVC	100	100	100	100	100	100	1
ADASYN	—	—	—	—	—	—	—	—	—
BorderlineSMOTE	1	SVC	100	100	100	100	100	100	1

TABLE 7.6
Classification Outcomes for the *Low* vs. *Severe* – Best *Acc, Rec, Prec,* F1–Score , *Spec,* AUC, and NPV Results for Each Over-Sampling Technique

Over-sampling Methods	# of Features	Algorithm	Acc (%)	Rec (%)	Prec (%)	Spec (%)	F1–Score (%)	NPV (%)	AUC
RandomOverSampler	14	KNN	100	100	100	100	100	100	1
SMOTE	12	LinDis	100	100	100	100	100	100	1
SVMSMOTE	17	LinDis	100	100	100	100	100	100	1
SMOTEN	70	RF	100	100	100	100	100	100	1
ADASYN	14	SVC	100	100	100	100	100	100	1
BorderlineSMOTE	10	SVC	100	100	100	100	100	100	1

TABLE 7.7
Classification Outcomes for the *Moderate* vs. *Severe* – Best *Acc, Rec, Prec,* F1–Score, *Spec,* AUC, and NPV Results for Each Over-Sampling Technique

Over-sampling Methods	# of Features	Algorithm	Acc (%)	Rec (%)	Prec (%)	Spec (%)	F1–Score (%)	NPV (%)	AUC
RandomOverSampler	2	KNN	100	100	100	100	100	100	1
SMOTE	2	SGD	100	100	100	100	100	100	1
SVMSMOTE	2	SVC	100	100	100	100	100	100	1
SMOTEN	5	LogRegCV	100	100	100	100	100	100	1
ADASYN	—	—	—	—	—	—	—	—	—
BorderlineSMOTE	2	ExTreeC	100	100	100	100	100	100	1

TABLE 7.8
Classification outcomes for the *All* vs. *All* – Best *Acc, Rec, Prec,*F1–Score (%), *Spec,* AUC, and NPV Results for Each Over-Sampling Technique

Over-sampling Methods	# of Features	Algorithm	Acc (%)	Rec (%)	Prec (%)	Spec (%)	F1–Score (%)	NPV (%)	AUC
RandomOverSampler	8	SVC	100	100	100	100	100	100	1
SMOTE	6	SVC	88.89	88.89	94.44	98.61	91.58	83.33	0.9722
SVMSMOTE	2	LogReg	100	100	100	100	100	100	1
SMOTEN	17	RF	88.89	88.89	79.37	77.78	83.86	98.77	0.8333
ADASYN	—	—	—	—	—	—	—	—	—
BorderlineSMOTE	10	SVC	100	100	100	100	100	100	1

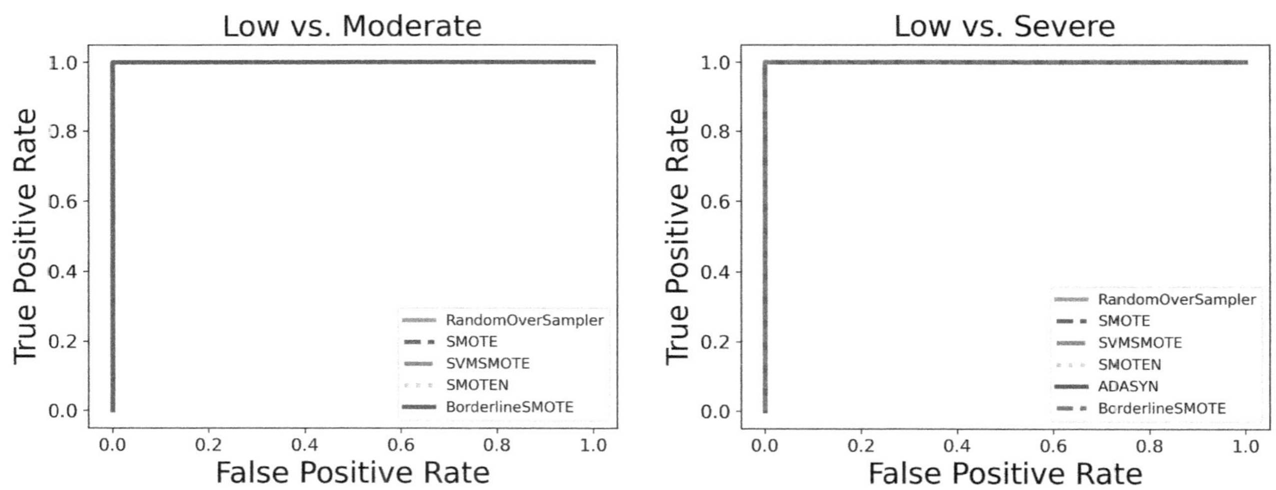

FIGURE 7.5 Best prediction results ROC Curves per study group comparison: (a) *Low* vs. *Moderate*, (b) *Low* vs. *Severe*, (c) *Moderate* vs. *Severe*, and (d) *All* vs. *All*.

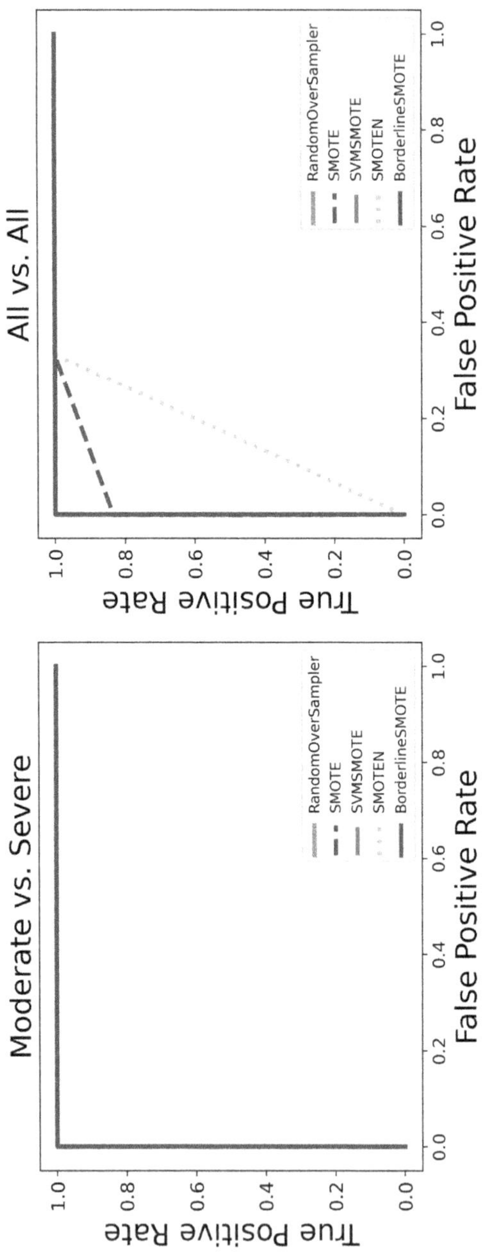

FIGURE 7.5 (Continued)

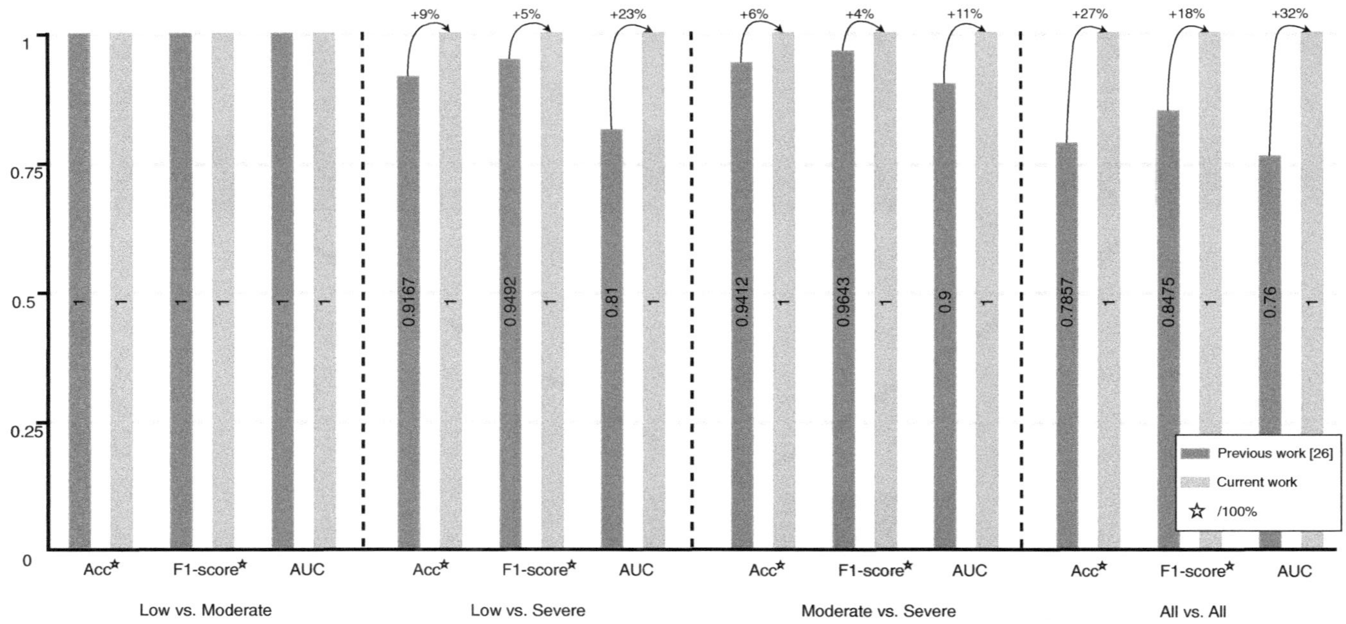

FIGURE 7.6 AUC, **F1 – Score**, *Acc* Comparison Results Between the Current Study and the Previous Study for Combined-Feature Power Analysis, Per Study Group: *Low* vs. *Moderate*, *Low* vs. *Severe*, *Moderate* vs. *Severe*, and *All* vs. *All*.

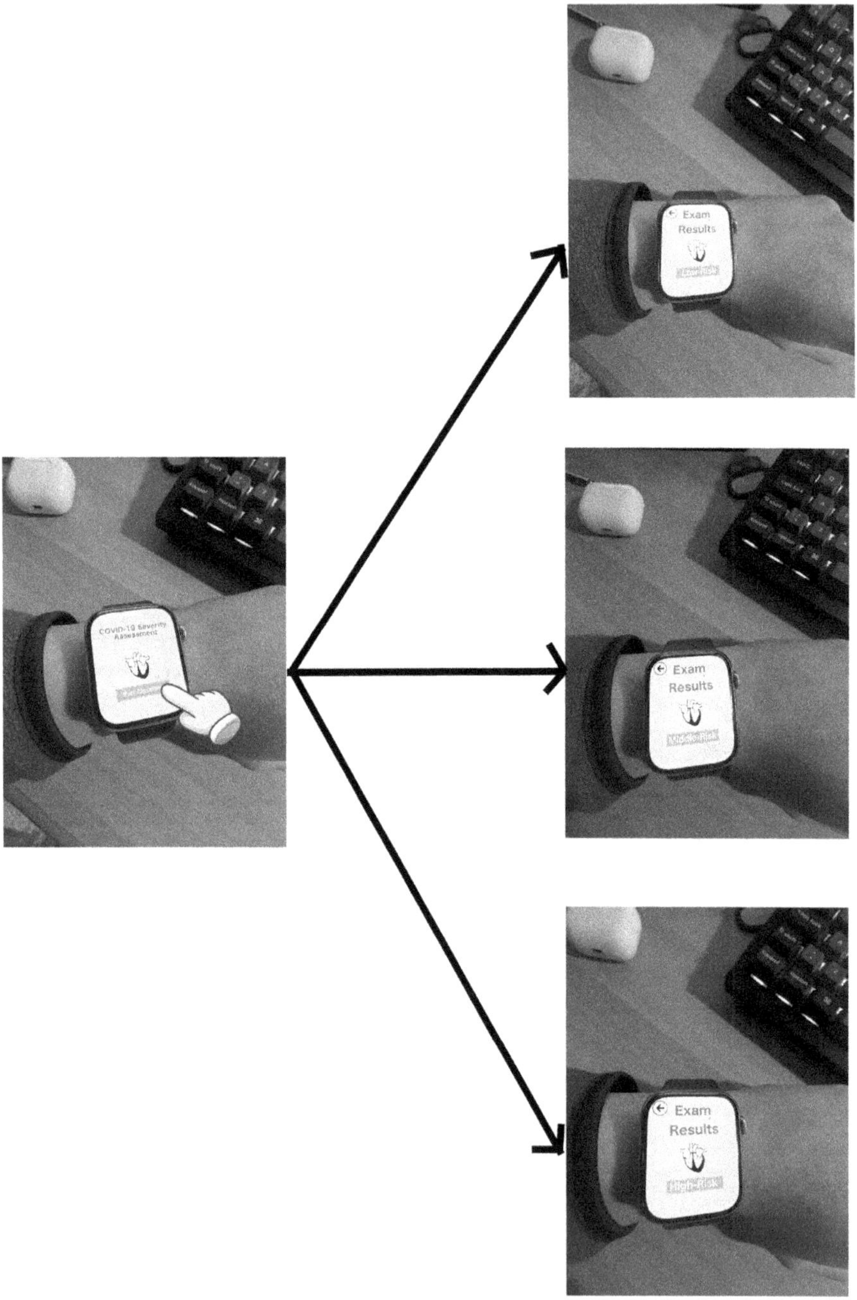

FIGURE 7.7 Apple Watch Application for COVID-19 Severity Assessment with the Possible Outcomes: (a) Application User Interface to Run the Algorithm, (b) Low-Risk Exam Results, (c) Middle-Risk Exam Results, and (d) High-Risk Exam Results.

of one. The SMOTE technique demonstrated the second-best performance, yielding 88.89% for both *Acc* and *Rec*, 94.44% for *Prec*, 91.58% for $F1-score$, 98.61% for *Spec*, and 83.33% for NPV, with an AUC of 0.9722. Finally, SMOTEN produced comparable results to SMOTE in terms of *Acc* and *Rec* (both at 88.89%) but exhibited reduced performance in other metrics: 79.37% *Prec*, 83.86% $F1-score$, 77.78% *Spec*, 98.77% NPV, and an AUC of 0.8333, positioning it as the least effective among the evaluated synthesizers.

Globally, among the six techniques employed for dataset balancing, only the ADASYN algorithm failed to produce results in 75% (three out of four) of the comparison groups because the database did not meet the imbalance threshold required by this technique. Regarding classifier performance, the Support Vector Machine (SVC) demonstrated superior effectiveness, appearing in 45% (11 out of 24) of the optimal results across all experimental configurations, making it the most robust classification algorithm in this comparative analysis.

7.4.1.1 Comparing Study Results with Previous Study Results for the Same Database

In our prior investigation (Ribeiro, Marques, et al. 2024), we implemented nonlinear feature extraction methodologies on broadband signals to analyze COVID-19 disease progression. The present research significantly expands upon this foundation by integrating sophisticated nonlinear feature extraction into a multiband analytical framework based on the DWT. Additionally, we enhance the robustness of our approach by augmenting the training set with advanced oversampling techniques, thereby mitigating the inherent limitations of limited sample sizes. Consequently, caution must be exercised when comparing our findings with earlier work, as this study employs a hold-out validation approach, whereas the previous study used cross-validation. These methodological refinements enhance our understanding of COVID-19 severity progression.

When directly comparing the two studies, the previous study already showed maximum performance results for *low* vs. *moderate*, as can be seen in Figure 7.6; however, the other group analyses were still far from reaching the maximum performance (0.81 of AUC for comparison *low* vs. *severe*, 0.9 of AUC for comparison *moderate* vs. *severe* and 0.76 of AUC for comparison *All* vs. *All*). With the integration of DWT and over-sampling techniques in this study, our results showed exponential improvement, achieving maximum performance (AUC = 1) across all three binary groups, improving by 23% compared to *low* vs. *severe* and 11% compared to *moderate* vs. *severe*. Regarding the *All* vs. *All* comparison, the current algorithm with DWT outperforms previous work by 32% in AUC, which is a notable improvement.

The *Acc* and *F1-score* also improved with the introduction of the DWT, while the *low* vs. *moderate* comparison already reached the maximum performance in the previous work. The *low* vs. *severe* group showed a performance boost of 9% and 5% for *Acc* and $F1-score$, respectively, when the DWT was used. The *Acc* improved 6% in the *moderate* vs. *severe*, with $F1-score$ improving 4% for the same Binary group. The *All* vs. *All* presented the most significant performance improvement when the DWT was used; the *Acc* improved 27%, and the $F1-score$ showed an 18% improvement.

Figure 7.5 shows that all oversampling techniques yielded optimal ROC curves for the binary classifications *low* vs. *moderate* and *moderate* vs. *severe*, except for ADASYN, which failed to produce a valid classification under the given conditions. Notably, all six methodologies yielded perfect ROC curves in the *low* vs. *severe* comparison scenario, indicating exceptional discriminative power for distinguishing between these distinct severity levels. In the more challenging multiclass classification context (*All* vs. *All*), illustrated in Figure 7.5.d, three methodologies (RandomOverSampler, SVMSMOTE, and BorderlineSMOTE) exhibited near-ideal performance characteristics, each attaining the maximum possible AUC value of one, thereby demonstrating their superior efficacy in this complex classification task.

Thus, our current analysis presents a finely tuned methodology compared with the previous study (Ribeiro, Marques, et al. 2024) by scrutinizing the diverse frequency scales inherent in the signal, particularly those intricately linked with heightened COVID-19 activity presented in ECG signals. Thus, a compelling inference emerges — crucial information about COVID-19 activity is embedded within the signal's entire broadband, and DWT is a good tool for helping to find the small and quick signal oscillations related to COVID-19 masked in the signal's broadband.

7.4.1.2 Comparing Study Results with State-of-the-Art Results – Other Databases

To benchmark our findings against the state of the art, we conducted a systematic literature review in Google Scholar from September to November 2025. We prioritized peer-reviewed articles from major publishers (e.g., Elsevier, Springer Nature, IEEE), guiding our search strategy with specific keywords: "COVID-19 severity classification", "COVID-19 severity DL", "COVID-19 disease severity", "COVID-19 severity scoring system", "prognostic models for COVID-19 severity", and "CT severity COVID-19 prediction". This process yielded 15 relevant studies (Yu et al. 2020; Yao et al. 2020; Booth, Abels, and McCaffrey 2020; Han et al. 2020; Meng et al. 2020; S. Sayed, Elkorany, and Mohammad 2021; Irmak 2021; Mahmud et al. 2021; Rahman et al. 2021; Cobre et al. 2021; Balaha, El-Gendy, and Saafan 2022; Taheriyan et al. 2022; Xiong et al. 2022; Sokhansanj and Rosen 2022; Ulukaya et al. 2023).

Among the 15 articles, 80% (12 out of 15 research papers) presented results in the form of Binary classifications, 46.67% (seven out of 15 research papers) used unbalanced datasets, and 40% (six out of 15 research papers) used small data samples. Our results align with the state-of-the-art findings in other databases. Among the selected literature, eight studies used classes that allow direct comparisons with our study. Specifically, in studies (Yu et al. 2020; Yao et al. 2020; Xiong et al. 2022; Mahmud et al. 2021; Cobre et al. 2021; Sokhansanj and Rosen 2022), where our binary groups *low* vs. *severe* and *moderate* vs. *severe* can be directly compared, our research demonstrated improvements in *Acc* ranging from 4.66% to 22.5%. Notably, the studies in (Sayed, Elkorany, and Mohammad 2021; Irmak 2021)—directly comparable to our *All* vs. *All* group—achieved identical *Acc* or exhibited an improvement of 4.5%. While direct comparisons require caution due to dataset heterogeneity, these metrics highlight the robustness of our proposed method.

Furthermore, our research appears to be unique in leveraging ECG signals to assess COVID-19 severity. Unlike the modalities used in previous studies, ECG is noninvasive, cost-effective, and ubiquitous in clinical settings. This accessibility makes our algorithm particularly suitable for bedridden patients and supports widespread adoption across diverse healthcare environments.

7.4.2 Cloud-coupled Architecture Discussion

The convergence of wearable devices, smartphones, and cloud computing has enabled a continuous-monitoring ecosystem capable of acquiring ECG data, processing it remotely, and predicting COVID-19 severity. Moreover, by offloading computation to the cloud, the system can be easily expanded to incorporate additional conditions or more sophisticated feature-extraction techniques. Nevertheless, several challenges remain, particularly the limited battery life of wearable devices and the dependence on stable, high-speed internet connectivity. Figure 7.8 shows the front-end diagram of the ecosystem created in this study.

7.5 CONCLUSION

This work presented a comprehensive wearable-to-cloud system designed for the early assessment of COVID-19 severity in critically ill patients. By adapting single-lead ECG recordings from consumer smartwatches (Apple watchOS and Android Wear OS), we established a seamless pipeline in which the wearable device handles secure signal acquisition and result display, while computationally intensive processing is offloaded to a cloud server.

The cloud-hosted algorithmic core employs a DWT to decompose raw ECG signals, extracting ten nonlinear dynamical features per frequency band. These features are compressed and analyzed by supervised ML classifiers. This specific configuration yielded exceptional performance: the system achieved 100% *Acc* and an AUC of 1.0 across all severity comparisons (*low*, *moderate*, and *severe*). Notably, the introduction of DWT enhanced signal detail, allowing our approach to outperform existing methods on the same dataset by significant margins—specifically, improving accuracy by 9% in *low* vs. *severe* cases and by 27% in the comprehensive *All* vs. *All* comparison.

These results validate the system as a powerful, noninvasive tool for resource-limited settings. By enabling electrode-free recording at the bedside, this solution empowers medical professionals to rapidly stratify patients and determine whether the severity of the disease allows the patient to remain in the current setting or requires transfer to a facility with more extensive care options (Popescu et al. 2023).

However, specific limitations regarding the underlying algorithm and data characteristics remain. Firstly, the use of nontraditional, nonlinear features poses challenges regarding clinical interpretability, as these metrics are not standard in routine cardiological assessment. Secondly, the reliance on oversampling techniques to balance the currently small dataset warrants caution regarding the model's generalizability to broader, unseen populations. Furthermore, while ECG analysis is

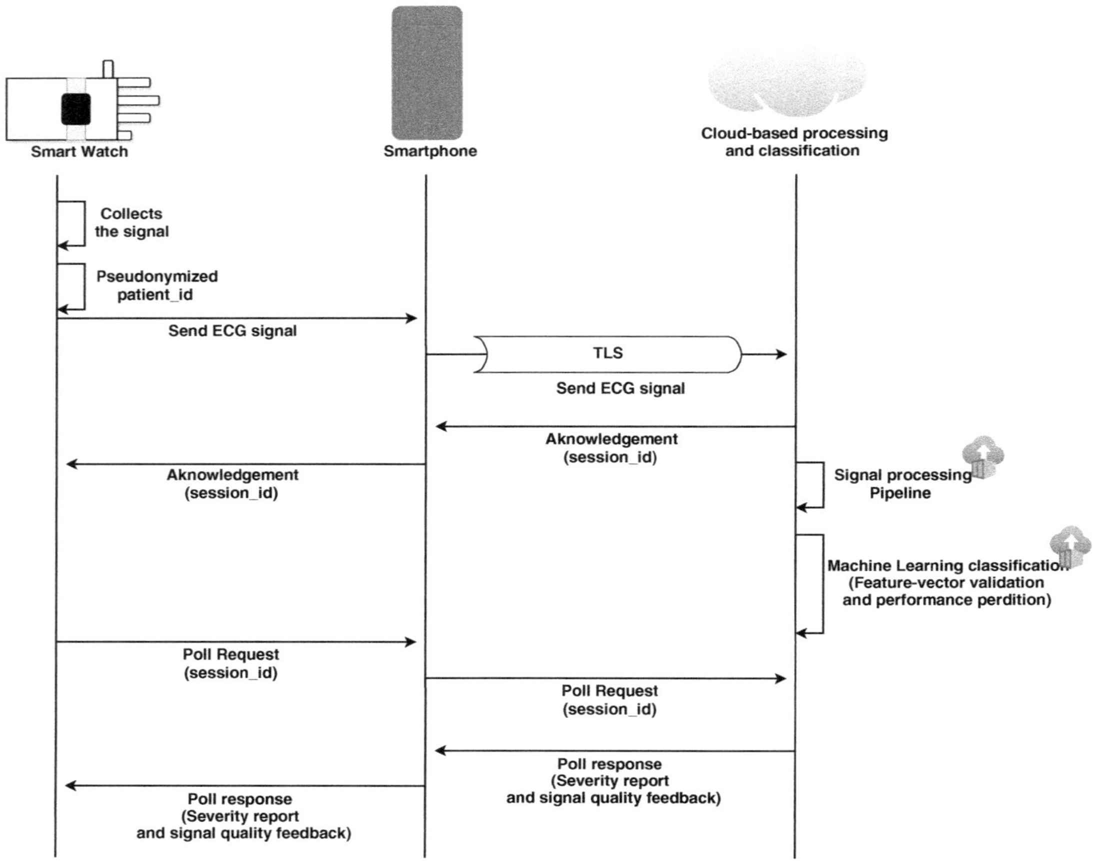

FIGURE 7.8 Front-End Diagram.

cost-effective, it inherently lacks the specificity of imaging modalities such as chest computed tomography; COVID-19-induced cardiac alterations used by our algorithm may mimic other cardiovascular disorders, potentially leading to confounding results (Ribeiro, Marques, and Rodrigues 2023; Santos et al. 2020).

Future work must prioritize validating this pipeline on larger, more diverse populations to ensure algorithmic robustness. The cloud-based architecture developed here offers significant potential for adaptation to classify other pulmonary disorders, such as chronic obstructive pulmonary disease (COPD), asthma, pneumonia, and pulmonary embolism. Finally, looking toward the next generation of the algorithm, integrating DL classifiers (Ismail Fawaz et al. 2020) and multi-agent explainable AI systems into this Internet of Things (IoT) framework represents a critical step. These advancements could reveal subtle disease-specific signatures that elude conventional analyses, thereby enhancing real-time monitoring and clinical confidence in automated diagnosis.

ACKNOWLEDGMENT

This work was supported by National Funds from FCT – Fundação para a Ciência e a Tecnologia through project UID/50016/2025 and by the National Council for Scientific and Technological Development (CNPq) via grant n°305517/2022-8.

João Paulo Madeiro thanks for the financial support of the Conselho Nacional de Desenvolvimento Científico e Tecnológico (CNPq), grants n. 420576/2023-1, 404683/2024-0, 200528/2025-4.

REFERENCES

Balaha, Hossam Magdy, Eman M El-Gendy, and Mahmoud M Saafan. 2022. "A Complete Framework for Accurate Recognition and Prognosis of COVID-19 Patients Based on Deep Transfer Learning and Feature Classification Approach." *Artificial Intelligence Review* 55 (6): 5063–5108. https://doi.org/10.1007/s10462-021-10127-8.

Barbosa, Maria Inês, Gabriel Silva, Pedro Ribeiro, Eduarda Vieira, André Perrotta, Patrícia Moreira, and Pedro Miguel Rodrigues. 2025. "Unraveling the Microbiome–Environmental Change Nexus to Contribute to a More Sustainable World: A Comprehensive Review of Artificial Intelligence Approaches." *Sustainability* 17 (16): 7209. https://doi.org/10.3390/su17167209.

Booth, Adam, Elizabeth Abels, and Peter McCaffrey. 2020. "Development of a Prognostic Model for Mortality in COVID-19 Infection Using Machine Learning." *Modern Pathology* 34 (3): 522–531.

Caesarendra, Wahyu, Buyung Kosasih, Kiet Tieu, and Craig A S Moodie. 2013. "An Application of Nonlinear Feature Extraction – A Case Study for Low Speed Slewing Bearing Condition Monitoring and Prognosis." In 2013 IEEE/ASME International Conference on Advanced Intelligent Mechatronics *(Wollongong), July 2013*, 1613–1618. IEEE. https://doi.org/10.1109/aim.2013.6584344.

Caldas, W. L., J. P. do Vale Madeiro, R. C. Pedrosa, J. P. P. Gomes, W. Du, and J. A. L. Marques. 2023. "Noise Detection and Classification in Chagasic ECG Signals Based on One-Dimensional Convolutional Neural Networks." In R. Lee (Ed.), *Computer and Information Science* (pp. 117–129). Switzerland: Springer International Publishing.

Cavalcante, C. H. L., P. E. O. Primo, C. A. F. Sales, W. L. Caldas, J. H. M. Silva, A. H. Souza, E. S. Marinho, R. C. Pedrosa, … and J. P. V. Madeiro. 2023. "Sudden Cardiac Death Multiparametric Classification System for Chagas Heart Disease's Patients based on Clinical Data and 24-Hours ECG Monitoring." *Mathematical Biosciences and Engineering* 20 (5): 9159–9178. https://doi.org/10.3934/mbe.2023402.

Cheong, S. H. R., Y. J. X. Ng, Y. Lau, and S.T. Lau. 2022. "Wearable technology for early detection of COVID-19: A systematic scoping review." Preventive Medicine 162, 107170.

Ciotti, Marco, Massimo Ciccozzi, Alessandro Terrinoni, Wen-Can Jiang, Cheng-Bin Wang, and Sergio Bernardini. 2020. "The COVID-19 Pandemic." *Critical Reviews in Clinical Laboratory Sciences* 57 (6): 365–388.

Cobre, Alexandre de Fátima, Dile Pontarolo Stremel, Guilhermina Rodrigues Noleto, Mariana Millan Fachi, Monica Surek, Astrid Wiens, Fernanda Stumpf Tonin, and Roberto Pontarolo. 2021. "Diagnosis and Prediction of COVID-19 Severity: Can Biochemical Tests and Machine Learning Be Used as Prognostic Indicators?" *Computers in Biology and Medicine* 134: 104531. https://doi.org/10.1016/j.compbiomed.2021.104531.

Cui, Jianfeng, Lixin Wang, Xiangmin He, Victor Hugo C De Albuquerque, Salman A AlQahtani, and Mohammad Mehedi Hassan. 2021. "Deep Learning-Based Multidimensional Feature Fusion for Classification of ECG Arrhythmia." *Neural Computing and Applications* 35 (22): 16073–16087. https://doi.org/10.1007/s00521-021-06487-5.

Daamouche, A., L. Hamami, N. Alajlan, and F. Melgani. 2012. "A Wavelet Optimization Approach for ECG Signal Classification." Biomedical Signal Processing and Control 7 (4): 342–349. https://doi.org/https://doi.org/10.1016/j.bspc.2011.07.001.

do Vale Madeiro, J. P., D. Barreto, J. A. L. Marques, and J. L. S. Júnior. 2019. "September. Evaluating Mathematical Models for Morphological Classification of the QRS Complex." In 2019 Computing in Cardiology (CinC) (pp. 1). IEEE. https://doi.org/10.23919/CinC49843.2019.9005790.

Duca, Ștefania, Adriana Chetran, Radu Miftode, Ovidiu Mitu, Alexandru Costache, Ana Nicolae, Dan Iliescu-Halițchi, Codruța-Olimpiada Halițchi-Iliescu, Florin Mitu, and Irina Costache. 2022. "Myocardial Ischemia in Patients with COVID-19 Infection: Between Pathophysiological Mechanisms and Electrocardiographic Findings." *Life* 12 (7): 1015.

Farshidfar, Farnaz, Navid Koleini, and Hossein Ardehali. 2021. "Cardiovascular Complications of COVID-19." *JCI Insight* 6 (13): 1504.

Ismail Fawaz, H., B. Lucas, G. Forestier, C. Pelletier, D. F. Schmidt, J. Weber, G. I. Webb, L. Idoumghar, P. A. Muller, and F. Petitjean. 2020. "Inceptiontime: Finding Alexnet for Time Series Classification." Data *M*ining and *K*nowledge *D*iscovery 34 (6): 1936–1962. https://doi.org/10.48550/ARXIV.1909.04939.

Fernandes, J. V. M. R., Alexandria, A. R. D., Marques, J. A. L., Assis, D. F. D., Motta, P. C., and Silva, B. R. D. S. 2024. "Emotion Detection from EEG Signals Using Machine Deep Learning Models." *Bioengineering* 11 (8): 782.

Garcia, Alejandro Antonio Torres, Carlos Alberto Reyes Garcia, Luis Villasenor-Pineda, and Omar Mendoza Montoya. 2022. *Biosignal Processing and Classification Using Computational Learning and Intelligence Principles, Algorithms, and Applications.* London: Academic Press.

Guido, Rodrigo. 2022. "Wavelets behind the Scenes: Practical Aspects, Insights, and Perspectives." *Physics Reports* 985 (November): 1–23. https://doi.org/10.1016/j.physrep.2022.08.001.

Santos, A. G., J. A. Marques, L. O. Rigo, and J. P. Madeir. 2023. "October. Exploring EEG Signal Features for Predicting Post Cardiac Arrest Prognosis." In 2023 Computing in Cardiology (CinC) (Vol. 50, pp. 1–4). IEEE. https://doi.org/10.22489/CinC.2023.312.

Han, R., Z. Liu, C. L. Philip Chen, L. Xu, and G. Peng. 2020, November. "Mortality Prediction for COVID-19 Patients via Broad Learning System." In 2020 7th International Conference on Information, Cybernetics, and Computational Social Systems (ICCSS) (pp. 837–842). IEEE. https://doi.org/10.1109/iccss52145.2020.9336835.

Hardstone, Richard, Simon-Shlomo Poil, Giuseppina Schiavone, Rick Jansen, Vadim V Nikulin, Huibert D Mansvelder, and Klaus Linkenkaer-Hansen. 2012. "Detrended Fluctuation Analysis: A Scale-Free View on Neuronal Oscillations." *Frontiers in Physiology* 3: 23105. https://doi.org/10.3389/fphys.2012.00450.

Hosseini, Elahe, Narjes Kashani, Hossein Nikzad, Javid Azadbakht, Hassan Bafrani, and Hamed Kashani. 2020. "The Novel Coronavirus Disease-2019 (COVID-19): Mechanism of Action, Detection and Recent Therapeutic Strategies." *Virology* 551 (December): 1–9.

Irmak, Emrah. 2021. "COVID-19 Disease Severity Assessment Using CNN Model." *IET Image Processing* 15 (8): 1814–1824. https://doi.org/10.1049/ipr2.12153.

Jiang, Joe-Air, Chih-Feng Chao, Ming-Jang Chiu, Ren-Guey Lee, Chwan-Lu Tseng, and Robert Lin. 2007. "An Automatic Analysis Method for Detecting and Eliminating ECG Artifacts in EEG." *Computers in Biology and Medicine* 37 (11): 1660–1671. https://doi.org/10.1016/j.compbiomed.2007.03.007.

Kalidas, Vignesh, and Lakshman Tamil. 2017. "Real-Time QRS Detector Using Stationary Wavelet Transform for Automated ECG Analysis." In 2017 IEEE 17th International Conference on Bioinformatics and Bioengineering (BIBE), October 2017, 457–461. IEEE. https://doi.org/10.1109/bibe.2017.00-12.

Klén, R., D. Purohit, R. Gómez-Huelgas, J. M. Casas-Rojo, J. M. Antón-Santos, J. M. Núñez-Cortés, C. Lumbreras, J.M. Ramos-Rincón, N. García Barrio, M. Pedrera-Jiménez, and A. Lalueza Blanco. 2022. "Development and Evaluation of a Machine Learning-Based in-Hospital COVID-19 Disease Outcome Predictor (CODOP): A Multicontinental Retrospective Study. Elife, 11: e75985. https://doi.org/10.7554/elife.75985.

Kotnis, Ashwin, Rishabh Mittal, Nidhi Chourasia, VivekK Bharti, Snigdha Singh, Poulami Sarkar, Amit Agrawal, Amrita Ghosh, Ranabir Pal, and JagatR Kanwar. 2022. "Blood-Based Biomarkers for Diagnosis, Prognosis, and Severity Prediction of COVID-19: Opportunities and Challenges." *Journal of Family Medicine and Primary Care* 11 (8): 4330. https://doi.org/10.4103/jfmpc.jfmpc_2283_21.

Kovačević, Martin Vetterli A N D Jelena. 1995. *Wavelets and Subband Coding*. Englewood Cliffs, New Jersey: Prentice Hall.

Kumar, Amit, and Mandeep Singh. 2015. "Optimal Selection of Wavelet Function and Decomposition Level for Removal of ECG Signal Artifacts." *Journal of Medical Imaging and Health Informatics* 5 (1): 138–146. https://doi.org/10.1166/jmihi.2015.1369.

Lai, Christopher, and Wilson Lam. 2021. "Laboratory Testing for the Diagnosis of COVID-19." *Biochemical and Biophysical Research Communications* 538 (January): 226–230.

Li, Cuiwei, Chongxun Zheng, and Changfeng Tai. 1995. "Detection of ECG Characteristic Points Using Wavelet Transforms." *IEEE Transactions on Biomedical Engineering* 42 (1): 21–28. https://doi.org/10.1109/10.362922.

Long, Brit, William Brady, Rachel Bridwell, Mark Ramzy, Tim Montrief, Manpreet Singh, and Michael Gottlieb. 2021. "Electrocardiographic Manifestations of COVID-19." *The American Journal of Emergency Medicine* 41 (March): 96–103.

Mahmud, Tanvir, Md. Jahin Alam, Sakib Chowdhury, Shams Nafisa Ali, Md. Maisoon Rahman, Shaikh Anowarul Fattah, and Mohammad Saquib. 2021. "CovTANet: A Hybrid Tri-Level Attention-Based Network for Lesion Segmentation, Diagnosis, and Severity Prediction of COVID-19 Chest CT Scans." *IEEE Transactions on Industrial Informatics* 17 (9): 6489–6498. https://doi.org/10.1109/tii.2020.3048391.

Malvar, Henrique. 1992. *Signal Processing with Lapped Transforms*. Norwood, Massachusetts: Artech House.

Marques, J. A. L., and S. Fong. (Eds.). 2022. *Epidemic Analytics for Decision Supports in COVID19 Crisis*. Switzerland: Springer.

Marques, J. A. L., and S. J. Fong. (Eds.). 2023. *Computerized Systems for Diagnosis and Treatment of COVID-19*. Switzerland: Springer.https://doi.org/10.1007/978-3-031-30788-1

Marques, J. A. L., F. N. B. Gois, J. P. do V. Madeiro, T. Li, and S. J. Fong. 2022. "Artificial Neural Network-Based Approaches for Computer-Aided Disease Diagnosis and Treatment." In A. K. Bhoi, V. H. C. de Albuquerque, P. N. Srinivasu, and G. Marques (Eds.), *Cognitive and Soft Computing Techniques for the Analysis of Healthcare Data* (pp. 79–99). Academic Press. https://doi.org/10.1016/B978-0-323-85751-2.00008-6

Marques, J. A. L., F. N. Bernardo Gois, J. A. Nunes da Silveira, T. Li, and S. J. Fong. 2022. "AI and Deep Learning for Processing the Huge Amount of Patient-Centric Data that Assist in Clinical Decisions." In A. K. Bhoi, V. H. C. de Albuquerque, P. N. Srinivasu, and G. Marques (Eds.), *Cognitive and Soft Computing Techniques for the Analysis of Healthcare Data* (pp. 101–121). United States: Academic Press. https://doi.org/10.1016/B978-0-323-85751-2.00001-3

Marques, J. A. L., P. C. Cortez, J. P. D. V. Madeiro, S. J. Fong, F. S. Schlindwein, and V. H. C. D. Albuquerque. 2019. "Automatic Cardiotocography Diagnostic System Based on Hilbert Transform and Adaptive Threshold Technique." *IEEE Access* 7: 73085–73094. https://doi.org/10.1109/ACCESS.2018.2877933

Marques, J. A. L., P. C. Cortez, J. P. V. Madeiro, V. H. C. Albuquerque, S. J. Fong, and F. S. Schlindwein. 2020. "Nonlinear characterization and complexity analysis of cardiotocographic examinations using entropy measures." *Journal of Supercomputing* 76 (2): 1305–1320. https://doi.org/10.1007/s11227-018-2570-8

Marques, J. A. L., T. Han, W. Wu, J. P. do V. Madeiro, A. V. L. Neto, R. Gravina, G. Fortino, and V. H. C. de Albuquerque. 2021. "IoT-Based Smart Health System for Ambulatory Maternal and Fetal Monitoring." *IEEE Internet of Things Journal* 8 (23): 16814–16824. https://doi.org/10.1109/JIOT.2020.3037759

Meng, Lingwei, Di Dong, Liang Li, Meng Niu, Yan Bai, Meiyun Wang, Xiaoming Qiu, Yunfei Zha, and Jie Tian. 2020. "A Deep Learning Prognosis Model Help Alert for COVID-19 Patients at High-Risk of Death: A Multi-Center Study." *IEEE Journal of Biomedical and Health Informatics* 24 (12): 3576–3584. https://doi.org/10.1109/jbhi.2020.3034296.

Mohamed Suhail, M., and T. Abdul Razak. 2022. "Cardiac Disease Detection from ECG Signal Using Discrete Wavelet Transform with Machine Learning Method." *Diabetes Research and Clinical Practice* 187 (May): 109852. https://doi.org/10.1016/j.diabres.2022.109852.

Mourad, Kholkhal, and Bereksi Reguig Fethi. 2016. "Efficient Automatic Detection of QRS Complexes in ECG Signal Based on Reverse Biorthogonal Wavelet Decomposition and Nonlinear Filtering." *Measurement* 94 (December): 663–670. https://doi.org/10.1016/j.measurement.2016.09.014.

Murray, C. P., A. P. Kenny, N. J. O'Sullivan, R. T. Murphy, and J.P. Curtain. 2025. "Efficacy of Wearable Devices Detecting Pulmonary Congestion in Heart Failure: A Systematic Review and Meta-Analysis." *Frontiers in Cardiovascular Medicine* 12: 1612545.

Nguyen Van, S., J. A. L. Marques, T. A. Biala, and Y. Li. 2021. "Identification of Latent Risk Clinical Attributes for Children Born Under IUGR Condition Using Machine Learning Techniques." *Computer Methods and Programs in Biomedicine* 200: 105842. https://doi.org/10.1016/j.cmpb.2020.105842

Pal, Saurabh, and Madhuchhanda Mitra. 2010. "Detection of ECG Characteristic Points Using Multiresolution Wavelet Analysis Based Selective Coefficient Method." *Measurement* 43 (2): 255–261. https://doi.org/10.1016/j.measurement.2009.10.004.

Peck, Roxy, Chris Olsen, and Jay L Devore. 2008. *Introduction to Statistics and Data Analysis*. Belmont: Cengage Learning.

Pedregosa, F., G. Varoquaux, A. Gramfort, V. Michel, B. Thirion, O. Grisel, M. Blondel, P. Prettenhofer, R. Weiss, V. Dubourg, and J. Vanderplas. 2011. "Scikit-Learn: Machine Learning in Python." *T*he Journal of *Machine* Learning *R*esearch 12: 2825–2830.

Perez, M. V., K.W. Mahaffey, H. Hedlin, J.S. Rumsfeld, A. Garcia, T. Ferris, V. Balasubramanian, A.M. Russo, A. Rajmane, L. Cheung, and G. Hung. 2019. "Large-Scale Assessment of a Smartwatch to Identify Atrial Fibrillation." *New England Journal of Medicine* 381 (20): 1909–1917.

Popescu, Irina-Maria, Madalin-Marius Margan, Mariana Anghel, Alexandra Mocanu, Sorina Maria Denisa Laitin, Roxana Margan, Ionut Dragos Capraru, et al. 2023. "Developing Prediction Models for COVID-19 Outcomes: A Valuable Tool for Resource-Limited Hospitals." *International Journal of General Medicine* 16 (July): 3053–3065. https://doi.org/10.2147/ijgm.s419206.

Pordeus, Daniel, Pedro Ribeiro, Laíla Zacarias, Adriel de Oliveira, João Alexandre Lobo Marques, Pedro Miguel Rodrigues, Camila Leite, Manoel Alves Neto, Arnaldo Aires Peixoto, and João Paulo do Vale Madeiro. 2023. "Training Strategies for Covid-19 Severity Classification." In I. Rojas, O. Valenzuela, F. Rojas Ruiz, L. J. Herrera, and F. Ortuño (Eds.), *Bioinformatics and Biomedical Engineering. IWBBIO 2023. Lecture Notes in Computer Science*, Vol. 13919. Cham: Springer. https://doi.org/10.1007/978-3-031-34953-9_40

Pordeus, Daniel, Pedro Ribeiro, Laíla Zacarias, João Paulo Madeiro, Joao Alexandre Lobo Marques, Pedro Miguel Rodrigues, Camila Leite, Manoel Alves Neto, Arnaldo Aires Peixoto Jr, and Adriel de Oliveira. 2023. "Classification of Severity of COVID-19 Patients Based on the Heart Rate Variability." In J. A. Lobo Marques and S. J. Fong (Eds.), *Computerized Systems for Diagnosis and Treatment of COVID-19* (pp. 155–177). Cham: Springer International Publishing. https://doi.org/10.1007/978-3-031-30788-1_10.

Rahman, Tawsifur, Amith Khandakar, Md Enamul Hoque, Nabil Ibtehaz, Saad Bin Kashem, Reehum Masud, Lutfunnahar Shampa, et al. 2021. "Development and Validation of an Early Scoring System for Prediction of Disease Severity in COVID-19 Using Complete Blood Count Parameters." *IEEE Access* 9: 120422–120441. https://doi.org/10.1109/access.2021.3105321.

Ribeiro, Pedro, Joana Sá, Daniela Paiva, and Pedro Miguel Rodrigues. 2024. "Cardiovascular Diseases Diagnosis Using an ECG Multi-Band Non-Linear Machine Learning Framework Analysis." *Bioengineering* 11 (1): 58. https://doi.org/10.3390/bioengineering11010058.

Ribeiro, Pedro, João Alexandre Lobo Marques, and Pedro Miguel Rodrigues. 2023. "COVID-19 Detection by Means of ECG, Voice, and X-Ray Computerized Systems: A Review." *Bioengineering* 10 (2): 198. https://doi.org/10.3390/bioengineering10020198.

Ribeiro, Pedro, João Alexandre Lobo Marques, Daniel Pordeus, Laíla Zacarias, Camila Ferreira Leite, Manoel Alves Sobreira-Neto, Arnaldo Aires Peixoto, Adriel de Oliveira, João Paulo do Vale Madeiro, and Pedro Miguel Rodrigues. 2024. "Machine Learning-Based Cardiac Activity Non-Linear Analysis for Discriminating COVID-19 Patients with Different Degrees of Severity." *Biomedical Signal Processing and Control* 87 (January): 105558. https://doi.org/10.1016/j.bspc.2023.105558.

Ribeiro, Pedro, Maria Inês Barbosa, Clara Sousa, and Pedro Miguel Rodrigues. 2025. "Near-Infrared Spectroscopy Machine-Learning Spectral Analysis Tool for Blueberries (Vaccinium Corymbosum) Cultivar Discrimination." *Foods* 14 (8): 1428. https://doi.org/10.3390/foods14081428.

Rioul, O., and M. Vetterli. 1991. "Wavelets and Signal Processing." *IEEE Signal Processing Magazine* 8 (4): 14–38. https://doi.org/10.1109/79.91217.

Rodrigues, Pedro Miguel, Diamantino Freitas, and João Paulo Teixeir. 2012. "Alzheimer Electroencephalogram Temporal Events Detection by K-Means." *Procedia Technology* 5 (2012): 859–864. https://doi.org/10.1016/j.protcy.2012.09.095.

Rodrigues, Pedro Miguel, Diamantino Freitas, João Paulo Teixeira, Bruno Bispo, Dílio Alves, and Carolina Garrett. 2018. "Electroencephalogram Hybrid Method for Alzheimer Early Detection." *Procedia Computer Science* 138 (2018): 209–214. https://doi.org/10.1016/j.procs.2018.10.030.

Rodrigues, Pedro Miguel, Diamantino Rui Freitas, and Joaquim Gabriel. 2014. "Portable Interface and Local Service Manager." *Procedia Computer Science* 27: 67–73. https://doi.org/10.1016/j.procs.2014.02.009.

Rodrigues, Pedro Miguel, Diamantino Rui Freitas, João Paulo Teixeira, Dílio Alves, and Carolina Garrett. 2018. "Electroencephalogram Signal Analysis in Alzheimer's Disease Early Detection." *International Journal of Reliable and Quality E-Healthcare* 7 (1): 40–59. https://doi.org/10.4018/IJRQEH.2018010104.

Rodrigues, Pedro Miguel, João Paulo Madeiro, and João Alexandre Lobo Marques. 2023. "Enhancing Health and Public Health through Machine Learning: Decision Support for Smarter Choices." *Bioengineering* 10 (7): 792. https://doi.org/10.3390/bioengineering10070792.

Safari, Saeed, Alireza Baratloo, Mohamed Elfil, and Ahmed Said Negida. 2018. "Part 2: Positive and Negative Predictive Values of Diagnostic Tests." *Archives of Academic Emergency Medicine* 3: 87. https://doi.org/10.22037/aaem.v3i3.274.

Santos, Marcus A. G,, Roberto Munoz, Rodrigo Olivares, Pedro P. Rebouças Filho, Javier Del Ser, and Victor Hugo C. de Albuquerque. 2020. "Online Heart Monitoring Systems on the Internet of Health Things Environments: A Survey, a Reference Model and an Outlook." *Information Fusion* 53 (January): 222–239. https://doi.org/10.1016/j.inffus.2019.06.004.

Sayed, Safynaz Abdel-Fattah, Abeer Mohamed Elkorany, and Sabah Sayed Mohammad. 2021. "Applying Different Machine Learning Techniques for Prediction of COVID-19 Severity." *Ieee Access* 9: 135697–135707. https://doi.org/10.1109/access.2021.3116067.

Sayed, Safynaz, Abeer Elkorany, and Sabah Mohammad. 2021. "Applying Different Machine Learning Techniques for Prediction of COVID-19 Severity." *Ieee Access* 9: 135697–135707.

Shen, Xiaoping, and Ahmed I Zayed, eds. 2014. *Multiscale Signal Analysis and Modeling*. 2013th ed. New York, NY: Springer.

Silva, G., P. Batista, and P. M. Rodrigues. 2025. "COVID-19 Activity Screening by a Smart-Data-Driven Multi-Band Voice Analysis." Journal of Voice 39 (3): 602–611. https://doi.org/10.1016/j.jvoice.2022.11.008.

Silva, Jackson Henrique Braga da, Paulo Cesar Cortez, Senthil K Jagatheesaperumal, and Victor Hugo C de Albuquerque. 2023. "ECG Measurement Uncertainty Based on Monte Carlo Approach: An Effective Analysis for a Successful Cardiac Health Monitoring System." *Bioengineering* 10 (1): 115. https://doi.org/10.3390/bioengineering10010115.

Singh, P., G. Chaudhary, and J. A. L. Marques. 2023. Medical information extraction of clinical notes and pictorial visualisation of electronic medical records summary interface. In Preeti Nagrath, Jafar A. Alzubi, Bhawna Singla, Joel J. P. C. Rodrigues and A. K. Verma

(Eds.), *Smart Distributed Embedded Systems for Healthcare Applications* (pp. 29–40). CRC Press.

Sivannarayana, N., and D. C. Reddy. 1999. "Biorthogonal Wavelet Transforms for ECG Parameters Estimation." *Medical Engineering & Physics* 21 (3): 167–174. https://doi.org/10.1016/s1350-4533(99)00040-5.

Smital, Lukáš, Martin Vítek, Jiří Kozumplík, and Ivo Provazník. 2013. "Adaptive Wavelet Wiener Filtering of ECG Signals." *IEEE Transactions on Biomedical Engineering* 60 (2): 437–445. https://doi.org/10.1109/tbme.2012.2228482.

Sokhansanj, Bahrad A., and Gail L. Rosen. 2022. "Predicting COVID-19 Disease Severity from SARS-CoV-2 Spike Protein Sequence by Mixed Effects Machine Learning." *Computers in Biology and Medicine* 149 (October): 105969. https://doi.org/10.1016/j.compbiomed.2022.105969.

Sundararajan, D. 2015. *Discrete Wavelet Transform a Signal Processing Approach.* 1st ed. New Jersey: Wiley.

Taheriyan, M., S. M. Ayyoubzadeh, M. Ebrahimi, S. R. N. Kalhori, A. H. Abooei, M. Gholamzadeh, and S. M. Ayyoubzadeh. 2022. "Prediction of COVID-19 patients' Survival by deep learning approaches." Medical journal of the Islamic Republic of Iran 36: 144. https://doi.org/10.47176/mjiri.36.144.

Ulukaya, Sezer, Ahmet Alp Sarıca, Oğuzhan Erdem, and Ali Karaali. 2023. "MSCCov19Net: Multi-Branch Deep Learning Model for COVID-19 Detection from Cough Sounds." *Medical & Biological Engineering & Computing* 61 (7): 1619–1629. https://doi.org/10.1007/s11517-023-02803-4.

Wang, Shuo, Yunfei Zha, Weimin Li, Qingxia Wu, Xiaohu Li, Meng Niu, Meiyun Wang, et al. 2020. "A Fully Automatic Deep Learning System for COVID-19 Diagnostic and Prognostic Analysis." *European Respiratory Journal* 56 (2): 2000775.

Xiong, Yibai, Yan Ma, Lianguo Ruan, Dan Li, Cheng Lu, and Luqi Huang. 2022. "Comparing Different Machine Learning Techniques for Predicting COVID-19 Severity." *Infectious Diseases of Poverty* 11 (1): 19. https://doi.org/10.1186/s40249-022-00946-4.

Yan, K., T. Li, J. A. L. Marques, J. Gao, S. J. Fong, K. Yan, T. Li, J. A. L. Marques, J. Gao, and S. J. Fong. 2023. "A Review on Multimodal Machine Learning in Medical Diagnostics." *Mathematical Biosciences and Engineering* 20 (5): 8708–8726. https://doi.org/10.3934/mbe.2023382

Yan, Xiquan, Xiaotong Han, Danhong Peng, Yong Fan, Zhixiong Fang, Da Long, Yu Xie, et al. 2020. "Clinical Characteristics and Prognosis of 218 Patients With COVID-19: A Retrospective Study Based on Clinical Classification." *Frontiers in Medicine* 7 (August): 485.

Yao, Haochen, Nan Zhang, Ruochi Zhang, Meiyu Duan, Tianqi Xie, Jiahui Pan, Ejun Peng, et al. 2020. "Severity Detection for the Coronavirus Disease 2019 (COVID-19) Patients Using a Machine Learning Model Based on the Blood and Urine Tests." *Frontiers in Cell and Developmental Biology* 8 (July): 683.

Yesudhas, Dhanusha, Ambuj Srivastava, and Michael Gromiha. 2020. "COVID-19 Outbreak: History, Mechanism, Transmission, Structural Studies and Therapeutics." *Infection* 49 (2): 199–213.

Yu, Zekuan, Xiaohu Li, Haitao Sun, Jian Wang, Tongtong Zhao, Hongyi Chen, Yichuan Ma, Shujin Zhu, and Zongyu Xie. 2020. "Rapid Identification of COVID-19 Severity in CT Scans through Classification of Deep Features." *BioMedical Engineering OnLine* 19 (1), 63. https://doi.org/10.1186/s12938-020-00807-x

Zacarias, H., J. A. L. Marques, V. Felizardo, M. Pourvahab, and N. M. Garcia. 2024. "ECG Forecasting System Based on Long Short-Term Memory." *Bioengineering* 11 (1): 89.

Zhao, T., F. N. B. Gois, J. A. L. Marques, B. R. dos Santos Silva, P. Cortez, S. K. Jagatheesaperumal, and V. H. C. de Albuquerque. 2025. "AutoML-Based EEG Signal Analysis in Neuro-Marketing Classification using Biclustering Method. Applied Soft Computing 181: 113412.

Zhi, Koh Yi, Oliver Faust, and Wenwei Yu. 2014. "Wavelet Based Machine Learning Techniques for Electrocardiogram Signal Analysis." *Journal of Medical Imaging and Health Informatics* 4 (5): 737–742. https://doi.org/10.1166/jmihi.2014.1314.

8 Electroencephalogram Wearable Platform for Stress Assessment and Reduction for Patients Submitted to Chronic Stress

João Alexandre Lobo Marques,
Francisco Sulivan Bastos Mota,
Camila Guerra, Pedro Miguel Rodrigues,
Paulo Cezar Nascimento Filho, and
Ganesh R. Naik

8.1 INTRODUCTION

Over the last century, the human brain has been studied in increasing detail by professionals from diverse scientific and clinical fields. Historically, however, this research has been predominantly oriented toward the identification, classification, and treatment of dysfunctions, whether physiological, anatomical, cognitive, or psychological. Within this paradigm, neuroscience was largely confined to a clinical and pathological framework, driven mainly by disciplines such as neurology, psychiatry, and psychology. As a result, the brain was often approached primarily as a site of disorder, and scientific inquiry focused on deficits, illnesses, or maladaptive behaviors rather than on its adaptive, regulatory, and self-organizing capacities.

This perspective has progressively shifted with the evolution of diagnostic technologies and, more recently, with the availability of low-cost, noninvasive systems for monitoring brain activity and other physiological processes linked to the nervous system (Marques, et al., 2021). Techniques such as electroencephalography (EEG), heart rate variability (HRV) analysis, and electrodermal activity (EDA) monitoring have enabled the investigation of neural and autonomic functioning in different contexts and in states of relative normality (Marques, et al., 2019). These advances have fostered a systemic understanding of the brain as a dynamic and adaptive organ that continuously regulates internal states in response to environmental demands.

DOI: 10.1201/9781003500445-8

Advancements in neuroscience have led to the conceptualization of the brain as a complex and dynamic system rather than a static organ of deficits (Bullmore & Sporns, 2009). Consequently, neuroscience has increasingly emphasized the study of healthy functioning, learning, resilience, and experience-dependent self-regulation processes, rather than focusing exclusively on pathology (Dayan & Cohen, 2011).

8.2 BRAIN MONITORING AND STRESS COPING AND REDUCTION

Recent advances in applied neuroscience have increasingly reframed the brain not as a static organ defined primarily by deficits, but as a dynamic, adaptive system capable of reorganizing itself in response to experience, learning, and environmental demands. Two relevant works that strongly support this paradigm shift are those of Dayan and Cohen (2011) and Bullmore and Sporns (2009). Together, these studies provide a robust theoretical and empirical foundation for the use of brain monitoring techniques, particularly EEG, in stress-coping and reduction interventions, which are discussed in the following subsections.

8.2.1 Neuroplasticity and Experience-Dependent Brain Reorganization

Dayan and Cohen (2011) conducted a comprehensive review of neuroplastic mechanisms underlying motor skill learning, integrating evidence from human and animal studies using neurophysiological recordings, neuroimaging, and behavioral paradigms. Their methodological approach synthesized findings from longitudinal learning experiments, including repeated training tasks combined with neural measurements such as EEG, magnetoencephalography (MEG), transcranial magnetic stimulation (TMS), and functional neuroimaging. Rather than focusing on pathology, the authors examined how repeated experience leads to durable changes in neural representations, synaptic efficacy, and functional connectivity.

A central result of their analysis is that learning induces measurable and progressive changes in neural oscillatory activity, cortical excitability, and network-level organization. Early stages of learning are associated with widespread neural engagement and increased cognitive effort, while later stages show more efficient, localized, and stable neural patterns. Importantly, these changes are not limited to motor domains; the same principles of experience-dependent plasticity apply to cognitive and emotional regulation processes. This indicates direct implications for stress coping, as chronic stress is known to disrupt neural efficiency, increase cognitive load, and impair executive control.

From an EEG perspective, the findings of Dayan and Cohen (2011) support the use of oscillatory markers, such as alpha, theta, and beta frequency bands activity, as indicators of learning, regulation, and adaptation. Stress reduction interventions based on EEG neurofeedback leverage precisely these plastic mechanisms: by repeatedly training individuals to modulate maladaptive neural patterns associated with stress (e.g., excessive beta activity or reduced alpha power), it becomes possible to promote long-term adaptive changes in neural functioning. Thus, EEG-based stress regulation is not merely symptomatic control, but an application of fundamental neuroplastic principles.

8.2.2 Brain Networks as Adaptive and Self-Organizing Systems

Complementing the plasticity-focused perspective, Bullmore and Sporns (2009) approached brain function from a systems neuroscience perspective, applying graph-theoretical methods to the study of structural and functional brain networks. Their work synthesized evidence from large-scale neuroimaging datasets, including EEG, MEG, and functional magnetic resonance imaging (fMRI), to characterize the brain as a complex network with non-random topology. Methodologically, they analyzed properties such as small-world organization, modularity, hubs, and efficiency, demonstrating that healthy brain function depends on a balance between functional integration and segregation.

One of the key findings of Bullmore and Sporns (2009) is that brain networks are inherently dynamic and can reconfigure in response to task demands, learning, and environmental stressors. Under conditions of stress, this balance can be disrupted, leading to either excessive segregation (rigidity) or excessive integration (noise and overload). Such dysregulation manifests as impaired cognitive control, emotional instability, and reduced resilience. Importantly, these network-level changes can be detected using EEG through measures such as coherence, phase synchronization, and functional connectivity between cortical regions.

This network-based framework strongly supports the use of EEG for stress monitoring and coping interventions. EEG is uniquely suited to capture the temporal dynamics of large-scale brain networks, enabling researchers and practitioners to observe how stress alters communication among frontal, limbic, and sensory regions in real time. EEG-based neurofeedback protocols can thus be designed not only to modulate local oscillatory power, but also to restore adaptive network configurations, promoting flexibility and resilience in the face of stress.

8.2.3 Implications for Electroencephalogram-Based Stress Reduction and Coping

Taken together, the contributions of Dayan and Cohen (2011) and Bullmore and Sporns (2009) provide complementary foundations for EEG-based stress mitigation. The former establishes that repeated, experience-driven modulation of neural activity leads to lasting plastic changes, validating the learning-based logic of neurofeedback and self-regulation training. The latter demonstrates that stress and adaptation must be understood at the level of interacting neural networks, reinforcing the importance of continuous brain monitoring rather than isolated measurements.

In practical terms, the use of wearable EEG systems operationalizes these principles by enabling real-time access to neural markers of stress and regulation. By monitoring oscillatory patterns and network dynamics associated with stress responses, individuals can learn to recognize and actively modulate their neural states. Over time, this process supports the development of more efficient, flexible, and resilient brain networks, contributing to sustained stress reduction and improved cognitive-emotional functioning.

Thus, EEG-based brain monitoring for stress coping is firmly grounded in contemporary neuroscience: it is an applied extension of well-established principles of neuroplasticity and network self-organization. Rather than addressing stress as a purely psychological phenomenon, this approach situates stress regulation within the brain's capacity for learning, adaptation, and systemic reconfiguration.

Over the last decade, this conceptual and technological evolution has led to a significant quantitative and qualitative expansion of applied neuroscience research. Neuroscience has increasingly intersected with other domains of knowledge, giving rise to interdisciplinary fields such as neurocardiology (focused on the interaction between the nervous system and cardiac regulation), neurocognition, affective neuroscience, and psychophysiology. In parallel, biofeedback and neurofeedback approaches have gained prominence as practical tools for promoting emotional regulation, learning optimization, and stress management in educational, occupational, and personal development settings. These approaches are grounded in the real-time monitoring of physiological and neural signals, allowing individuals to develop awareness of their internal states and to intentionally modulate stress-related responses.

Within this applied framework, EEG has emerged as one of the most effective and accessible techniques for studying and regulating stress. EEG enables the real-time recording of cortical electrical activity with high temporal resolution, making it particularly well suited to capturing rapid neural fluctuations associated with arousal, attention, and emotional regulation. Unlike neuroimaging techniques such as functional magnetic resonance imaging or positron emission tomography, EEG is noninvasive, comparatively low-cost, and increasingly portable, facilitating its use beyond laboratory and clinical environments and enabling the development of wearable solutions for a variety of applications.

From a neurophysiological standpoint, stress is consistently associated with specific EEG patterns. Elevated stress levels tend to be reflected in EEG frequency bands, such as:

- increased beta-band activity,
- reduced alpha power,
- alterations in frontal asymmetry.

These changes indicate heightened vigilance, cognitive load, and emotional tension. In contrast, states of relaxation and effective self-regulation are often characterized by increased alpha and theta activity, particularly in frontal and central regions, reflecting reduced sympathetic activation and improved emotional balance. These neural signatures provide objective markers for assessing stress and evaluating the effectiveness of regulatory interventions (Davidson, 2004; Klimesch, 1999).

8.2.4 Wearable Electroencephalograms

The emergence of wearable EEG technologies represents a decisive step in translating neuroscience research into practical stress-mitigation applications. Advances in dry electrodes, wireless communication, miniaturized electronics, and embedded signal processing have enabled the development of lightweight, user-friendly EEG headsets capable of continuous monitoring in everyday settings. These wearable systems support real-time applications, enabled by neurofeedback paradigms that provide users with immediate information about their brain activity, facilitating learning processes that promote voluntary self-regulation. Through repeated exposure and practice, users can harness neuroplastic mechanisms to develop more adaptive neural patterns, contributing to sustained reductions in stress and improvements in cognitive and emotional functioning.

Wearable EEG-based interventions are particularly relevant in educational and professional environments characterized by high cognitive and emotional demands, where chronic stress negatively affects attention, memory, executive functioning, and well-being. Empirical evidence suggests that EEG-based neurofeedback can contribute to reductions in perceived stress, improvements in emotional regulation, and enhanced cognitive performance, reinforcing a shift from reactive or pharmacological approaches toward preventive and self-empowering strategies (Hammond, 2011; Micoulaud-Franchi et al., 2015).

The increasing prevalence of stress-related conditions in contemporary societies has intensified the demand for wearable EEG technologies capable of providing objective, continuous, and noninvasive assessment of cognitive and affective states in everyday environments. Wearable EEG systems, combined with advances in artificial intelligence (AI), enable the real-time acquisition and analysis of neurophysiological signals associated with stress, emotional regulation, mental workload, and adaptive coping processes. AI and deep learning (DL) methods have proven essential for processing large volumes of patient-centric EEG data, transforming complex neural dynamics into interpretable biomarkers that support stress detection, monitoring, and personalized intervention strategies (Marques, Bernardo Gois, et al., 2022; Marques, Gois, et al., 2022). Recent research demonstrates that machine learning (ML) approaches—including nonlinear signal analysis, deep neural networks, recurrent architectures, and automated learning pipelines—can effectively capture latent EEG patterns related to emotional states, cognitive load, and stress responses, enabling scalable and wearable-compatible stress classification and forecasting systems (Fernandes et al., 2024; Guilherme Cunha Santos et al., 2023; Marques et al., 2020; Zhao et al., 2025). In parallel, multimodal decision-support frameworks that integrate EEG-derived features with contextual, behavioral, and physiological data have shown strong potential to enhance stress coping and mitigation by enabling timely feedback, adaptive interventions, and data-driven self-regulation strategies (Nguyen Van et al., 2021; Rodrigues et al., 2023; Yan et al., 2023). These developments are further reinforced by advances in medical information extraction, digital well-being analytics, and intelligent health platforms, which facilitate the integration of wearable EEG-based stress monitoring into personalized, interpretable, and resilient mental-health ecosystems (Li et al., 2020; Singh et al., 2023).

Moreover, wearable EEG devices can be integrated with other physiological sensors, such as HRV and EDA, enabling a multimodal assessment of stress using indicators from both the central and the autonomic nervous systems. This integrative approach aligns with contemporary conceptions of stress as a systemic phenomenon involving continuous interaction between neural, cardiac, and autonomic processes.

By combining EEG-derived neural markers with autonomic measures, it becomes possible to construct individualized neurophysiological profiles and to design adaptive interventions tailored to the user's specific regulatory patterns.

Within this broad range of applications, interventions supporting cognitive development and emotional regulation stand out as particularly promising. Understanding how stress interferes with attention, learning, memory consolidation, and executive functions has become increasingly central in both educational and occupational neuroscience. Brain monitoring technologies, and EEG in particular, offer objective and scalable tools for identifying maladaptive stress responses and for guiding personalized interventions grounded in neuroplasticity—the brain's capacity to reorganize synaptic connections in response to experience and learning.

In this context, international organizations have emphasized the importance of neuroscience-informed practices for improving learning and well-being. The Organisation for Economic Co-operation and Development (OECD) highlights that advances in neuroscience shed new light on long-standing questions about human learning and suggest evidence-based strategies through which educational systems and training environments can better support learners across the lifespan (OECD, 2002). Extending this perspective, integrating wearable EEG-based monitoring and neurofeedback technologies represents a powerful, scalable approach to mitigating stress, enhancing cognitive resilience, and promoting sustainable performance across educational, professional, and societal contexts.

8.2.5 Neurofeedback as a Nonclinical, Self-Regulatory, and Educational Intervention

Although neurofeedback emerged historically within clinical and experimental neuroscience, its contemporary applications extend well beyond the domain of diagnosis and treatment of neurological or psychiatric disorders. It is therefore essential to clearly distinguish neurofeedback used as a self-regulation and cognitive training tool from clinical interventions, both conceptually and operationally.

Clinical interventions are typically embedded within a medical or mental health framework and are initiated following a formal diagnosis based on standardized diagnostic criteria (e.g., the Diagnostic and Statistical Manual of Mental Disorders (DSM) or the International Classification of Diseases (ICD) classifications). Their primary objective is symptom reduction, functional restoration, or disease management, often through pharmacological treatment, psychotherapy, or structured rehabilitation protocols. In contrast, neurofeedback, when applied in educational, social, or preventive contexts, is not intended to diagnose or treat pathology. Instead, it operates as a learning-based intervention designed to enhance self-regulatory capacities, attentional control, emotional balance, and stress resilience in individuals who may experience transient or context-dependent difficulties rather than clinically defined disorders (Hammond, 2011; Sitaram et al., 2017).

From a neuroscientific perspective, neurofeedback is grounded in principles of operant conditioning and experience-dependent neuroplasticity. Individuals receive real-time feedback about specific features of their brain activity—most commonly EEG oscillatory patterns—and gradually learn to modulate these patterns through repetition and reinforcement. Importantly, this process does not impose an external "normalization" of brain activity; instead, it facilitates the exploration and stabilization of neural states associated with improved attention, emotional regulation, or relaxation (Ros et al., 2014; Gruzelier, 2014). This distinguishes neurofeedback from clinical treatments that aim to correct or compensate for dysfunction.

In nonclinical applications, neurofeedback is typically framed as a preventive and developmental strategy, particularly relevant in populations exposed to chronic stress, psychosocial vulnerability, or adverse environmental conditions. Stress-related attentional lapses, emotional dysregulation, and learning difficulties are often adaptive responses to context rather than indicators of intrinsic neurological pathology. In such cases, neurofeedback offers a means of strengthening regulatory mechanisms without labelling individuals as disordered or deficient. This approach aligns with contemporary critiques of the overdiagnosis of cognitive issues in education and mental health, which caution against conflating contextual learning difficulties with neurodevelopmental disorders (McEwen, 2007; Relvas, 2010).

Another fundamental distinction lies in the role of the participant. Clinical interventions often position the individual as a patient receiving treatment administered by a professional. Neurofeedback training, by contrast, emphasizes active participation, autonomy, and self-observation. Participants learn to recognize internal states of focus or calm and to intentionally access them, fostering an internal locus of control. This participatory dimension is particularly relevant in educational and community-based contexts, as it supports empowerment, self-efficacy, and long-term resilience rather than dependence on external therapeutic agents (Sitaram et al., 2017).

Ethically, this differentiation is crucial when working with vulnerable populations in contexts of social risk with chronic stress scenarios. Framing neurofeedback as a training and self-regulation tool reduces the risk of stigma, avoids unnecessary medicalization, and respects developmental variability. At the same time, it does not preclude referral to clinical services when clear indicators of neurological or psychiatric disorders are present. Neurofeedback, in this sense, functions as a complementary, upstream intervention that supports well-being and cognitive readiness while remaining distinct from clinical care.

Table 8.1 presents a list of multiple dimensions for comparing clinical interventions and nonclinical neurofeedback training approaches.

Figure 8.1 presents a graphical representation of the overall application of neurofeedback for stress coping and mitigation.

8.3 STRESS COPING AND REDUCTION USING WEARABLE ELECTROENCEPHALOGRAM NEUROFEEDBACK SYSTEM

Within the context presented in the previous sections, the main objective of this Chapter is to present a pilot study focused on the use of neurophysiological monitoring with wearable EEG devices with the aim of proposing nonclinical methodologies/protocols for stress coping and reduction at the Instituto da Primeira Infância (IPREDE) Institute, in Brazil, validating an intervention for mothers under chronic stress.

TABLE 8.1
Identification of Different Aspects of Clinical Interventions Compared to Nonclinical Neurofeedback Training Approaches, Considering Multiple Dimensions

Dimension	Clinical Interventions	Neurofeedback-Based Training
Primary goal	Diagnosis, treatment, or remediation of disorders	Development of self-regulation, attention, and stress coping
Entry criterion	Formal clinical diagnosis (DSM/ICD)	No diagnosis required; based on functional or contextual needs
Conceptual framework	Pathology-oriented, symptom-focused	Learning-oriented, neuroplasticity-based
Role of participant	Patient, often a passive recipient of treatment	Active learner and self-regulator
Main mechanisms	Pharmacological, psychotherapeutic, or rehabilitative	Operant conditioning and experience-dependent neuroplasticity
Use of electroencephalogram (EEG)	Diagnostic support or clinical monitoring	Real-time feedback for training and learning
Time horizon	Often short- to medium-term symptom management	Medium- to long-term skill acquisition and resilience
Stigmatization risk	Higher (linked to diagnosis and disorder labels)	Lower (focus on skills and capacities)
Typical settings	Hospitals, clinics, mental health services	Schools, community centers, educational or NGO programs
Ethical framing	Medical treatment	Educational and psychosocial support
Relationship to clinical care	Primary mode of intervention	Complementary or preventive; does not replace clinical care

8.3.1 Instituto da Primeira Infância – First Infancy Institute, Fortaleza – Brazil

The Institute of the First Infancy, widely known as IPREDE, was established in Fortaleza in 1986 by a dedicated group of healthcare professionals who sought to combat the devastating rates of severe childhood malnutrition and social vulnerability then prevalent. There were only 100 children out of every thousand born with the possibility of reaching one year of age, and where 30% of malnourished children had growth sequelae. Over the years, the situation has changed significantly; the child malnutrition rate is still high, between 6% and 7%, and the mortality rate is below 20 per thousand births, prompting the institution to evolve its mission.

Originally founded as the Institute for the Prevention of Malnutrition and Exceptionality (Instituto de Prevenção à Desnutrição e à Excepcionalidade or IPREDE), the organization has undergone a profound transformation over nearly four decades, evolving its mission as the landscape of public health shifted. While its early

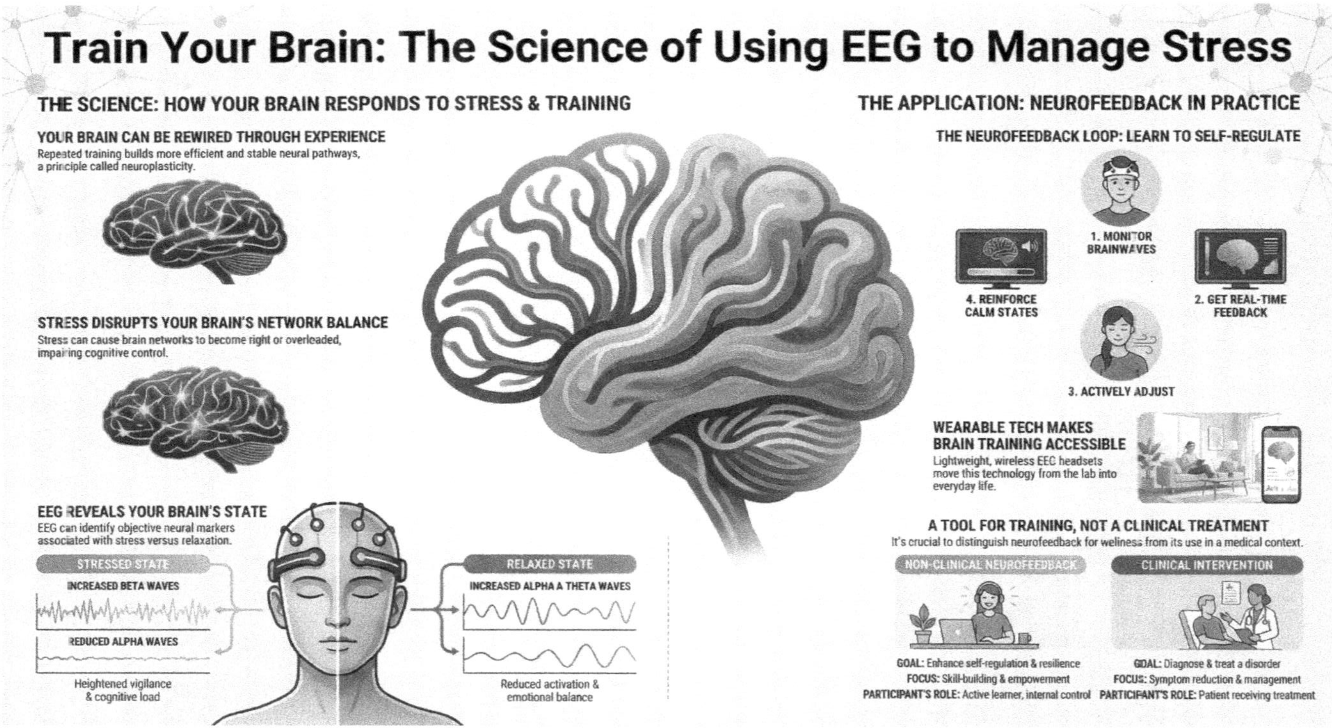

FIGURE 8.1 Graphical Representation of the Overall Application of Neurofeedback for Stress Coping and Mitigation.

years were defined by a clinical battle against absolute hunger, the institution eventually transitioned into its current identity as a holistic center for early childhood development, reflecting a broader commitment to the physical, cognitive, and psychosocial growth of children during their most formative years.

Today, IPREDE operates as an international benchmark for excellence, providing integrated care through a unique systemic methodology that treats the family unit as the foundation for a child's future. By utilizing an approach inspired by the concept of welcoming environments, the institute transforms its clinical spaces into warm, home-like settings featuring toy libraries, reading rooms, and theatres. This nurturing atmosphere is supported by a vast multidisciplinary team comprising dozens of professional specialties, ranging from pediatricians and nutritionists to psychologists and social workers, all dedicated to ensuring that children from zero to six years old reach their full potential.

Understanding the responsibility for the child's cause and the ethical commitment to society, IPREDE took a new step, becoming a reference center for early childhood, a space for the production, teaching, and dissemination of the theme to society at large. The Institute develops programs, projects, and services in articulation with the various sectors of society, with public purposes, focusing on nutrition and development in early childhood, as well as working on the generation and dissemination of technical-scientific knowledge from these acquired experiences, the production and promotion of culture and art as an instrument of awareness and appreciation of the citizen.

Beyond its medical and developmental interventions, the institute places a significant emphasis on social inclusion and the empowerment of women, offering professional training and psychological support to mothers who are often the sole providers for their households. Within this approach, the application of neurophysiological monitoring as a tool to reduce stress in mothers under chronic stress due to a high social risk situation was considered to evaluate feasibility and practical outcomes.

This comprehensive social impact has earned IPREDE numerous prestigious accolades, including multiple recognitions from the Criança Esperança program and the Medalha Iracema, the city of Fortaleza's highest honor. As it continues to advocate for the rights of the most vulnerable populations in Ceará, the official IPREDE website remains the primary resource for those looking to support or learn more about their life-changing work in 2025.

8.4 BRAIN MONITORING AND STRESS REDUCTION IN VULNERABLE POPULATIONS

The need to implement structured interventions aimed at cognitive assessment and management, and at stress reduction, is highly relevant for improving the quality of life of the population assisted by IPREDE, including children, mothers, and other family members. These groups are frequently exposed to adverse social, emotional, and environmental conditions that directly affect cognitive performance, emotional regulation, and overall well-being. In this context, interventions grounded in applied neuroscience—particularly neurofeedback—offer promising, noninvasive, and empowering strategies to support attention regulation, emotional balance, and cognitive resilience.

Stress is widely recognized as a critical factor influencing quality of life, as it interferes with motivation, emotional stability, and the capacity to cope with daily challenges. Prolonged exposure to stressors often leads to feelings of inefficacy and helplessness, contributing to decreased self-esteem and reduced engagement in learning and social activities. From a physiological standpoint, stress is associated with profound alterations in multiple biological systems, including the endocrine, immune, and nervous systems, as well as in behavioral, emotional, and cognitive functioning (Pacak & Palkovits, 2001; McEwen, 2007). These systemic effects highlight the importance of interventions that address stress not only as a psychological experience but as a neurobiological and regulatory process.

In early childhood, the impact of stress is particularly critical. Longitudinal research has shown that children exposed to high levels of parental emotional stress present increased vulnerability to physical illness and emotional dysregulation over time. A longitudinal study conducted at the University of Rochester, which followed children across several years, demonstrated higher rates of illness and emotional difficulties among children whose caregivers experienced elevated and persistent stress levels (Essex et al., 2002). Such findings reinforce the notion that stress operates as a transgenerational and systemic factor, affecting both physical health and cognitive-emotional development.

From the perspective of cognitive development in Brazilian children, large-scale educational assessments further reveal significant learning challenges. Data from the 2013 Avaliação Brasileira do Ciclo de Alfabetização (ABC Test), conducted by the non-governmental organization (NGO) Todos pela Educação with the support of the Instituto Nacional de Estudos e Pesquisas Educacionais Anísio Teixeira (INEP) and the Instituto Paulo Montenegro, revealed alarming results. Among approximately 54,000 students from over 1,200 public and private schools, nearly 70% demonstrated writing performance below the expected level, and 66.7% failed to reach adequate learning outcomes in mathematics for their grade level (Anuário Brasileiro da Educação Básica, 2013). Regional disparities were particularly evident: in the Northeast, 86.4% of third-grade students showed insufficient mathematical knowledge, while even in the Southeast—the best-performing region—this figure reached 57%. In writing, more than 86% of students nationwide failed to achieve satisfactory performance (Anuário Brasileiro da Educação Básica, 2013).

These results point to substantial difficulties in teaching and learning processes within Brazilian classrooms, deeply embedded in social, familial, emotional, and individual contexts. Importantly, such difficulties should not be automatically classified as learning disorders. As emphasized by Relvas (2010), the literature often uses terms such as difficulties, disorders, disturbances, and disabilities interchangeably and inappropriately. Learning difficulties may be transient, context-dependent, and unrelated to structural or functional alterations of the central nervous system. Emotional distress, stress exposure, or environmental instability can temporarily compromise attention, memory, and executive functions, without constituting a neurodevelopmental disorder. The term learning disorder should therefore be reserved for primary and specific conditions associated with documented neurological alterations (Relvas, 2010).

Within this framework, neurofeedback emerges as a particularly relevant intervention. Neurofeedback is a form of biofeedback that uses real-time monitoring of brain activity via (EEG, enabling individuals to learn to regulate their neural states. By providing immediate feedback on specific brain patterns associated with attention, relaxation, or emotional regulation, neurofeedback allows users to engage in a learning process that gradually modifies neural activity through operant conditioning mechanisms (Hammond, 2011; Sitaram et al., 2017).

From a cognitive modeling perspective, neurofeedback does not aim to "correct" deficits, but rather to support the development of adaptive neural strategies for attention control and stress regulation. Protocols targeting attentional processes often focus on enhancing sensorimotor rhythm (SMR) or beta-band regulation to support sustained attention and executive functioning, while relaxation-oriented protocols commonly promote increased alpha and theta activity associated with calm, internally regulated states (Gruzelier, 2014; Ros et al., 2014). Through repeated training sessions, individuals learn to recognize internal states of focus or relaxation and to voluntarily access them, fostering neuroplastic changes that extend beyond the training context.

For populations assisted by IPREDE, including children exposed to psychosocial vulnerability and caregivers experiencing chronic stress, neurofeedback offers several advantages: it is noninvasive, does not rely on verbal mediation, respects individual rhythms, and emphasizes self-regulation rather than diagnosis. By supporting attentional stability and emotional regulation, neurofeedback-based cognitive modeling can contribute to improved learning readiness, reduced stress reactivity, and enhanced well-being, without reinforcing stigmatizing labels or pathologizing normal developmental variability.

In this sense, neurofeedback aligns with contemporary educational and health perspectives that prioritize prevention, resilience, and empowerment. Rather than framing cognitive or emotional difficulties solely as deficits, neurofeedback situates them within a dynamic model of brain regulation, learning, and adaptation—one that is particularly suited to complex social contexts where stress plays a central role.

8.5 RESEARCH PROJECT

8.5.1 INFRASTRUCTURE

The research project was conducted using the IPREDE's existing infrastructure, which provides an integrated environment suitable for applied neuroscience research, clinical support activities, and technological development. The institution provides a range of physical spaces that support participant reception, data acquisition, interdisciplinary collaboration, and system development.

The facilities made available for the project include:

* Clinical service areas comprising reception, waiting rooms, and auxiliary support rooms.
* Dedicated rooms for individualized participant assessment and intervention.

* Specialized rooms for physiological and neurophysiological signal acquisition.
* A software development laboratory for data processing and system integration.
* A basic electronics laboratory bench for hardware testing and integration.
* Meeting rooms for interdisciplinary coordination.
* A videoconference room enabling interaction with remote research teams.

In addition to the physical infrastructure, the project benefited from a diverse set of neurophysiological monitoring equipment and software resources, enabling multimodal data acquisition and analysis. The available instrumentation included:

a) Emotiv EPOC brain monitoring systems with 15 EEG sensors.
b) Emotiv Insight brain monitoring systems with five EEG sensors.
c) Q-Wiz professional EEG systems supporting configurations from four to 20 channels.
d) Brainlink Pro EEG systems with two channels.
e) Brainlink Light EEG systems with a single channel.
f) Proprietary and open-source software for EEG data acquisition and storage, including libraries for application development.
g) Cardiac monitoring systems and sensors for galvanic skin response and respiratory rate, based on open-architecture hardware.
h) A HRV analysis system supporting time-domain, frequency-domain, phase-based, geometric, and nonlinear analyses, as well as graphical visualization tools.

This infrastructure enabled the implementation of an integrated experimental platform capable of supporting real-time monitoring, signal processing, AI analysis, and visualization of stress-related physiological markers.

8.5.2 Proposed Methodology

The research methodology was structured into two complementary components. First, the procedural workflow defining participant engagement, assessment phases, and intervention activities is described. Second, the computational and technological framework underpinning data acquisition, processing, and analysis is detailed, including the equipment and analytical methods employed.

This dual structure ensured coherence between the experimental protocol and the technological system, enabling both ecological validity in participant interactions and methodological rigor in data analysis.

8.5.3 Sample Size and Characterization

A total of 16 women assisted by IPREDE were recruited for this pilot study using a purposive sampling strategy, consistent with the exploratory nature of the research and the targeted social context. Participants were allocated into three subgroups as follows:

- Subgroup 1 – EEG neurofeedback intervention group: eight participants.
- Subgroup 2 – Placebo group with EEG system: four participants.
- Subgroup 3 – Control group: four participants.

All participants received detailed information regarding the objectives, procedures, and ethical aspects of the study and provided written informed consent prior to participation.

As part of the institutional protocol, the IPREDE multidisciplinary team conducted a standardized anamnesis process based on the IRDI methodology (Clinical Risk Indicators for Child Development), adapted for use with children and family contexts. Although the present study focused on adult participants, this process ensured a comprehensive understanding of familial and psychosocial conditions relevant to stress exposure.

To address the research objectives, both subjective and objective measures of stress were employed. Subjective stress perception was assessed using the Perceived Stress Scale (PSS), while objective neurophysiological evaluation was performed using quantitative electroencephalography (qEEG).

Inclusion Criteria

- Female participants assisted by IPREDE.
- Age between 20 and 40 years.
- Voluntary participation with informed consent.

Exclusion Criteria

- Prior diagnosis of psychopathology.
- Emergence of clinical indicators of psychopathology during the study period;
- Voluntary withdrawal from the study at any stage.

Participants meeting exclusion criteria were withdrawn from the study and, when appropriate, referred to relevant clinical services.

8.5.4 Experimental Protocol

The experimental protocol was organized into assessment and intervention phases distributed over time, allowing both cross-sectional and longitudinal analysis of stress-related neurophysiological patterns. The protocol consisted of the following stages:

A1 – Initial Assessment: qEEG recording and administration of the PSS;
T1 – Intervention Phase 1: 16 neurofeedback sessions conducted over eight weeks.
A2 – Intermediate Assessment: qEEG recording.

T2 – Intervention Phase 2: 16 additional neurofeedback sessions conducted over 8 weeks.
A3 – Final Assessment: qEEG recording and administration of the PSS.

Neurofeedback protocols were defined by a neuropsychology specialist and collaboratively validated by an interdisciplinary team comprising pediatricians, neuropediatricians, psychologists, biomedical engineers, and data scientists. This collaborative approach ensured that intervention strategies were scientifically grounded, ethically appropriate, and aligned with the study's nonclinical objectives.

8.6 PROJECT MODELING

The project was modeled considering the integrated technological platform composed of three parts, as presented in Figure 8.2:

(i) Cognitive and Relaxation Subsystem
(ii) AI Classifiers and Clustering,
(iii) Data Analysis and Visualization.

8.6.1 Cognitive and Relaxation Activities Subsystem

The first part of the platform is the cognitive and relaxation activities subsystem. The subsystem integrates digital applications with physiological monitoring devices, enabling synchronized stimulation and data acquisition. Validation tests confirmed the correct functioning of the applications and their compatibility with cerebral monitoring sensors, demonstrating readiness for experimental use. A representation is shown in Figure 8.3.

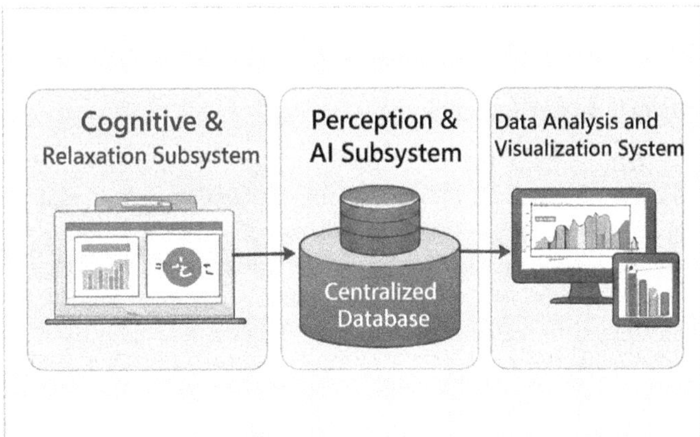

FIGURE 8.2 Technology Platform Divided into Three Parts.

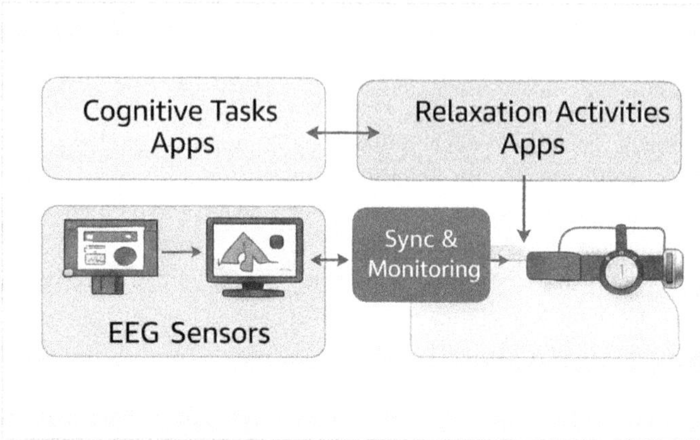

FIGURE 8.3 Cognitive and Relaxation Activities Subsystem Integrating Activities and Electroencephalogram Monitoring.

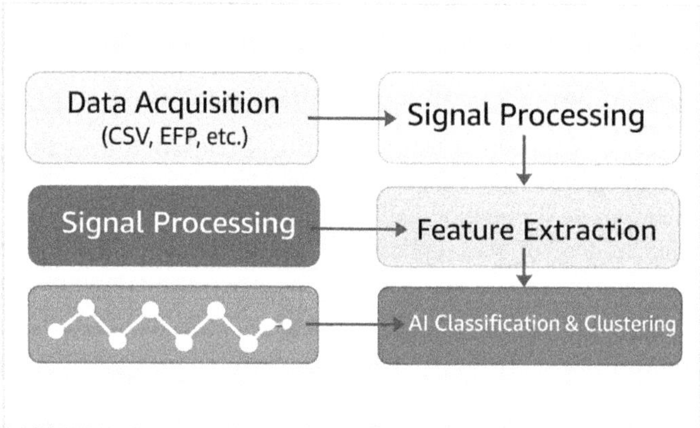

FIGURE 8.4 Block Diagram of the Artificial Intelligence Subsystem, from Data Acquisition, Going Through Feature Extraction and Implementation of Artificial Intelligence Techniques.

8.6.2 Artificial Intelligence Subsystem

The AI Subsystem enabled the acquisition, processing, and interpretation of biometric signals. Results include the successful implementation of multi-format data ingestion routines (e.g., comma-separated values (CSV), electrical fingerprint (EFP)) and AI algorithms for signal classification and Automated Clustering, as presented in Figure 8.4. These components provided reliable identification of physiological patterns, supporting both real-time monitoring and post-hoc analysis.

8.6.3 Data Analysis and Visualization Subsystem

The Data Analysis and Visualization Subsystem translated data into meaningful analytical outputs, including interactive dashboards and intelligent reports, incorporating

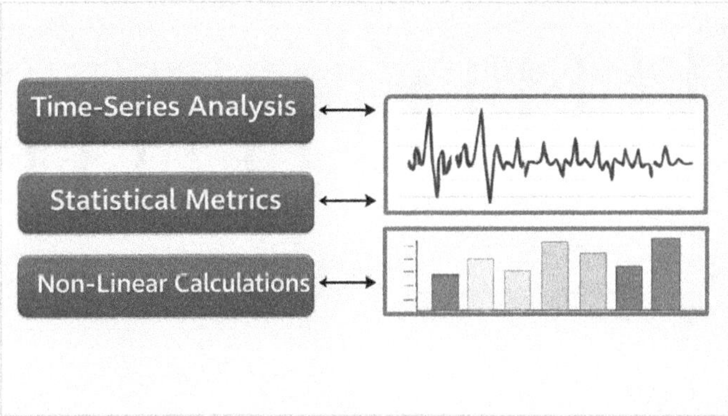

FIGURE 8.5 Data Analysis and Visualization Subsystem with Dashboards and Intelligent Reports.

time-series visualizations, statistical and nonlinear metrics, and outputs from AI techniques. A graphical representation is presented in Figure 8.5. This subsystem enhanced interpretability and facilitated scientific decision-making, confirming the system's analytical maturity.

8.7 SYSTEM IMPLEMENTATION

The first part of this section presents a robust frequency-domain EEG signal analysis pipeline. The system operationalized a set of technical requirements to extract reliable spectral features associated with stress and relaxation states. EEG signals were processed through a dedicated filtering layer, which included (i) outlier removal to reduce artifacts and noise intrinsic to wearable EEG acquisition, and (ii) bandpass filtering focused on alpha (8–12 Hz) and beta (12–30 Hz) frequency bands.

8.7.1 Preprocessing

To analyze the data correctly in the frequency domain, it was necessary to implement a sequence of filters to enable optimal signal analysis, including outlier filtering and bandpass filters for the alpha (8–12Hz) and beta (12–30Hz) frequency bands. In Figure 8.6, a box plot of the EEG spectrum across different frequencies is presented as a technique for detecting and filtering outliers.

Following that, bandpass filters were implemented for both the alpha (8–12Hz) and beta (12–30Hz) frequency bands, as presented in Figure 8.7.

8.7.2 Spectral Analysis

To analyze across different intervals, the system generated a 3D (i.e., three-dimensional) plot of the EEG spectrum for the same subject at different points in the data collection, as shown in Figure 8.8.

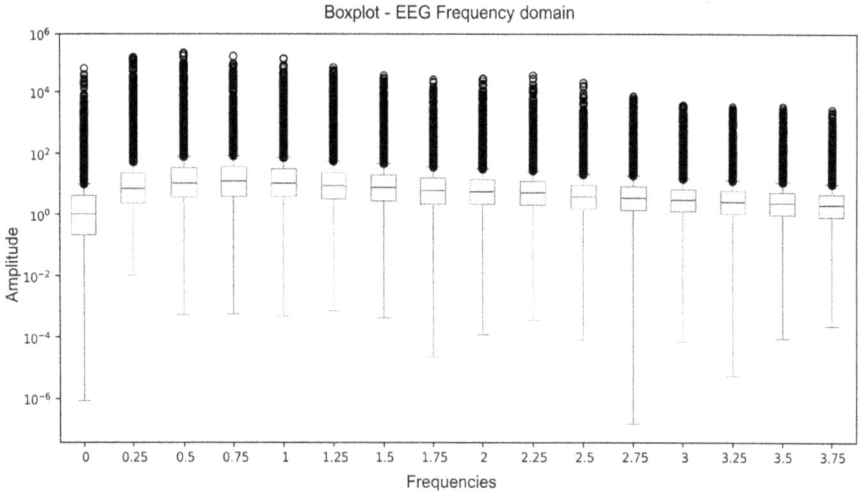

FIGURE 8.6 Boxplot from Electroencephalogram in the Frequency Domain for Detection and Filtering of Outliers.

From a methodological standpoint, the successful implementation of inter-participant 3D comparisons and statistical metrics across participants confirms that the system meets its initial design requirements for exploration and comparative EEG analysis. Clinically, these results suggest that wearable EEG devices, when combined with appropriate filtering and spectral analysis, can yield interpretable biomarkers relevant to chronic stress monitoring.

Beyond static frequency-domain representations, the system implemented time-evolving spectral analysis in three dimensions. The resulting figures show how EEG power across frequency bands changes over time during a monitoring session. These visualizations provide a dynamic perspective on stress-related brain activity, enabling clinicians to observe transient increases or decreases in alpha and beta power.

The results indicate that this temporal–spectral representation is particularly valuable for stress management applications, as it supports the identification of moments of heightened arousal or relaxation within a session. This capability is essential for linking neurophysiological patterns to specific activities or interventions proposed by the system, such as breathing exercises, cognitive tasks, or relaxation techniques.

8.7.3 Unsupervised Clustering and Profiles Identification

The frequency-spectrum plots for each participant, segmented into three temporal sections per session, enabled a fine-grained analysis of intra-session dynamics. Additionally, 3D spectral visualizations provided an effective means of simultaneously comparing multiple participants, highlighting inter-individual variability in alpha and beta activity. This analysis illustrates how alpha-band dominance is associated with relaxation-related states, whereas increased beta activity reflects heightened cognitive load and stress-related activation.

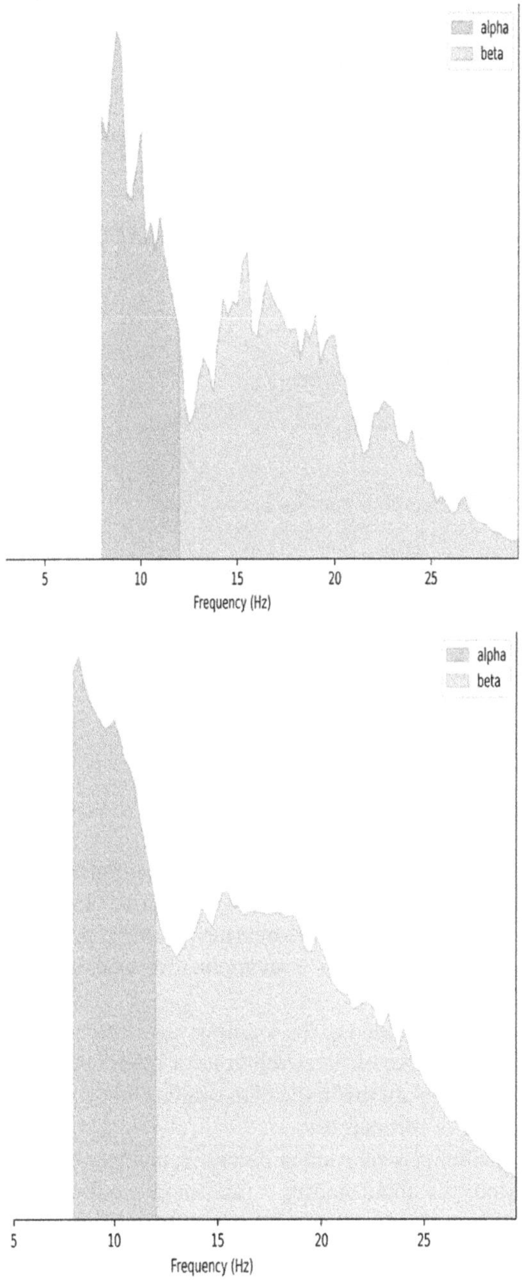

FIGURE 8.7 Visualization of Alpha and Beta Electroencephalogram Spectrum for Two Subjects After Bandpass Filtering.

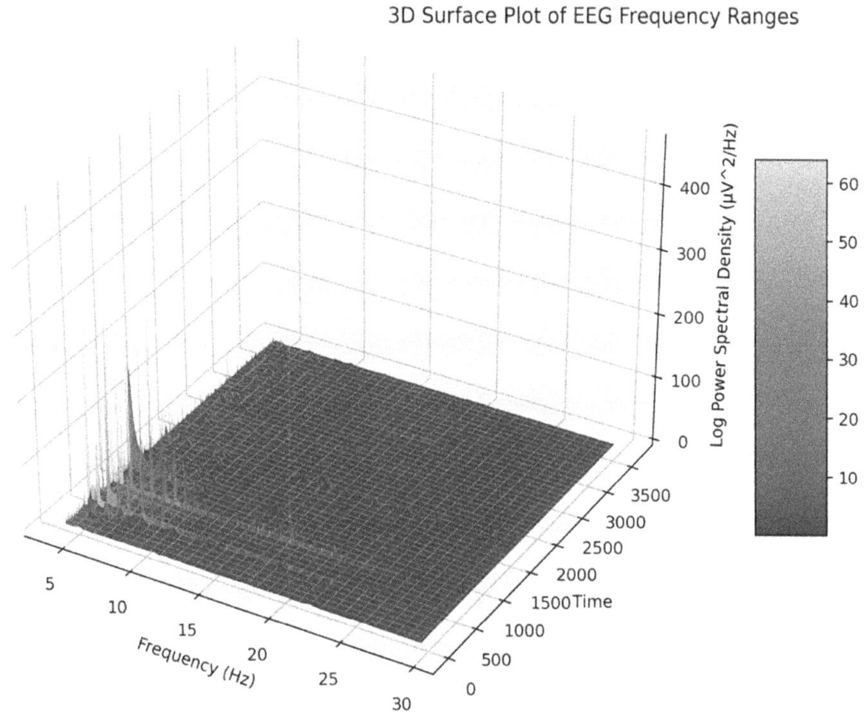

FIGURE 8.8 Three-Dimensional Plot of the Electroencephalogram Spectrum for the Same Subject in Different Moments of the Data Collection.

One of the main requirements for the desired computerized diagnostic support system is the ability to learn from new data without prior classification or labels; that is, the techniques must take the data set, measure multiple possible comparisons, and eventually divide it into clusters. This is an application of the concept of unsupervised learning.

In these, no labels are provided to the learning algorithm in advance, allowing it to evaluate the data and try to establish correlations or other similarities, which can lead to the discovery of hidden patterns in the data sources that could not be established at the time, the beginning of the analysis.

Clustering is considered a relevant problem in unsupervised learning; like other problems of this kind, it's about finding structure in a collection of unlabeled data. Given a set of points, with a notion of distance between points, group the points into some number of clusters, so that within the cluster the distances must be small, i.e., the members of the clusters are close/similar to each other, while externally the distances must be large, i.e., members of different clusters are different.

It is thus necessary to define a measure of proximity between two data points, which can be a measure of similarity or dissimilarity, and some potential techniques include: cosine distance between vectors; Jaccard distance for subsets; and Euclidean distance for points. The definition of the distance measure is strongly dependent on the application under analysis and should be validated accordingly.

The proposed solution is the Centroid Clustering technique, which, in addition to grouping, also reduces dimensionality within the subspaces of the variables. It is based on a popular technique called K-Means, which is simple and efficient. The algorithm aims to classify a given dataset into k clusters. It starts by defining k centers, one for each cluster. These centroids must be placed effectively, as different locations can yield different results. A good option is to place them as far apart as possible. The next step is to assign each point in each data set to its nearest centroid. When there are no outstanding points, the first stage is completed, and an early groupage is made.

At this point, we need to recalculate "k" new centroids as barycenter's of the clusters resulting from the previous step. Once we have "k" new centroids, a new link must be established between each point in the dataset and its nearest new centroid. A loop has been generated. As a result of this loop, the k centroids move iteratively until no further changes occur.

Finally, K-Means aims to minimize an objective function, in this case, a quadratic error function.

The algorithm can be expressed in the following steps:

i. Let X = {x1,x2,x3,........,xn} be the data set and V = {v1,v2,.......,vc} the center set.
ii. Randomly select 'c' clustering centers.
iii. Calculate the distance between each point and the center of a cluster.
iv. Assign a point from data X as the center of the cluster whose distance from the center of the cluster is as small as possible for all cluster centers.
v. Recalculate the new cluster center
vi. Recalculate the distance between each data point and the new centers of determined clusters.
vii. Stop when no new points of data X are determined as cluster scepter, otherwise repeat from step iii.

The procedure will always end, but the k-Means algorithm does not necessarily find the most optimal setting, corresponding to the minimum of the global objective function. As mentioned earlier, the algorithm is significantly sensitive to randomly selected initial cluster centers. The strategy to reduce this effect is to run the algorithm multiple times and determine the model with the best performance.

8.8 RESULTS AND DISCUSSION

This section presents and interprets the results from implementing the wearable EEG-based stress-monitoring and neurofeedback system. The analysis integrates spectral EEG features, Unsupervised Clustering, and supervised ML classifiers to characterize stress-related neurophysiological profiles and their temporal evolution.

Rather than adopting a diagnostic or pathology-oriented framework, the results are interpreted from a functional and regulatory perspective, consistent with the non-clinical objectives of the proposed methodology. The system was designed to identify patterns of neural activation associated with different modes of stress regulation, to track intra-individual changes across sessions, and to support personalized stress-coping strategies grounded in neuroplasticity and learning.

The combination of exploratory (unsupervised) and confirmatory (supervised) AI techniques allowed the system to (i) discover latent neurophysiological profiles without predefined labels, (ii) assess the stability and evolution of these profiles across sessions, and (iii) evaluate the feasibility of automated classification based on EEG features. The following subsections describe these results in detail, emphasizing their neurophysiological meaning, methodological relevance, and translational implications for stress management in vulnerable populations.

8.8.1 Unsupervised Clustering and Identification of Stress-Related Profiles

Unsupervised Clustering was employed as a central analytical strategy to explore the structure of EEG-derived features without imposing predefined categories or clinical labels. This choice reflects the study's exploratory nature and its commitment to avoiding premature pathologization of stress responses.

Using Centroid-based Clustering (k-Means), the system identified four distinct clusters, hereafter referred to as Cluster Types 1-4. Each cluster represents a neurophysiological regulation profile, characterized by specific distributions of alpha and beta band activity, as well as complementary time-domain and nonlinear features.

Importantly, clustering was performed on feature sets extracted from wearable EEG recordings acquired in real-world conditions, demonstrating that meaningful structure can emerge even from low-density, portable neurophysiological data. The resulting clusters should not be interpreted as fixed individual traits, but rather as dynamic functional states reflecting different modes of stress-related brain regulation.

The clustering results, illustrated through dedicated visualization interfaces, demonstrate that the system can differentiate patients with varying levels of stress-related neural activation. Importantly, inter-session clustering analyses showed that the same patient could be consistently grouped across multiple monitoring sessions, while also revealing changes in cluster membership when stress regulation improved or deteriorated over time.

These findings are particularly relevant from a clinical and translational perspective. They suggest that unsupervised AI can function as a powerful exploratory tool for identifying patient subtypes, monitoring longitudinal changes, and supporting personalized stress management strategies. Rather than imposing rigid diagnostic categories, the system allows stress-related profiles to emerge directly from the data.

The frequency-spectrum plots for each participant, segmented into three temporal sections per session, enabled a fine-grained analysis of intra-session dynamics. Additionally, D spectral visualizations provided an effective means of simultaneously comparing multiple participants, highlighting inter-individual variability in alpha and beta activity. This analysis illustrates how alpha-band dominance is associated with relaxation-related states, whereas increased beta activity reflects heightened cognitive load and stress-related activation.

8.8.2 Cluster Type 1 – Low Beta Activity and Reduced Cognitive Arousal

Cluster Type 1 is primarily characterized by low beta-band activity, suggesting reduced cortical activation associated with cognitive effort, vigilance, or stress-related arousal. From a neurophysiological standpoint, this profile may reflect a state of low engagement or hypo-activation, which can be observed in contexts of fatigue, emotional withdrawal, or reduced attentional mobilization.

In the context of chronic stress, such a pattern may emerge not as relaxation per se, but as a protective or disengagement response following prolonged exposure to stressors. This interpretation aligns with models of stress regulation in which individuals oscillate between hyper-arousal and hypo-arousal as adaptive, though potentially maladaptive in the long-term, coping strategies.

The identification of this cluster highlights the system's capacity to detect not only heightened stress activation but also attenuated regulatory states, which are equally relevant for tailoring intervention strategies.

A visualization of three participants of the cluster is presented in Figure 8.9.

8.8.3 Cluster Type 2 – Mixed Alpha and Beta Activation

Cluster Type 2 exhibits simultaneously elevated alpha and beta activity, indicating a mixed pattern of cortical engagement. This profile suggests a state in which cognitive effort and regulatory mechanisms co-occur, potentially reflecting active coping, task engagement under stress, or transitional states between tension and relaxation.

From a functional perspective, this cluster may correspond to individuals who remain cognitively engaged despite stress exposure, mobilizing executive resources while attempting to regulate emotional arousal. Such a profile is particularly informative in stress management contexts, as it may indicate adaptive engagement that can be optimized through targeted neurofeedback strategies.

The presence of this mixed activation pattern underscores the importance of moving beyond simplistic dichotomies of "stressed vs. relaxed" and recognizing gradual, context-dependent regulatory states.

A visualization of three participants of the cluster is presented in Figure 8.10.

8.8.4 Cluster Type 3 – Dominant Alpha Activity and Relaxation-Related Regulation

Cluster Type 3 is characterized by dominant alpha-band activity, a pattern consistently associated in the literature with relaxation, internalized attention, and reduced sympathetic arousal. In the context of the proposed system, this cluster represents a neurophysiological profile aligned with effective stress regulation.

The emergence of this cluster provides empirical support for the system's ability to detect neural signatures compatible with relaxed and self-regulated states using

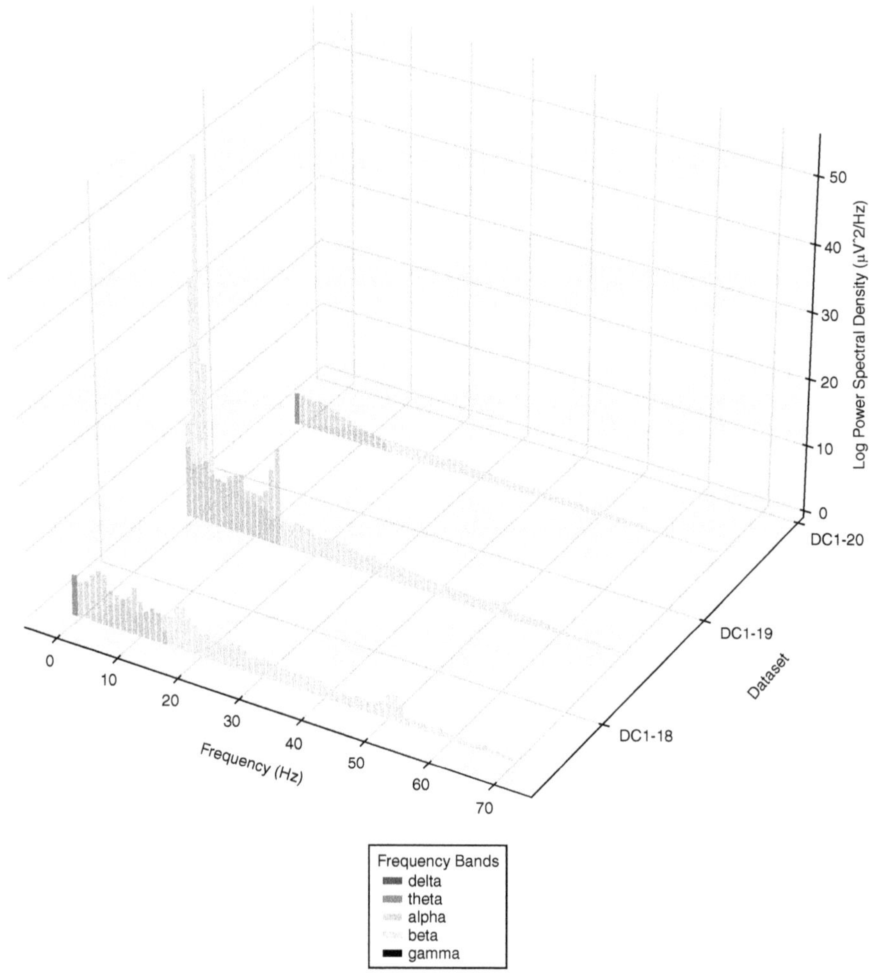

FIGURE 8.9 Cluster Type 1 – Characterized by Low Beta Activity.

wearable EEG devices. Importantly, this profile does not imply the absence of stressors, but rather reflects the individual's capacity to maintain neural regulation despite environmental or emotional challenges.

This cluster serves as a functional reference profile within the system, supporting the evaluation of intervention effects across sessions.

A visualization of three participants of the cluster is presented in Figure 8.11.

8.8.5 Cluster Type 4 – Lower Beta Peaks and Heightened Arousal

Cluster Type 4 is distinguished by peaks in the lower beta frequency range, suggesting increased cognitive load, vigilance, or stress-related activation. This profile is commonly associated with heightened arousal and sustained attentional demand, often observed during acute stress or emotionally charged situations.

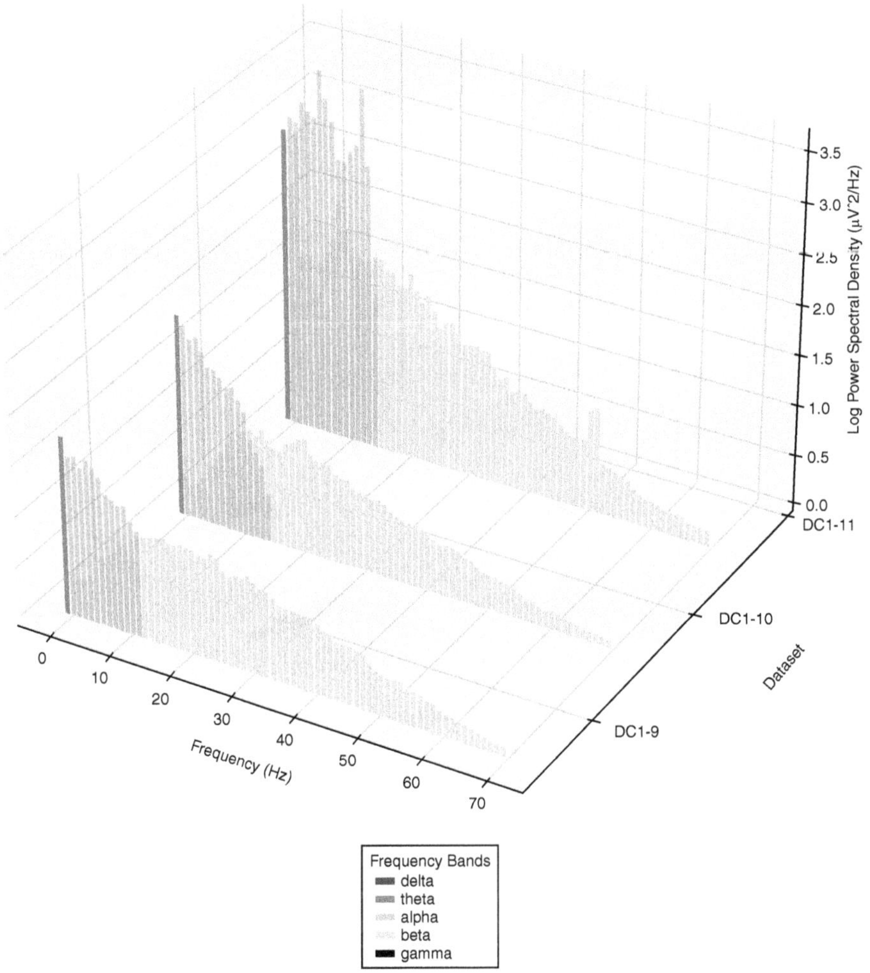

FIGURE 8.10 Cluster Type 2 – Characterized by Higher Activity in Alpha and Beta Bands.

In chronic stress contexts, persistent expression of this profile may reflect ongoing cognitive and emotional strain. However, as with other clusters, this pattern should not be interpreted pathologically. Instead, it represents a state-dependent regulatory configuration that may fluctuate in response to context, intervention, and learning.

The identification of this cluster reinforces the system's sensitivity to stress-related activation patterns that are relevant for monitoring and guiding self-regulation strategies.

This cluster is presented in Figure 8.12.

8.8.6 Inter-Session Clustering and Longitudinal Regulation Dynamics

A particularly relevant result of the proposed system lies in its ability to track inter-session changes in cluster membership for the same participant. Longitudinal analyses revealed that individuals could transition between clusters across sessions, reflecting improvements or deteriorations in stress regulation over time.

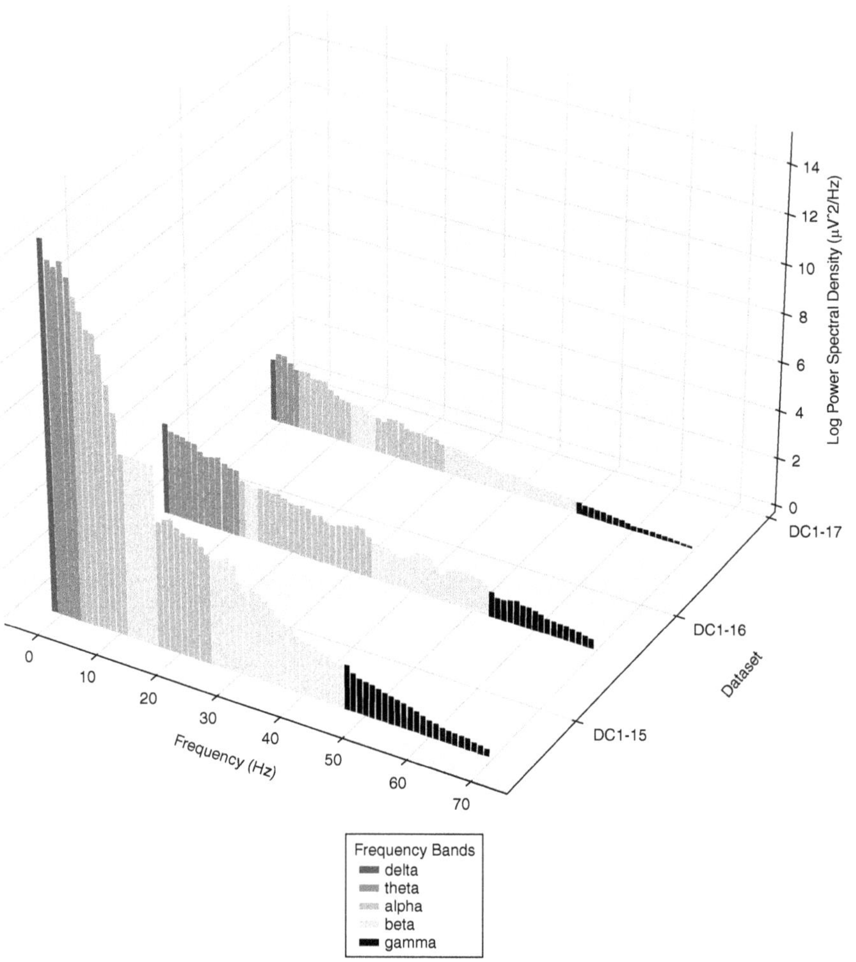

FIGURE 8.11 Cluster Type 3 – Characterized by Dominant Alpha Activity.

Figures illustrating inter-session spectral changes demonstrate that increases in alpha activity and reductions in beta dominance often accompany progression toward more regulated profiles, whereas inverse patterns may signal heightened stress or reduced regulatory capacity. These transitions provide objective markers of learning-dependent neuroplastic changes, consistent with the principles underlying neurofeedback and self-regulation training.

From a methodological standpoint, these results validate the use of Unsupervised Clustering for monitoring trajectories rather than assigning static labels. Clinically and socially, this dynamic perspective is essential when working with vulnerable populations, as it respects individual variability and avoids deterministic interpretations.

Examples of two patients are presented in Figures 8.13 and 8.14.

Overall, the results from Sections 8.2 to 8.6 demonstrate that the proposed wearable EEG system can identify meaningful stress-related neurophysiological profiles,

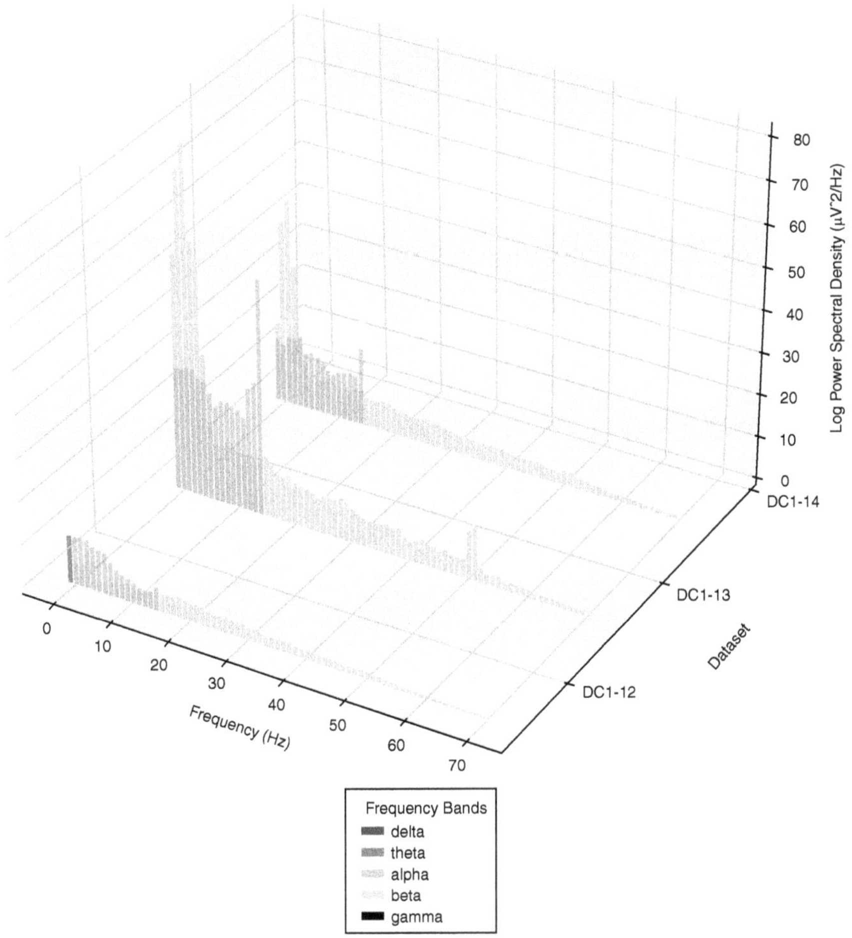

FIGURE 8.12 Cluster Type 4 – Characterized by Peaks in the Lower Beta Band.

track their temporal evolution, and support a personalized, nonclinical approach to stress coping and reduction.

8.8.7 Machine Learning Classifiers

This section evaluates the performance of ML classifiers on EEG data within the context of the Stress Management System. The widespread use of AI techniques for classification tasks across domains has gained immense popularity. However, due to the complexity and opacity of AI algorithms, there is a growing demand for tools that explain how they arrive at their results. In response to this demand, explaining how the system works is necessary, given the various approaches to analyzing AI techniques. In this way, the selected techniques can also generate explanations of the models under analysis without compromising their performance. This empowers humans to understand and trust the tasks performed by AI systems.

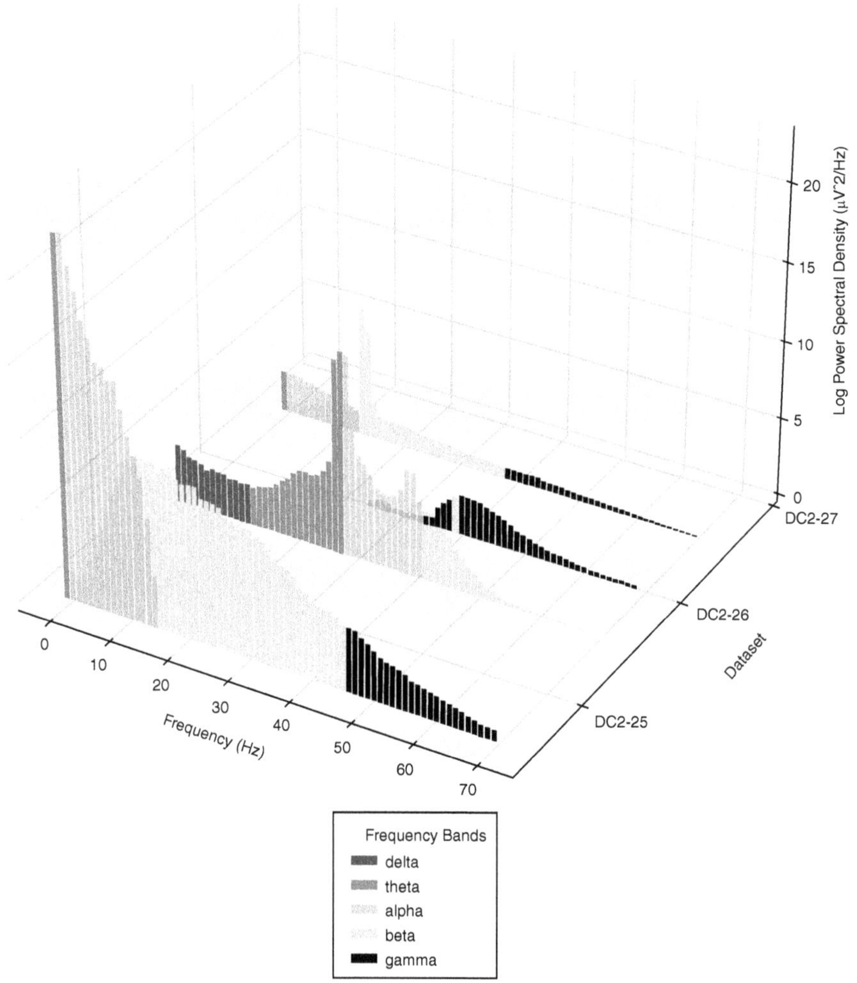

FIGURE 8.13 Spectral Analysis of Three Sessions of the Same Participant, Indicating a Decrease in Alpha and Beta Bands.

Various ML techniques have been widely used to provide comprehensive analytics across multiple data types. This Chapter proposes the use of three algorithms, based on different classification approaches, which are briefly defined below:

(i) K-Nearest Neighbors (KNN) is an instance-based classifier with no training model in its formulation. Instances are stored during the training phase, and predictions are made by majority voting over the distances to neighbors.
(ii) Support Vector Machine (SVM): The SVM classifier relies on information extracted from the training data, known as support vectors, which is used for class separation. This classifier works well with large databases due to its high computational complexity.

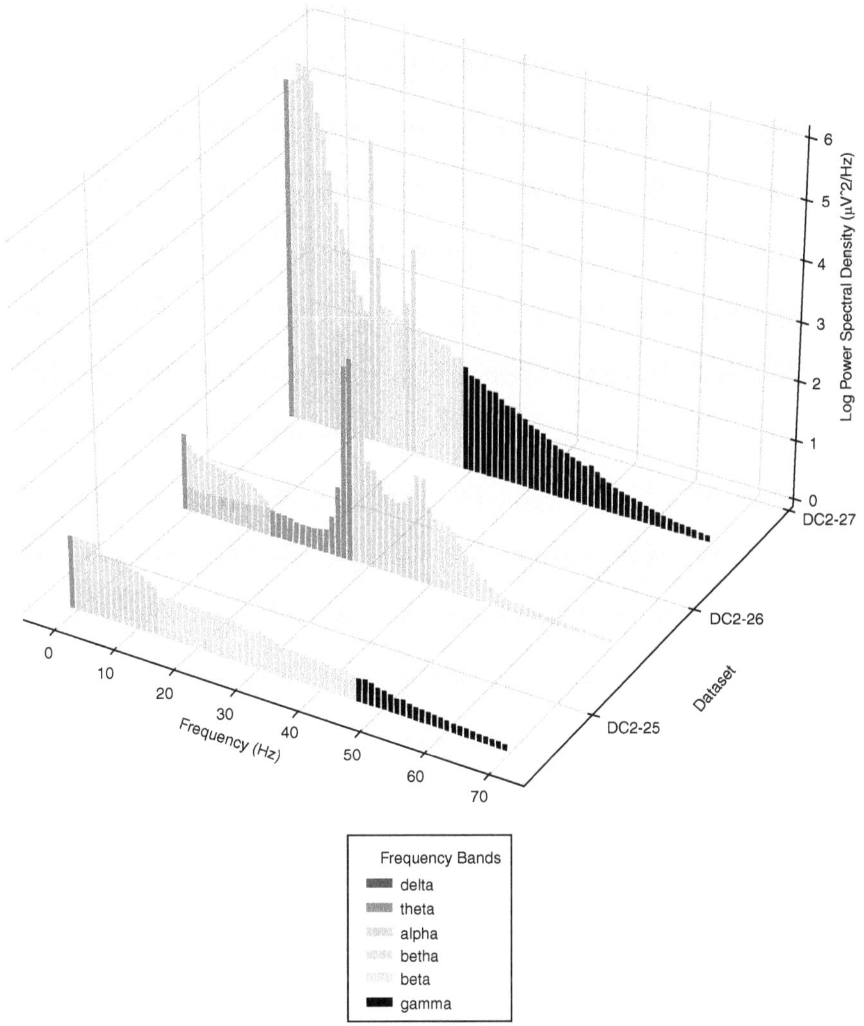

FIGURE 8.14 Spectral Analysis of Three Sessions of the Same Participant, Indicating an Increase in Alpha and Beta Bands.

(iii) Random Forrest (RF): adopts decision trees as a classification approach and is an ensemble bagging method, where predictions are generated from the combination of multiple decision tree classifiers.

To evaluate the performance of the proposed AI system, we consider four metrics presented in Equations one to four, as follows:

Accuracy (Acc): Calculates the percentage of correct predictions, considering all possible cases.

$$Acc = \frac{TP+TN}{TP+FP+TN+FN} \quad (1)$$

Precision (P): Estimates performance based on the correct positive prediction rate.

$$P = \frac{TP}{TP + FP} \tag{2}$$

Recall (R): Estimates performance based on the correct negative prediction rate.

$$R = \frac{TP}{TP + FN} \tag{3}$$

F1-score (F1): This is the harmonic mean of the P and R metrics, giving a general idea about both performances.

$$\mathrm{F1} = \frac{2 \times \mathrm{P} \times \mathrm{R}}{\mathrm{P} + \mathrm{R}} \tag{4}$$

Where:

TP – Total number of true positive cases
TN – Total number of true negative cases
FP – Total number of false positive cases
FN – Total number of false negative cases

TABLE 8.2
Results of Machine Learning Techniques for Electroencephalogram Signals in the Time Domain

Technique	Accuracy (Acc)	Precision (P)	Recall (R)	F1-score (F1)
K-Nearest Neighbors (KNN)	0.59	0.62	0.63	0.62
Support Vector Machine (SVM)	0.67	0.78	0.62	0.69
Random Forest (RF)	0.80	0.81	0.77	0.78

TABLE 8.3
Results of Machine Learning Techniques for Electroencephalogram Signals in the Frequency Domain

Technique	Accuracy (Acc)	Precision (P)	Recall (R)	F1-score (F1)
K-Nearest Neighbors (KNN)	0.67	0.63	0.64	0.63
Support Vector Machine (SVM)	0.81	0.83	0.79	0.80
Random Forest (RF)	0.85	0.88	0.81	0.84

TABLE 8.4
Results of Machine Learning Techniques for Electroencephalogram Signals in the Combined Time and Frequency Domain

Technique	Accuracy (Acc)	Precision (P)	Recall (R)	F1-score (F1)
K-Nearest Neighbors (KNN)	0.44	0.50	0.43	0.41
Support Vector Machine (SVM)	0.71	0.75	0.69	0.71
Random Forest (RF)	0.78	0.82	0.78	0.80

8.8.8 Electroencephalogram Time-Domain Features

The results in Table 8.2 indicate that the random forest (RF) technique performed satisfactorily on the time-domain EEG data.

The P of 0.81 for the RF technique, the R of 0.77, and the Acc of 0.80 indicate good classifier performance, especially given the clinical analysis of the signs.

8.8.9 EEG Frequency-Domain Features

The results presented in Table 8.3 indicate that the RF and SVM techniques achieved satisfactory performance on the frequency-domain EEG data.

The P of the RF technique of 0.88 and the R of 0.81, in addition to the Acc of 0.85, indicate a classifier of good performance, especially considering the clinical analysis of the signals. Similar analyses can be made for the SVM technique's P of 0.83, R of 0.79, and Acc of 0.81, indicating good classifier performance, especially given the clinical analysis of the signals.

8.8.10 EEG Time and Frequency-Domain Features Combined

The results in Table 8.4 indicate that the RF technique also performed best, followed by SVM. The P of the RF technique of 0.82 and the R of 0.78, in addition to the Acc of 0.78, indicate a classifier of good performance, especially considering the clinical analysis of the signs. It is worth noting that in this case, the KNN technique performed very poorly, indicating that it is not suitable for this combined set of features.

For EEG signals in the time domain, RF achieved an accuracy of 0.80, with balanced precision and recall. These results indicate that temporal EEG features already contain meaningful information for stress-related classification. However, the strongest performance was obtained using EEG signals in the frequency domain. In this case, RF achieved an accuracy of 0.85, with high precision (0.88) and recall (0.81), while SVM also performed well.

Combining time- and frequency-domain features did not improve classifier performance, suggesting that increased feature complexity may introduce redundancy rather than provide additional discriminative power. These findings indicate that frequency-domain EEG features—particularly alpha and beta band metrics may indicate the most informative inputs for stress detection in the proposed system.

As a conclusion, RF is the classification algorithm with the best performance. This choice reflects a deliberate design decision that prioritizes performance, robustness, and interpretability, key requirements for clinical decision-support systems. The results reinforce the notion that, in applied healthcare contexts, classical ML methods may outperform more complex models when data volume and variability are constrained. Future studies to improve these metrics may consider new classification techniques, such as XGBoost, or AutoML (automated ML) approaches.

8.9 CONCLUSION

This chapter presents the design, implementation, and evaluation of a wearable EEG-based system for stress assessment and coping, developed and validated in the real-world context of the IPREDE in Fortaleza, Brazil. The project was motivated by the high and sustained demand for scalable, nonclinical interventions capable of supporting mothers exposed to chronic psychosocial stress, a population whose emotional regulation directly impacts early childhood development and family well-being.

One of the main contributions of this work is the successful development and deployment of a comprehensive neurophysiological monitoring and analysis system within an institution characterized by high service demand and social vulnerability. The system demonstrated feasibility in terms of usability, robustness, and integration into IPREDE's multidisciplinary workflow, reinforcing its potential applicability in nonclinical, community-based environments. Importantly, the proposed solution was designed not as a diagnostic tool, but as a decision-support and self-regulation platform, aligned with ethical principles that avoid medicalization and stigma.

From a systems engineering perspective, the chapter introduced a modular architecture composed of three dynamically interacting subsystems: (i) the Cognitive and Relaxation Activities Subsystem, responsible for delivering structured neurofeedback and stimulation tasks; (ii) the AI Subsystem, dedicated to signal preprocessing, feature extraction, Unsupervised Clustering, and supervised classification; and (iii) the Data Analysis and Visualization Subsystem, which translated complex neurophysiological data into interpretable dashboards and reports. This modular design enhances scalability, transparency, and future extensibility, allowing individual components to evolve independently as new sensors, algorithms, or intervention strategies are incorporated.

A central scientific contribution of the study was the application of unsupervised learning techniques to identify stress-related neurophysiological profiles directly from wearable EEG data. Using Centroid-based Clustering, the system consistently identified four distinct cluster types, each representing a functional mode of stress regulation rather than a fixed or pathological category. These clusters captured meaningful variations in alpha and beta band dynamics, ranging from hypoactivation and disengagement (Cluster Type 1) to mixed regulatory engagement (Cluster Type 2), effective relaxation-related regulation (Cluster Type 3), and heightened arousal associated with sustained cognitive load (Cluster Type 4). The ability to observe inter-session transitions between clusters further demonstrated that these profiles are dynamic and sensitive to learning-dependent neuroplastic changes, reinforcing the suitability of the approach for longitudinal stress monitoring.

In parallel, the evaluation of supervised ML classifiers provided important insights into the discriminative power of different EEG feature sets. The results showed that frequency-domain features, particularly alpha and beta band metrics, yielded the most informative representations for stress-related classification. Among the evaluated algorithms, RF consistently achieved the best overall performance, balancing accuracy, precision, recall, and interpretability across time-domain, frequency-domain, and combined feature sets. These findings support the use of classical ensemble learning methods in applied neuroscience contexts where dataset size and variability are constrained, and where transparency and robustness are essential.

Despite these positive outcomes, several limitations and areas for improvement should be acknowledged. First, the study was conducted as a pilot with a relatively small sample size, which limits generalizability and motivates replication with larger, more diverse cohorts. Second, the EEG recordings relied primarily on low-density wearable devices, which, while suitable for ecological settings, constrain spatial resolution and advanced connectivity analyses. Third, although clustering and classification results were consistent, further validation against additional psychophysiological markers (e.g., HRV and EDA) would strengthen the multimodal interpretation. Finally, while the system demonstrated sensitivity to stress-related dynamics, long-term follow-up studies are needed to assess the durability of neurofeedback-induced regulatory changes.

Future development avenues naturally emerge from these findings. Planned directions include: (i) expansion of the study to larger populations and extended intervention periods; (ii) integration of multimodal physiological data fusion, combining EEG with autonomic and contextual signals; (iii) incorporation of advanced ML approaches such as XGBoost, AutoML, and explainable AI frameworks to enhance adaptability and transparency; and (iv) refinement of personalized intervention protocols based on individual regulatory trajectories rather than static profiles. Additionally, the modular architecture enables the system to adapt to other educational, occupational, and community settings characterized by chronic stress exposure.

In conclusion, this work demonstrates that wearable EEG technology, when combined with carefully designed system modeling and data-driven AI methods, can support meaningful, ethical, and scalable approaches to stress coping in nonclinical environments. By framing stress regulation as a dynamic learning and self-regulatory process, rather than a diagnostic condition, the proposed system contributes to applied neuroscience, digital health, and social innovation, offering a robust foundation for future research and real-world deployment.

REFERENCES

Anuário Brasileiro da Educação Básica. (2013). *Todos pela educação*. Moderna.

Bullmore, E., & Sporns, O. (2009). Complex brain networks: Graph theoretical analysis of structural and functional systems. *Nature Reviews Neuroscience*, 10(3), 186–198. https://doi.org/10.1038/nrn2575

Davidson, R. J. (2004). What does the prefrontal cortex "do" in affect: Perspectives on frontal EEG asymmetry research. *Biological Psychology*, 67(1–2), 219–234. https://doi.org/10.1016/j.biopsycho.2004.03.008

Dayan, E., & Cohen, L. G. (2011). Neuroplasticity subserving motor skill learning. *Neuron*, 72(3), 443–454. https://doi.org/10.1016/j.neuron.2011.10.008

Essex, M. J., Klein, M. H., Cho, E., & Kalin, N. H. (2002). Maternal stress beginning in infancy may sensitize children to later stress exposure: effects on cortisol and behavior. *Biological Psychiatry*, 52(8), 776–784.

Fernandes, J. V. M. R., Alexandria, A. R. D., Marques, J. A. L., Assis, D. F. D., Motta, P. C., & Silva, B. R. D. S. (2024). Emotion detection from EEG signals using machine deep learning models. *Bioengineering*, 11(8), 782.

Gruzelier, J. H. (2014). EEG-neurofeedback for optimising performance. I: A review of cognitive and affective outcome in healthy participants. *Neuroscience & Biobehavioral Reviews*, 44, 124–141. https://doi.org/10.1016/j.neubiorev.2013.09.015

Guilherme Cunha Santos, A., Marques, J. A.L., Rigo Jr., L., & Paulo Madeiro, J. (2023). Exploring EEG signal features for predicting post cardiac arrest prognosis. In *2023 Computing in Cardiology Conference*. https://doi.org/10.22489/CinC.2023.312

Hammond, D. C. (2011). What is neurofeedback: An update. *Journal of Neurotherapy*, 15(4), 305–336. https://doi.org/10.1080/10874208.2011.623090

Klimesch, W. (1999). EEG alpha and theta oscillations reflect cognitive and memory performance: A review and analysis. *Brain Research Reviews*, 29(2–3), 169–195. https://doi.org/10.1016/S0165-0173%2898%2900056-3

Li, G., Huang, S., Xu, W., Jiao, W., Jiang, Y., Gao, Z., & Zhang, J. (2020). The impact of mental fatigue on brain activity: A comparative study both in resting state and task state using EEG. *BMC Neuroscience*, 21(1), 20.

Marques, J. A. L., Bernardo Gois, F. N., Nunes da Silveira, J. A., Li, T., & Fong, S. J. (2022). AI and deep learning for processing the huge amount of patient-centric data that assist in clinical decisions. In A. K. Bhoi, V. H. C. de Albuquerque, P. N. Srinivasu, & G. Marques (Eds.), *Cognitive and Soft Computing Techniques for the Analysis of Healthcare Data* (pp. 101–121). Academic Press. https://doi.org/10.1016/B978-0-323-85751-2.00001-3

Marques, J. A. L., Cortez, P. C., Madeiro, J. P. D. V., Fong, S. J., Schlindwein, F. S., & Albuquerque, V. H. C. D. (2019). Automatic cardiotocography diagnostic system based on Hilbert transform and adaptive threshold technique. *IEEE Access*, 7, 73085–73094. https://doi.org/10.1109/ACCESS.2018.2877933

Marques, J. A. L., Cortez, P. C., Madeiro, J. P. V., Albuquerque, V. H. C., Fong, S. J., & Schlindwein, F. S. (2020). Nonlinear characterization and complexity analysis of cardiotocographic examinations using entropy measures. *Journal of Supercomputing*, 76(2), 1305–1320. https://doi.org/10.1007/s11227-018-2570-8

Marques, J. A. L., Gois, F. N. B., Madeiro, J. P. do V., Li, T., & Fong, S. J. (2022). Artificial neural network-based approaches for computer-aided disease diagnosis and treatment. In A. K. Bhoi, V. H. C. de Albuquerque, P. N. Srinivasu, & G. Marques (Eds.), *Cognitive and Soft Computing Techniques for the Analysis of Healthcare Data* (pp. 79–99). Academic Press. https://doi.org/10.1016/B978-0-323-85751-2.00008-6

Marques, J. A. L., Han, T., Wu, W., Madeiro, J. P. do V., Neto, A. V. L., Gravina, R., Fortino, G., & de Albuquerque, V. H. C. (2021). IoT-based smart health system for ambulatory maternal and fetal monitoring. *IEEE Internet of Things Journal*, 8(23), 16814–16824. https://doi.org/10.1109/JIOT.2020.3037759

McEwen, B. S. (2007). Physiology and neurobiology of stress and adaptation: Central role of the brain. *Physiological Reviews*, 87(3), 873–904. https://doi.org/10.1152/physrev.00041.2006

Micoulaud-Franchi, J. A., McGonigal, A., Lopez, R., Daudet, C., Kotwas, I., & Bartolomei, F. (2015). Electroencephalographic neurofeedback: Level of evidence in mental and brain disorders and suggestions for good clinical practice. *Neurophysiologie Clinique/Clinical Neurophysiology*, 45(6), 423–433. https://doi.org/10.1016/j.neucli.2015.10.077

Nguyen Van, S., Marques, J. A. L., Biala, T. A., & Li, Y. (2021). Identification of latent risk clinical attributes for children born under IUGR condition using machine learning techniques. *Computer Methods and Programs in Biomedicine*, 200, 105842. https://doi.org/10.1016/j.cmpb.2020.105842

Organisation for Economic Co-operation and Development. (2002). *Understanding the Brain: Towards a New Learning Science*. OECD Publishing.

Pacak, K., & Palkovits, M. (2001). Stressor specificity of central neuroendocrine responses: implications for stress-related disorders. *Endocrine Reviews*, 22(4), 502–548.

Relvas, M. P. (2010). *Dificuldades de aprendizagem: Uma abordagem psicopedagógica*. Wak Editora.

Ros, T., Munneke, M. A. M., Ruge, D., Gruzelier, J. H., & Rothwell, J. C. (2014). Endogenous control of waking brain rhythms induces neuroplasticity in humans. *European Journal of Neuroscience*, 39(12), 2081–2093. https://doi.org/10.1111/ejn.12530

Singh, P., Chaudhary, G., & Marques, J. A. L. (2023). Medical information extraction of clinical notes and pictorial visualisation of electronic medical records summary interface. In Preeti Nagrath, Jafar A. Alzubi, Bhawna Singla, Joel J. P. C. Rodrigues, & A. K. Verma (Eds.), *Smart Distributed Embedded Systems for Healthcare Applications* (pp. 29–40). CRC Press.

Sitaram, R., Ros, T., Stoeckel, L., Haller, S., Scharnowski, F., Lewis-Peacock, J., … & Sulzer, J. (2017). Closed-loop brain training: The science of neurofeedback. *Nature Reviews Neuroscience*, 18(2), 86–100. https://doi.org/10.1038/nrn.2016.164

Yan, K., Li, T., Marques, J. A. L., Gao, J., Fong, S. J., Yan, K., Li, T., Marques, J. A. L., Gao, J., & Fong, S. J. (2023). A review on multimodal machine learning in medical diagnostics. *Mathematical Biosciences and Engineering*, 20(5), 8708–8726. https://doi.org/10.3934/mbe.2023382

Zhao, T., Gois, F. N. B., Marques, J. A. L., dos Santos Silva, B. R., Cortez, P., Jagatheesaperumal, S. K., & de Albuquerque, V. H. C. (2025). AutoML-based EEG signal analysis in neuromarketing classification using biclustering method. *Applied Soft Computing*, 181, 113412.

9 Explainable Artificial Intelligence for Wearable Multimodal Stress Detection

Deep Learning Interpretation and High-Accuracy Evaluation on the WESAD Dataset

Vitor Emmanuel Andrade, Roney Malaguti, Francisco Nauber Bernardo Gois, Ganesh R. Naik, and João Alexandre Lobo Marques

9.1 INTRODUCTION

Chronic psychological stress has consolidated itself as one of the most insidious challenges of contemporary public health, driving a silent crisis that places an increasing burden on healthcare systems worldwide. Far from being a transient emotional response, stress initiates a complex cascade of neuroendocrine reactions that, when persistently dysregulated, contribute directly to the etiology of cardiovascular diseases, immune suppression, and severe neuropsychiatric disorders.

Historically, clinical assessment of stress-related conditions has relied almost exclusively on self-reported psychometric instruments or on sporadic physiological measurements conducted in controlled laboratory environments. While methodologically convenient, these approaches fail to capture the temporal, contextual, and dynamic nature of physiological responses as they unfold in daily life, significantly limiting their ecological validity.

The recent convergence of affective computing and the Internet of Medical Things (IoMT) has enabled a paradigm shift in mental health monitoring. The widespread adoption of wearable devices has enabled continuous, noninvasive acquisition of biomarkers associated with the autonomic nervous system (ANS), opening new

 DOI: 10.1201/9781003500445-9

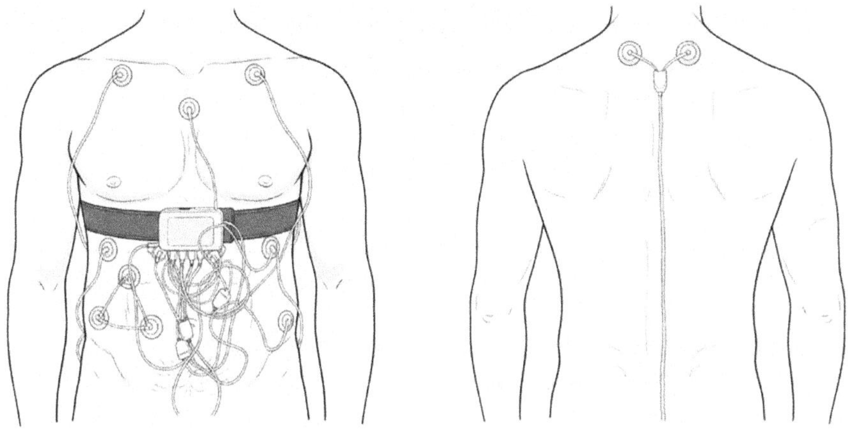

FIGURE 9.1 Wrist-Worn Empatica E4 Sensor Placement for Real-Time Multimodal Physiological Signal Acquisition in the Wearable Stress and Affect Detection Stress and Affect Detection Protocol. (Schmidt et al., 2018.)

avenues for real-world stress detection. Within this context, the wearable stress and affect detection (WESAD) dataset has emerged as a benchmark in the literature, providing high-fidelity multimodal physiological recordings that capture the autonomic response to experimentally induced stress under standardized conditions (Schmidt et al., 2018).

Figure 9.1 illustrates the sensor configuration adopted in the WESAD protocol, highlighting the Empatica E4 device on the wrist and its role in enabling unobtrusive, continuous monitoring. The figure illustrates the inherent complexity of multimodal data acquisition for affective state recognition, as multiple physiological subsystems are measured simultaneously through a single wearable form factor. By focusing on wrist-based sensing, the experimental setup mirrors realistic deployment scenarios in which user compliance, comfort, and long-term wearability are critical constraints, thereby reinforcing the dataset's ecological relevance.

In this study, we restrict the analysis to the wrist-worn Empatica E4 signals to emulate a ubiquitous monitoring scenario. This configuration captures heterogeneous physiological modalities—optical (blood volume pulse (BVP) for heart rate (HR) estimation), electrodermal activity (EDA for sympathetic activation), thermal (skin temperature reflecting vasomotor regulation), and mechanical (accelerometry or ACC, for movement). The synchronous acquisition of these channels is essential because stress manifests systemically: activation of the hypothalamic-pituitary-adrenal (HPA) axis induces concurrent tachycardia, peripheral vasoconstriction, and phasic increases in skin conductance. However, as implicitly suggested by the wrist placement shown in Figure 9.1, this convenience comes at the cost of increased susceptibility to motion artifacts, which can confound physiological interpretations by introducing behavioral noise that overlaps with stress-induced responses.

To address the high dimensionality, nonlinearity, and temporal dependencies inherent in such physiological time series, the literature has progressively shifted from

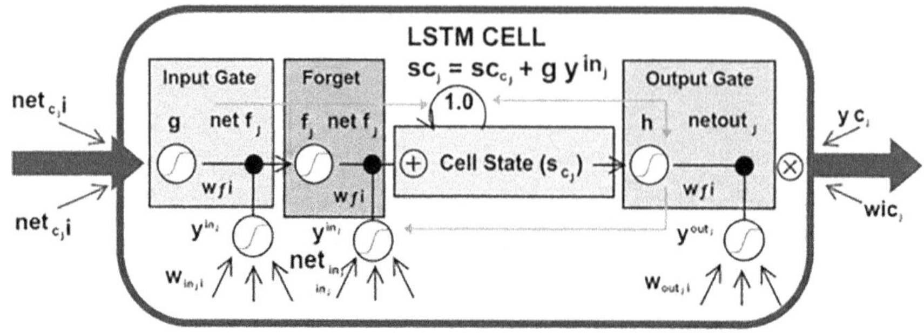

FIGURE 9.2 Internal Structure of an Long Short-Term Memory Cell With Its Gating Mechanisms. (Hochreiter & Schmidhuber, 1997.)

classical statistical approaches toward deep learning (DL) architectures (Fawaz et al., 2019). Among these, long short-term memory (LSTM) networks have demonstrated superior performance in modeling sequential biosignals, particularly in stress and affect recognition tasks. Their architectural design enables end-to-end learning directly from raw signals, allowing the model to capture both short-term fluctuations and long-range temporal dependencies.

Figure 9.2 depicts the internal structure of an LSTM memory cell, detailing the gating mechanisms—input, forget, and output gates—that regulate the flow of information across time. This architecture explains why LSTMs are well-suited for physiological signal processing: the gates selectively preserve or discard historical information, enabling the network to retain traces of prior stressors and contextualize the current physiological state. In theory, this temporal memory enables the model to distinguish transient artifacts from sustained autonomic responses, a property particularly relevant in noisy wearable data streams.

Despite these advantages, the same architectural complexity illustrated in Figure 9.2 also underpins a major limitation of LSTM-based models: their opacity. The layered nonlinear transformations obscure the causal pathways linking physiological inputs to classification outputs, effectively rendering the model a "black box" (Rudin, 2019). In healthcare applications, this opacity introduces a critical epistemological risk, as models may achieve high accuracy by exploiting spurious correlations—such as repetitive wrist movements captured by accelerometers—rather than learning genuine markers of autonomic stress dysregulation (London, 2019).

As a consequence, predictive accuracy alone is insufficient for clinical validation. Regulatory agencies increasingly emphasize transparency, auditability, and explainability as mandatory requirements for artificial intelligence-based (AI-based) medical systems. In response, this chapter proposes a comparative investigation between two modeling paradigms: (i) a deep LSTM architecture trained on raw multimodal time series and (ii) a multilayer perceptron (MLP) trained on engineered physiological features. To interrogate the decision-making processes of both models, we employ explainable artificial intelligence (XAI) techniques, specifically integrated gradients (IG) (Sundararajan, Taly, & Yan, 2017).

Research Question:

RQ: *Do high-performing DL models for stress detection learn physiologically meaningful markers of autonomic stress, or do they primarily rely on behavioral correlates such as motion artifacts?*

Research Hypotheses:

- **H1:** The LSTM model trained on raw signals achieves predictive performance comparable to or superior to the feature-based MLP model.
- **H2:** Explainability analysis reveals that both models assign significant importance to motion-related features, particularly ACC.
- **H3:** IG enables discrimination between models driven by true autonomic physiology (EDA, HR, temperature) and those relying on spurious behavioral cues.

The remainder of this chapter is organized as follows. Section 9.3 provides a comprehensive review of related work on wearable-based stress detection, with particular emphasis on DL architectures and the role of XAI in physiological computing. Section 9.4 details the experimental framework, including the dataset description, preprocessing pipeline, model architectures, and validation protocol. Section 9.5 presents the quantitative results alongside the explainability analysis, highlighting how different physiological and behavioral signals contribute to model decisions. Section 9.6 discusses the findings from clinical, methodological, and regulatory perspectives, emphasizing their implications for trustworthy AI in health applications. Finally, Section 9.7 concludes the chapter by summarizing the main contributions and outlining directions for future research.

Figure 9.3 provides a comprehensive overview of the research framework established in this study, spanning from data acquisition to final implications. The diagram delineates the methodological pipeline, commencing in the upper-left quadrant with the use of the multimodal WESAD dataset, which provides physiological and motion signals collected exclusively from the Empatica E4 wrist-worn device, including BVP, electrodermal activity (EDA), skin temperature (TEMP), and tri-axial ACC. These signals feed into the core methodology illustrated in the upper-right quadrant, where two complementary modeling paradigms are evaluated: an end-to-end LSTM trained on raw multimodal time series and a feature-based MLP leveraging physiologically informed descriptors. To ensure transparency and physiological validity, XAI techniques are integrated to interpret model decisions and assess the contribution of individual modalities and features. As summarized in the bottom-left quadrant, the experimental results demonstrate high classification performance while identifying key predictive factors. In particular, the analysis highlights the dominant role of autonomic markers derived from BVP and EDA, along with contextual information from motion signals, in stress prediction. Finally, the bottom-right quadrant emphasizes the study's conclusion that incorporating explainability is essential not only for achieving robust performance but also for establishing trust, interpretability, and feasibility in real-world wearable stress monitoring applications.

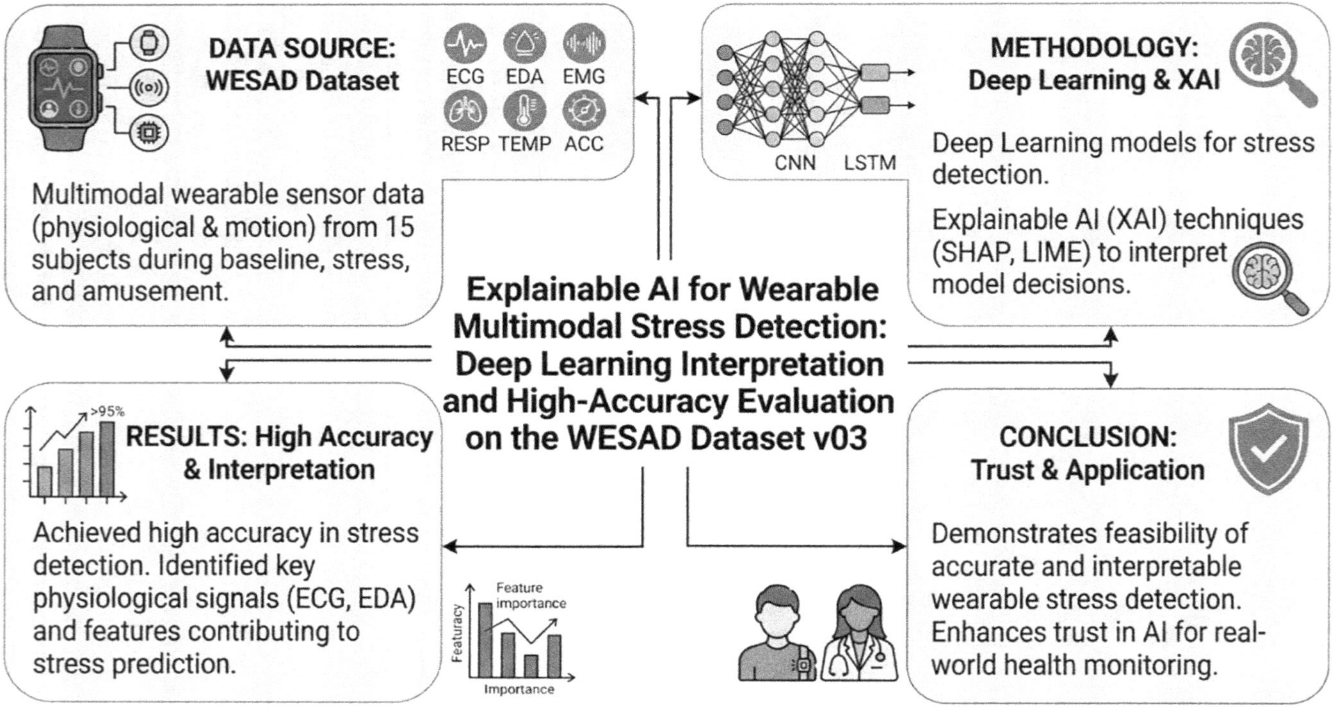

FIGURE 9.3 A Visual Overview of the Research Framework, Methodology, and Key Findings Presented in the Study "Explainable Artificial Intelligence for Wearable Multimodal Stress Detection".

9.2 THEORETICAL BACKGROUND

The development of a robust and explainable stress detection system requires the synergistic integration of multiple domains of knowledge, bridging the traditional boundaries between biomedicine and computer science. This section establishes the multidisciplinary foundation necessary for understanding the present study and is structured around four interconnected pillars. First, we examine the physiological mechanisms underlying stress and their manifestation in signals captured by wearable devices, thereby justifying the selection of the biomarkers employed. Second, we describe the characteristics of the WESAD dataset, which serves as the controlled experimental environment for this work. Third, we ground the DL architectures applied to time-series data, with particular emphasis on LSTM networks. Finally, we introduce the principles of XAI, which are essential for ensuring the clinical transparency and trustworthiness of the proposed models.

Figure 9.4 illustrates the comprehensive theoretical framework underpinning this study, demonstrating the synergistic integration of biomedicine and computer science required for robust stress detection. The framework is structured around four interconnected foundational pillars visualized in the diagram. The first pillar, *Stress physiology and wearable sensors*, establishes the biomedical foundation by depicting how the ANS orchestrates the stress response through the antagonistic balance of the sympathetic ("fight-or-flight") and parasympathetic ("rest-and-digest") branches. It highlights how wearable sensors capture manifestations of acute stress, such as increased EDA, driven solely by sympathetic innervation, and altered heart rate variability (HRV), reflecting autonomic interplay, while ACC provides crucial contextual information on physical movement versus mental stress. The second pillar outlines the WESAD Dataset as the controlled experimental environment. It illustrates the rigorous protocol for acquiring data using sensing devices such as the Empatica E4, ensuring reliable ground-truth labels by segmenting recordings into distinct affective states: baseline, amusement, acute stress induction (via the Trier Social Stress Test or TSST), and recovery via meditation. The third pillar focuses on DL architectures for time-series modeling. The figure contrasts traditional feature-based approaches relying on manual engineering with end-to-end representation learning architectures, specifically highlighting LSTM networks. LSTMs are well-suited to modeling long-range temporal dependencies in raw physiological signals through specialized memory cells and gating mechanisms. Finally, the fourth pillar addresses XAI for clinical transparency and trust. It demonstrates the application of post-hoc techniques to interpret the "black box" LSTM model. The resulting feature attribution heatmaps enable validation of model decisions, ensuring that predictions are driven by genuine high-relevance autonomic markers (such as EDA and HRV) rather than low-relevance artifacts or noise from ACC.

9.2.1 Stress Physiology and Wearable Sensors

Wearable and Internet of things-based (IoT-based) health monitoring systems have been widely investigated for continuous physiological assessment in real-world environments. Prior studies have demonstrated the feasibility of ambulatory monitoring

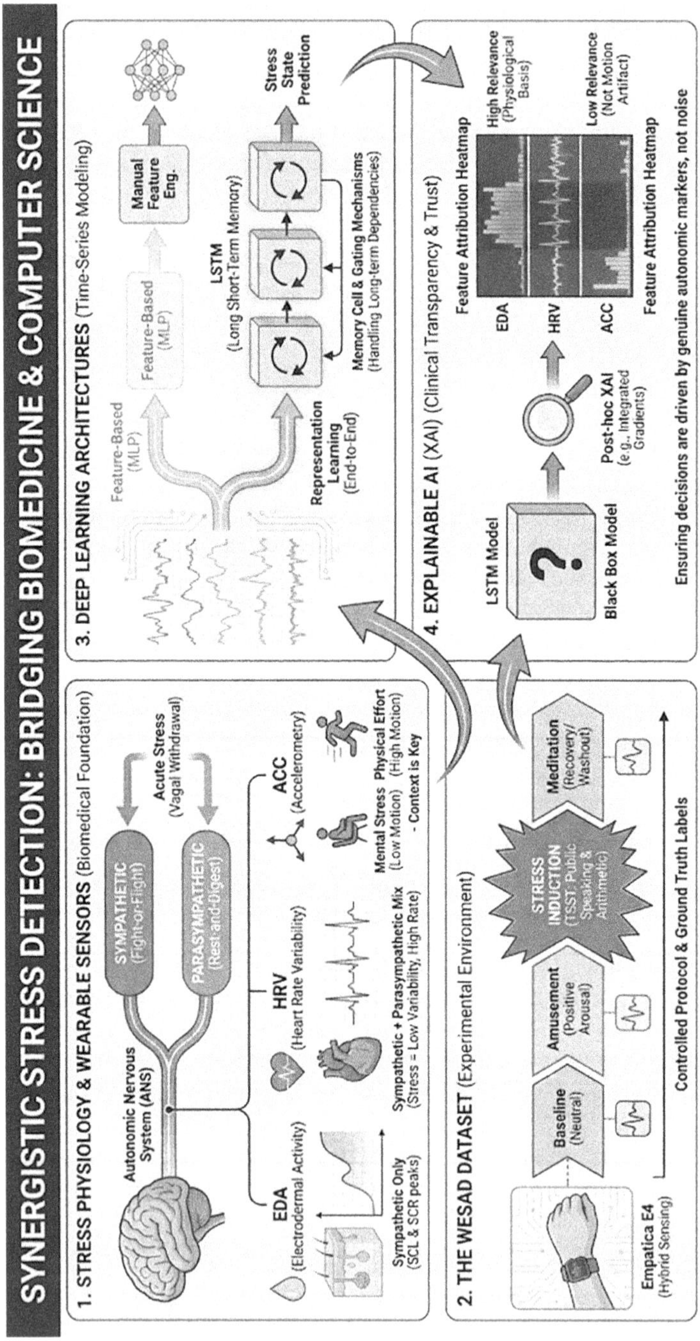

FIGURE 9.4 Bridging Biomedicine and Computer Science: A Four-Pillar Framework for Stress Detection Combining Physiological Sensing, Controlled Data Acquisition, Deep Learning, and Explainable Artificial Intelligence.

using electrocardiogram-centered (ECG-centered) architectures for maternal health, cardiac risk assessment, and long-term cardiovascular surveillance, highlighting the potential of connected wearable platforms for clinical decision support (Nguyen Van et al., 2021; Cavalcante et al., 2023).

In parallel, advances in DL have enabled robust noise detection and signal quality assessment in ECG streams collected from wearable devices, further strengthening the reliability of such systems in uncontrolled environments (Caldas et al., 2023). Although ECG-based solutions remain central in many clinical applications, recent trends increasingly favor wrist-worn devices due to their practicality, scalability, and user adherence, motivating this study's focus on multimodal pulse-based sensing.

Automated detection of affective states requires a deep understanding of the biological mechanisms underlying the stress response, which should not be interpreted as an isolated event but rather as a systemic reaction orchestrated by the ANS. The ANS functions as a rapid control interface between the brain and peripheral organs and is functionally divided into two antagonistic branches. The first is the sympathetic nervous system (SNS), which mobilizes energy in response to perceived threats, thereby characterizing the classic fight-or-flight response. The second is the parasympathetic nervous system (PNS), which promotes energy conservation and physiological recovery and is associated with rest-and-digest states.

During an episode of acute stress, a phenomenon known as vagal withdrawal occurs, characterized by inhibition of parasympathetic activity and marked activation of the sympathetic branch. This coordinated response leads to immediate changes in physiological parameters that can be measured by noninvasive wearable sensors.

EDA, historically known as the galvanic skin response (GSR), is widely regarded as one of the most robust biomarkers for stress detection due to its exclusive sympathetic innervation. Unlike the heart, which is modulated by both the sympathetic and para SNSs, eccrine sweat glands are activated solely by the SNS. When an individual perceives a stressor, hypothalamic activation triggers the release of acetylcholine at sudomotor nerve endings, causing the filling of sweat gland ducts. This process increases the skin's electrical conductance even before sweat becomes visible on the surface.

The EDA signal comprises two distinct components. The first is the skin conductance level (SCL), which reflects tonic baseline activity and varies slowly over time. The second is the skin conductance response (SCR), which appears as rapid, transient peaks in response to discrete stimuli or stressors (Greco et al., 2016).

In parallel with the electrodermal response, the cardiovascular system undergoes immediate adaptations to support anticipated metabolic demands. HRV is considered the gold-standard metric for quantifying the dynamic interaction between the sympathetic and parasympathetic branches at the sinoatrial node of the heart. Under resting conditions, parasympathetic dominance induces high beat-to-beat variability. During stress, increased sympathetic dominance elevates the mean HR and reduces variability, resulting in a more rigid, regular cardiac rhythm. Modern wearable devices capture these dynamics through photoplethysmography (PPG), enabling continuous, real-time monitoring of cardiovascular responses.

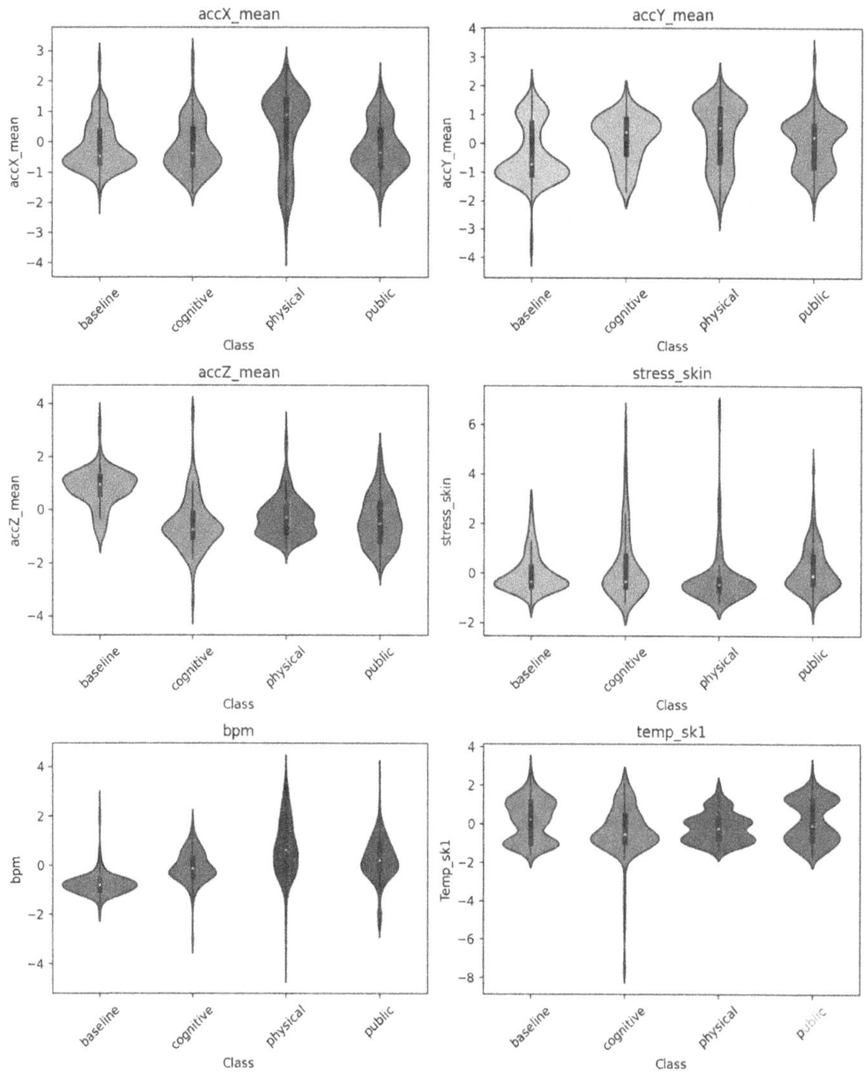

FIGURE 9.5 Violin Plots of Physiological Feature Distributions Across Baseline, Cognitive Load, Socio-Evaluative Stress, and Physical Effort Conditions.

The distribution of these physiological signals under different experimental stress conditions is illustrated in Figure 9.5.

The HR (bpm) plots show a progressive increase in median values from baseline through cognitive and social stress conditions, reaching their maximum during physical effort. This confirms that while psychological stress elevates HR, physical exercise induces a substantially stronger cardiovascular response, which may confound classification algorithms that rely exclusively on this metric.

In contrast, the electrodermal activity plots reveal a distinct pattern. Skin conductance responses are notably higher and more variable during cognitive load and socio-evaluative stress than during physical exertion or rest. This observation reinforces the specificity of EDA as a marker of psychological arousal, as it is less influenced by muscular metabolic demand than HR.

Additionally, the ACC signals (accX, accY, accZ) indicate that mental stress conditions (cognitive and public) exhibit movement profiles that closely resemble the baseline state, characterized by low variance, and differ sharply from those in the physical effort condition. This distinction is fundamental to the present study, as it suggests that a well-trained multimodal model should leverage motion data not merely to detect activity, but to contextualize physiological changes—discriminating, for example, between an increase in HR driven by anxiety (low movement) and one driven by physical exercise (high movement).

9.2.2 The Wearable Stress and Affect Detection Dataset

The rapid growth of patient-centric medical data has driven the adoption of AI techniques capable of handling large-scale, heterogeneous, and multimodal information streams. DL models have been extensively applied to support clinical decision-making, disease diagnosis, and prognostic analysis across diverse medical domains.

Recent advances further emphasize the importance of multimodal learning strategies that integrate physiological signals, clinical records, and behavioral data to improve robustness and generalization in medical diagnostics (Yan et al., 2023). However, the increasing complexity of such models has raised concerns regarding transparency and trustworthiness, reinforcing the need for XAI approaches in healthcare systems (Rodrigues et al., 2023).

The validation of stress detection algorithms requires data that capture high-quality physiological signals and provide reliable ground-truth labels synchronized with well-defined stress-inducing events. In this context, the WESAD dataset has established itself as a reference benchmark in the affective computing literature and is widely used to evaluate and compare DL models for stress recognition (Schmidt et al., 2018). Released by the University of Siegen, the dataset comprises multimodal recordings from 15 participants (mean age 27.5 ± 2.4 years) who were exposed to a rigorously designed experimental protocol intended to elicit three distinct affective states: neutral, stress, and amusement (Schmidt et al., 2018).

A key strength of the WESAD dataset lies in its hybrid sensing approach, which combines clinical-grade chest-mounted sensors (RespiBAN) with a commercial wrist-worn wearable device (Empatica E4). This dual configuration enables researchers to benchmark consumer-grade wearable measurements against medical-grade physiological signals, thereby assessing the feasibility and limitations of ubiquitous stress monitoring in real-world settings (Schmidt et al., 2018; Siirtola, 2019).

The WESAD experimental protocol was carefully structured to ensure internal validity and to isolate psychological stress from other forms of physiological arousal. Each recording session lasted approximately two hours and began with a 20-minute baseline phase, during which participants remained seated and relaxed while reading neutral magazines. This phase establishes individual physiological reference levels under resting conditions (Schmidt et al., 2018).

Stress induction was achieved using the TSST, a gold-standard paradigm in experimental psychology that combines cognitive load with socio-evaluative threat (Schmidt et al., 2018; Gedam & Paul, 2021). In the WESAD protocol, the TSST consists of two consecutive tasks: a simulated public speaking task, in which participants are asked to present their personal qualifications to an evaluative panel, followed by a mental arithmetic task requiring rapid serial subtraction under time pressure. Together, these tasks reliably elicit acute psychological stress and robust autonomic responses (Schmidt et al., 2018).

Unlike studies that focus solely on a stress-rest dichotomy, WESAD includes an additional "Amusement" condition, induced by humorous video clips. This phase plays a critical role in training classifiers capable of discriminating between stress (negative valence, high arousal) and amusement (positive valence, high arousal), as both affective states can elevate HR and skin conductance, potentially leading to false positives in simplistic models (Schmidt et al., 2018).

The temporal organization of the protocol, including intermediate recovery phases labeled as "Meditation," is designed to ensure that physiological signals return toward baseline levels before the introduction of a new stimulus. This temporal separation is essential for minimizing carry-over effects and preserving the separability of affective states, as illustrated in Figure 9.6.

Figure 9.6 details the temporal segmentation used to generate the class labels that support supervised model training. Each temporal block (Baseline, Amusement, TSST) corresponds to a specific target class in the stress classification task. The inclusion of meditation periods between stimuli serves as a physiological washout mechanism, allowing the ANS to recover from prior activation and reducing the risk that residual effects contaminate subsequent conditions (Schmidt et al., 2018; Siirtola, 2019).

In the present study, we focus exclusively on data acquired from the wrist-worn Empatica E4 device during the active experimental phases. The device, worn on the nondominant wrist, samples PPG at 64 Hz, EDA and TEMP at 4 Hz, and tri-axial

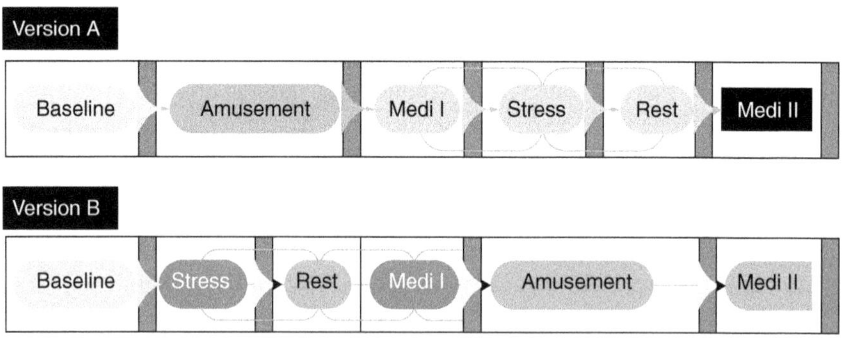

FIGURE 9.6 Timeline of the Wearable Stress and Affect Detection Experimental Protocol: Alternating Phases of Baseline Calibration, Amusement Induction, Trier Social Stress Test, and Meditation Recovery With Self-Report Assessment Intervals. (Schmidt et al., 2018.)

ACC at 32 Hz. This sampling configuration provides sufficient temporal resolution for analyzing cardiac variability and phasic electrodermal responses, while simultaneously capturing motion-related artifacts relevant to real-world wearable deployments (Schmidt et al., 2018).

The consistency and reliability of the WESAD labels are further reinforced by subjective self-reports collected after each protocol phase. Participants completed standardized questionnaires, including the self-assessment manikin (SAM), to rate valence, arousal, and dominance dimensions (Schmidt et al., 2018). These subjective assessments serve as a cross-validation mechanism for the experimentally assigned labels, confirming that participants experienced the intended affective states. Statistical analyses reported by the dataset authors demonstrate that the stress condition (TSST) elicited significant increases in HR and electrodermal responses relative to baseline, thereby physiologically validating the protocol and supporting the use of these signals for training deep neural networks (DNNs) (Schmidt et al., 2018).

9.2.3 Explainable and Interpretable Artificial Intelligence in Biomedical Signals

Explainability has become a critical requirement in biomedical signal analysis, particularly in applications involving DL models trained on complex and high-dimensional physiological data. While DNNs have demonstrated remarkable performance across a wide range of medical tasks, their inherent opacity poses significant challenges in safety-critical domains, where clinical decisions must be justified, audited, and aligned with established physiological knowledge. As a result, XAI has emerged not merely as a complementary analytical tool, but as a foundational requirement for trustworthy AI-driven healthcare systems.

Recent studies have explored explainable and AutoML-based approaches in electroencephalogram (EEG) signal analysis for emotion recognition, neuromarketing, and clinical prognosis, highlighting the capacity of transparent models to extract physiologically meaningful insights from nonstationary biosignals. For instance, explainability-driven analyses in EEG-based emotion recognition have demonstrated how attribution methods can uncover frequency bands, cortical regions, and temporal patterns associated with affective states, thereby bridging the gap between predictive performance and neurophysiological interpretability (Zhao et al., 2025; Fernandes et al., 2024). Similarly, AutoML frameworks combined with explainability techniques have been shown to mitigate model selection bias while preserving interpretability, particularly in scenarios involving heterogeneous patient populations and limited labeled data.

Beyond EEG, the relevance of XAI extends across multiple biosignal modalities, including cardiovascular, electrodermal, and multimodal wearable data. In these contexts, explainability enables the identification of whether model predictions are grounded in legitimate autonomic markers or driven by spurious correlations related to motion, noise, or data imbalance. This distinction is especially critical in wearable sensing, where behavioral confounders are intrinsically coupled with physiological responses and can lead to misleading performance gains under optimistic validation protocols.

Moreover, explainability plays a pivotal role in supporting subject-independent generalization, a key requirement for real-world deployment of wearable health monitoring systems. By revealing how different models weight physiological versus behavioral inputs, XAI provides mechanistic insight into generalization failures that remain invisible to aggregate performance metrics alone. Consequently, explainability facilitates not only post-hoc interpretation, but also model auditing, comparative evaluation, and informed design choices throughout the development lifecycle.

Taken together, these findings reinforce the broader relevance of XAI techniques in biomedical signal analysis and motivate their systematic application in wearable stress-detection systems. In such applications, clinical interpretability is essential not only for user trust and ethical accountability but also for regulatory compliance and patient safety. By embedding explainability at the core of the analytical pipeline, wearable affective computing systems can move beyond black-box prediction toward transparent, auditable, and clinically meaningful decision support.

9.2.4 Affective Computing and Emotion Recognition

Beyond physiological sensing, affective computing research has extensively explored facial expression analysis and imaging-based approaches for emotion recognition. Advances in DL architectures, including convolutional and transformer-based models, have enabled robust emotion classification from facial data under controlled laboratory conditions and in real-time applications, demonstrating high discriminative performance across multiple benchmark datasets. Such approaches have been successfully applied in domains ranging from human-computer interaction and digital marketing to mental health screening, underscoring the versatility of vision-based affective computing.

Despite these advances, facial expression-based emotion recognition systems remain inherently sensitive to a variety of external and contextual factors. Variations in illumination, head pose, occlusions, camera quality, and cultural expression patterns can substantially degrade performance outside controlled environments. In addition, vision-based methods raise significant concerns related to privacy, data protection, and user acceptance, particularly in continuous monitoring scenarios where explicit consent and sustained user compliance cannot be guaranteed.

In contrast, wearable physiological sensing offers a more discreet, privacy-preserving, and continuous alternative for affective state monitoring. Physiological signals captured via wrist-worn devices can be collected unobtrusively over extended periods, enabling longitudinal assessment of stress and emotional dynamics in naturalistic settings. Unlike facial analysis, which depends on visual availability and user engagement, wearable sensing operates independently of environmental visibility and minimizes behavioral disruption, making it especially suitable for real-world stress detection and health monitoring applications.

These considerations motivate the present study's focus on multimodal wearable data rather than on vision-based affective computing. By leveraging physiological signals reflecting ANS activity, the proposed approach aims to achieve robust stress detection while addressing the practical, ethical, and operational limitations of imaging-based emotion recognition systems.

In addition, bibliometric and methodological analyses have shown rapid growth in facial- and gesture-based affective computing research over the past decade, driven largely by advances in DL and computer vision (Qian & Marques, 2023).

9.2.5 Deep Learning Architectures for Time-Series Data

The processing of physiological signals acquired via wearable sensors poses distinct challenges due to the sequential and temporal characteristics of the data. Unlike static images, which are dominated by spatial correlations, biosignals such as EDA and BVP exhibit inherent temporal dependencies, in which the current physiological state is substantially conditioned by antecedent events (Fawaz et al., 2019). To address this complexity, the extant literature has coalesced around two principal modeling paradigms: feature-based approaches, which depend on manually engineered descriptors and conventional neural architectures such as the MLP; and representation-learning (end-to-end) approaches, which employ deep architectures—notably convolutional neural networks (CNNs) and LSTM networks—to extract discriminative patterns directly from raw time-series data.

9.2.5.1 Multilayer Perceptron and the Need for Feature Engineering

The MLP represents the quintessential architecture of artificial neural networks ANNs), consisting of fully connected layers arranged in a feedforward structure. However, when applied to time-series data, MLPs exhibit a fundamental architectural limitation: they are inherently agnostic to the sequential order of the input data (Bobade & Vani, 2020). If raw temporal samples are directly fed into an MLP, each time point is treated as an independent feature, causing the model to disregard temporal dynamics and lose the contextual information embedded in signal evolution over time (Gedam & Paul, 2021).

To mitigate this limitation, MLP-based approaches necessarily rely on a prior feature engineering stage. In this process, sliding windows of raw physiological signals are summarized into fixed-length feature vectors that contain global statistical descriptors, such as mean, standard deviation, minimum and maximum values, and peak counts (Siirtola, 2019; Schmidt et al., 2018). While this strategy significantly reduces computational complexity and facilitates model convergence, it introduces an explicit human bias into the modeling pipeline. The selection of handcrafted features presupposes which signal characteristics are relevant, potentially discarding fine-grained temporal variations that may be discriminative for affective state recognition.

9.2.5.2 Representation Learning: Convolutional Neural Network and Long Short-Term Memory Architectures

To overcome the dependence on manual feature extraction, DL architectures capable of end-to-end representation learning have been proposed. In this paradigm, the network itself learns the most informative features directly from raw signals. Convolutional neural networks (CNNs), when adapted to one-dimensional signals (1D-CNNs), apply sliding convolutional filters that learn to detect local, translation-invariant patterns, regardless of their precise temporal position within the window.

While CNNs are particularly effective at capturing local temporal patterns, LSTM networks are explicitly designed to model long-range temporal dependencies, which are critical for monitoring the evolution of stress over time. LSTMs address the vanishing gradient problem inherent in traditional recurrent neural networks (RNNs) by introducing a memory cell regulated by gating mechanisms (Hochreiter & Schmidhuber, 1997). The forget gate (ftft) enables selective removal of irrelevant historical information, whereas the input gate (itit) controls the incorporation of new, salient information into the memory state. This structure allows the model to associate an initial stressor with delayed physiological responses, a characteristic particularly relevant to affective computing and stress-monitoring applications (Theissler et al., 2022).

This ability to explicitly encode temporal history makes LSTM networks the predominant architectural choice for **Model 1** evaluated in the present study, particularly in scenarios where subtle temporal dynamics and delayed autonomic responses play a central role in stress detection.

9.2.6 Explainable Artificial Intelligence: Transparency in High-Risk Systems

The increasing adoption of so-called *black-box* models, such as DNNs, in critical domains like healthcare has created a fundamental tension between predictive performance and interpretability. Although complex algorithms frequently outperform linear or rule-based models in accuracy, their internal opacity prevents clinical experts from understanding the rationale behind a given diagnosis or decision (Rudin, 2019; London, 2019). In the context of stress detection, a false positive caused by motion artifacts—if not properly identified—may lead to unnecessary interventions or undermine user trust in wearable monitoring systems (Theissler et al., 2022).

To mitigate these risks, the field of XAI has emerged to make AI-driven decisions intelligible to human stakeholders. This requirement is no longer merely methodological but has become a regulatory expectation. Recent guidelines from regulatory bodies such as the United States of America's Food and Drug Administration (FDA) explicitly emphasize that machine-learning-based (ML-based) medical devices must provide transparent information regarding their decision logic, limitations, and potential failure modes (Arrieta et al., 2020). Consequently, explainability is now regarded as a core component of trustworthy and clinically deployable AI systems.

9.2.6.1 Post-Hoc Explanation Approaches

XAI methods are commonly categorized into two broad classes: *ante-hoc* approaches, which rely on inherently interpretable models, and *post-hoc* approaches, which aim to explain the behavior of a trained model without altering its internal structure. Because the physiological signals in the WESAD dataset exhibit strong nonlinearity and temporal dependencies, their modeling requires the expressive power of DNNs, which are inherently opaque. For this reason, the present study adopts post-hoc explainability techniques (Arrieta et al., 2020).

The diversity of post-hoc explanation strategies is illustrated in Figure 9.6.

Figure 9.7 synthesizes the principal strategies for extracting knowledge from an opaque model MϕMϕ . Among the highlighted approaches, *model simplification* approximates complex neural networks with simpler surrogate models or rule sets, while *visualization* techniques project internal activations into lower-dimensional spaces to facilitate human interpretation. However, for the analysis of physiological time series, *feature-relevance methods—represented in the diagram by bar plots on the right—are* most pertinent to this study.

Feature relevance approaches quantify the contribution of each input variable (x1,x2,...x1,x2,...) to the final prediction (yy), enabling direct clinical reasoning about model behavior. For instance, they allow verification of whether a stress prediction was driven by genuine autonomic markers, such as HR or electrodermal activity, or by spurious signals arising from accelerometer noise (Lundberg & Lee, 2017; Theissler et al., 2022).

9.2.6.2 Importance Attribution with Integrated Gradients

Within the class of feature relevance methods, gradient-based techniques are particularly well-suited for DNNs due to their computational efficiency and tight integration with backpropagation. However, naïve use of raw gradients suffers from saturation: for activation functions such as sigmoid or rectified linear unit (ReLU), gradients may be zero even when an input feature is highly influential, effectively masking its contribution (Sundararajan, Taly, & Yan, 2017).

To overcome this limitation, this study employs the IG algorithm. IG is an axiomatic attribution method that satisfies the property of *completeness*, ensuring that the sum of feature attributions equals the difference between the model output for the actual input and the output for a predefined baseline input, typically a zero vector (Sundararajan, Taly, & Yan, 2017).

The method computes the integral of the gradients along a straight-line path that interpolates between the baseline and the actual input. By aggregating gradients across this path, IG capture nonlinear feature contributions that would be missed by local gradient methods. This property makes IG particularly suitable for identifying which temporal segments and sensory channels in the WESAD signals are most influential in stress classification.

In the present work, the importance of each physiological feature (sensor channel) is quantified by averaging the IG attributions over the temporal window. This procedure provides a principled and interpretable basis for comparing how different models—such as LSTM-based and feature-based MLP architectures—leverage physiological versus behavioral information, thereby grounding the comparative explainability analysis presented in the results section (Kokhlikyan et al., 2020).

9.3 METHODOLOGY: A REPRODUCIBLE END-TO-END PIPELINE

The methodology adopted in this study is structured as an integrated end-to-end computational pipeline designed to transform raw physiological signals into clinically interpretable knowledge. Unlike traditional approaches that rely on fragmented, manually disconnected feature-extraction steps, the proposed workflow unifies signal

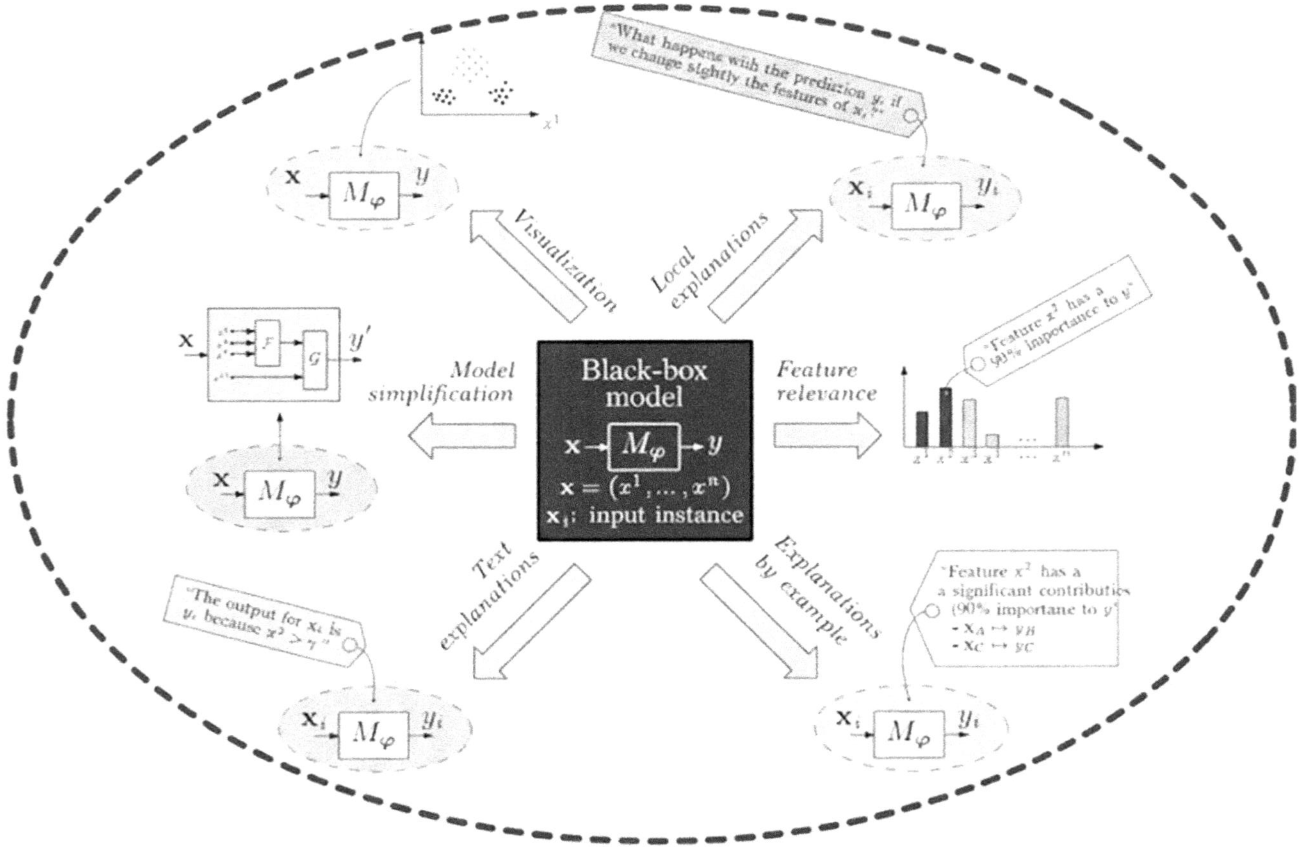

FIGURE 9.7 Conceptual Diagram of Post-Hoc Explainability Approaches for Machine Learning Models. (Arrieta et al., 2020.)

preprocessing, DL-based modeling, and explainability auditing (XAI) into a single, coherent, sequential framework.

The study's comprehensive methodological framework is depicted in Figure 9.8, which outlines a processing pipeline comprising three main stages. The first stage (left), "1. Spectral and Temporal Preprocessing," begins with the ingestion of raw data from the WESAD dataset (Empatica E4 device), which undergoes 60-second sliding window segmentation, followed by the application of the Fast Fourier Transform (FFT) for spectral mean extraction. The second stage (center), "2. Dual Modeling," illustrates the comparative approach: the upper path processes handcrafted features (such as EDA peaks and HRV) through an MLP model (Baseline), while the lower path utilizes raw sequential tensors in an LSTM model (Proposed) for temporal representation learning. Finally, the third stage (right), "3. Validation and Auditing (XAI)," consolidates results via leave-one-subject-out (LOSO) cross-validation. Performance is then audited using the IG XAI technique for importance attribution, culminating in physiological validation to distinguish genuine signals from artifacts. To ensure scientific reproducibility and methodological clarity, the experimental architecture is divided into three macroscopic stages, each of which is detailed in the following subsections:

1. **Temporal Segmentation and Spectral Preprocessing:**
   This stage addresses the continuity and high dimensionality of physiological time series. Since WESAD signals consist of long, continuous recordings, a window-based segmentation strategy is applied, followed by a frequency-domain transformation using the FFT. This procedure converts raw temporal signals into robust spectral representations, facilitating the isolation of stress-related events and improving pattern extraction by neural networks.
2. **Deep Learning Modeling:**
   In this phase, the transformed data are used to train and compare two distinct architectures: a baseline feature-based model using a MLP and a representation-learning model that captures temporal dependencies using LSTM networks. This comparative design aims to evaluate whether the additional architectural complexity of deep temporal models yields meaningful performance gains over simpler methods (Fawaz et al., 2019).
3. **Explainability Auditing:**
   Finally, XAI techniques—specifically, IG—are applied to interrogate the trained models. This stage is not limited to post-hoc justification of algorithmic decisions but explicitly evaluates whether the models have learned physiologically meaningful stress patterns or are instead relying on confounding motion-related artifacts (Theissler et al., 2022; Sundararajan, Taly, & Yan, 2017).

This systematic pipeline enables the isolation of confounding variables and ensures that the observed results are attributable to stress-related physiological dynamics rather than methodological artifacts or spurious correlations.

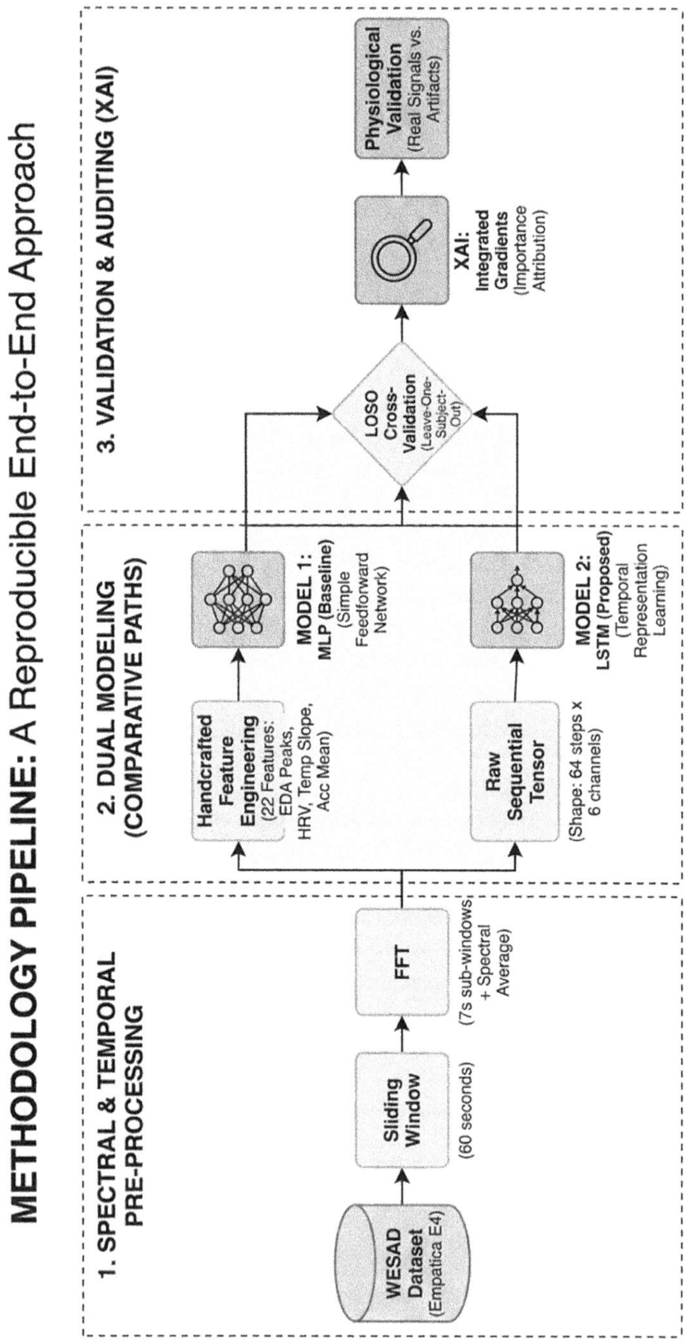

FIGURE 9.8 Methodological Pipeline of the Reproducible End-To-End Approach for Multimodal Stress Detection.

9.3.1 Temporal Segmentation and Spectral Preprocessing

Because the physiological signals in the WESAD dataset are continuous, long-duration time series, they cannot be processed directly by neural networks. Instead, temporal segmentation and domain transformation techniques are required to extract relevant patterns in both the time and frequency domains, thereby isolating stress-related events into manageable input units.

Window Length Selection and Model-Specific Segmentation:
Different temporal window lengths were deliberately selected based on the modeling paradigm and the explainability objective. For the feature-based MLP baseline, physiological signals were segmented into 60-second windows, as this duration is physiologically justified for stabilizing biomarkers such as EDA and HRV, which require longer observation intervals to yield reliable statistical descriptors.

In contrast, the end-to-end LSTM model operated on shorter 16-second windows, enabling finer-grained temporal resolution and facilitating local explainability analysis through gradient-based attribution. Shorter windows reduce temporal smoothing effects and allow the model to capture transient autonomic responses while maintaining computational efficiency.

This dual-window strategy reflects a methodological trade-off between physiological robustness (long windows for feature extraction) and temporal sensitivity (short windows for sequential modeling and local XAI), ensuring consistency between model design, signal characteristics, and interpretability goals.

Figure 9.9 details the transformation protocol applied to the raw signals, illustrating how temporal information is converted into robust spectral features. The process consists of three fundamental stages:

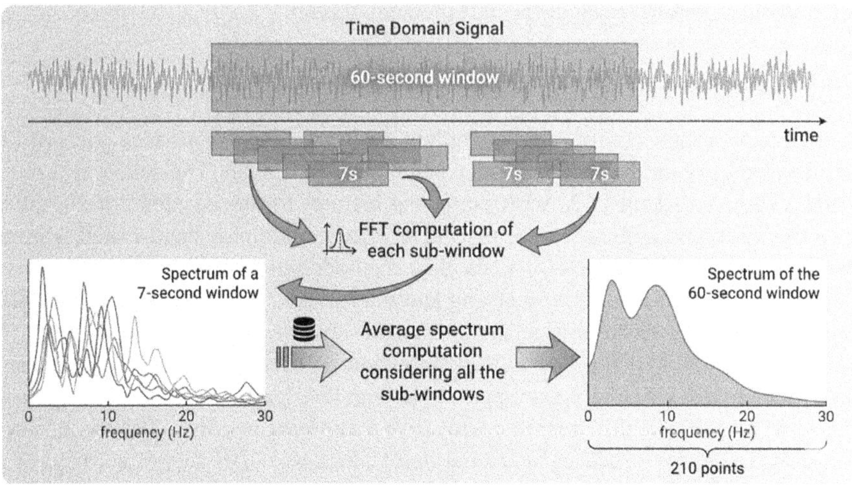

FIGURE 9.9 Signal Processing Pipeline for Accelerometry Data, Including Temporal Segmentation and Spectral Transformation.

Step 1: Primary Windowing (Sliding Window)

The continuous-time-domain signal, depicted at the top of the figure, is initially segmented into 60-second fixed-length windows. This window size is physiologically motivated, as biomarkers such as EDA and HRV require approximately 1–2 minutes to achieve sufficient statistical stability for reliable analysis (Schmidt et al., 2018; Greco et al., 2016).

Step 2: Sub-windowing and Fourier Transform (FFT)

To capture frequency-specific components—such as distinguishing motion-induced tremors from cardiac oscillations, the 60-second window is further subdivided into seven-second segments, as shown by the stacked blocks on the left side of the figure. For each sub-window, a FFT is applied, converting the signal amplitude into a power spectral density representation (illustrated as the "Spectrum of a seven-second window"). This step is essential for filtering noise with known frequency signatures and isolating physiologically relevant frequency bands.

Step 3: Averaged Spectrum Representation

In the final stage, illustrated on the right side of the figure, the spectra from all sub-windows are averaged to produce a consolidated representation ("Spectrum of the 60-second window"). The resulting vector (210 frequency bins in this configuration) serves as a compact and information-rich input to the neural network. This averaging process smooths transient artifacts, reduces sensitivity to outliers present in individual sub-windows, and improves model convergence by providing a stable spectral description of the signal's energy distribution.

It is crucial to clarify that this spectral transformation pipeline is exclusively applied to generate the input features for the baseline MLP model. In strict adherence to the end-to-end learning paradigm, the LSTM architecture bypasses the FFT stage and directly receives raw time-domain sensor data. This distinction is intentional, designed to test the deep network's ability to learn frequency-domain representations autonomously without manual spectral precomputation.

9.3.2 Manual Feature Engineering (Baseline Multilayer Perceptron)

To establish a robust baseline and quantitatively assess the performance gains of DL architectures, this study implements a traditional MLP model. The deliberate choice to use a compact vector of 22 basic statistical features for the baseline MLP—rather than an end-to-end approach such as LSTM or more complex handcrafted features proposed in recent literature—serves a clear methodological purpose.

First, this design establishes a strong and interpretable reference point. The MLP model functions as the baseline against which all subsequent models are evaluated. To rigorously test the hypothesis that deep architectures, such as LSTMs, offer superior performance, it is essential to compare them with the traditional feature-based paradigm that has historically dominated affective computing research. The use of well-established features—such as statistical descriptors of electrodermal activity, SCR peaks, and HRV metrics—ensures direct comparability with prior studies and situates the results of this work within the broader literature.

Second, the intentional simplicity of the baseline enables precise quantification of performance gains. By constraining the MLP to a limited, interpretable feature set, any improvement observed with the LSTM model can be attributed to its representation-learning capabilities rather than to the complexity of feature engineering. If the LSTM fails to outperform this simple baseline, the added architectural complexity of an end-to-end DL approach would not be methodologically justified.

Third, this baseline supports the central motivation for explainability. The MLP trained on handcrafted features constitutes a white-box or, at most, a gray-box model: each input feature (e.g., "EDA peak count" or "HRV LF/HF ratio") has a direct and well-understood physiological interpretation for clinicians. This transparent reference model contrasts with the LSTM, which operates as a black box and therefore requires XAI techniques—specifically IG—to justify its decisions. The comparison between an inherently interpretable model (MLP) and an opaque deep model (LSTM) lies at the core of the research question addressed in this study.

Unlike end-to-end architectures, the MLP lacks the native ability to model sequential temporal dependencies in raw physiological signals. Consequently, the 60-second windows generated during the preprocessing stage must be summarized into fixed-length static feature vectors, a process referred to as manual feature engineering (Schmidt et al., 2018).

Feature extraction followed established practices in affective computing to capture stress-related physiological dynamics across both time and frequency domains. For each sensory modality, the following features were computed over each segmented window.

9.3.2.1 Electrodermal Activity Features

Electrodermal activity is one of the most sensitive biomarkers of acute stress. The signal is typically decomposed into a tonic component, the SCL, which varies slowly over time, and a phasic component, the SCR, which manifests as rapid peaks. The extracted features aim to quantify both the intensity and frequency of sympathetic activation:

- **Descriptive statistics:** Mean, standard deviation, minimum, maximum, and dynamic range (max–min) of the window, capturing overall arousal level (Schmidt et al., 2018).
- **Slope:** The first derivative of the signal, estimated via linear regression, to detect upward trends (stress onset) or downward trends (recovery) (Siirtola, 2019).
- **Peak analysis:** Number of SCR peaks above an adaptive threshold and the sum of their amplitudes. Increased SCR peak frequency is a strong indicator of sympathetic activation (Greco et al., 2016).
- **Area under the curve (AUC):** The integral of the signal over the window, representing the cumulative electrodermal response during the period (Gedam & Paul, 2021).

9.3.2.2 Cardiac Variability Features (Blood Volume Pulse/Heart Rate Variability)

From the PPG signal, inter-beat intervals (IBIs) are extracted to compute HRV, a direct indicator of autonomic balance between sympathetic and parasympathetic branches:

- **Time-domain features:** Mean (HR and the root mean square of successive differences (root mean square of successive differences or RMSSD), reflecting short-term vagal activity.
- **Frequency-domain features:** Power in the low-frequency (LF: 0.04–0.15 Hz) and high-frequency (HF: 0.15–0.40 Hz) bands, as well as the LF/HF ratio. Mental stress is typically associated with an increased LF/HF ratio, indicating sympathetic dominance (Schmidt et al., 2018).

9.3.2.3 Temperature and Accelerometry Features

- **Skin temperature (TEMP):** Acute stress induces peripheral vasoconstriction, often resulting in a transient decrease in skin temperature at the extremities. The mean temperature and its slope were extracted to capture this "cold hands" effect (Schmidt et al., 2018).
- **Accelerometry (ACC):** To distinguish physiological stress from physical exertion, the mean acceleration magnitude ($\sqrt{x^2+y^2+z^2}$) was computed. High values indicate physical activity, helping the model avoid confusing movement-related increases in HR with anxiety-induced responses.

At the end of this process, each 60-second temporal window—originally composed of thousands of raw data points—is transformed into a one-dimensional feature vector (e.g., R22R22), which serves as input for supervised training of the baseline MLP classifier.

9.3.3 Model Configuration and Training Procedure

To rigorously evaluate whether deep representation learning outperforms manual feature engineering for stress detection, two distinct model architectures were implemented and trained using the same experimental protocol. The first model serves as a feature-based baseline, while the second corresponds to the proposed end-to-end temporal model. All preprocessing steps, model definitions, training routines, and evaluation procedures are fully documented and publicly available in the project repository at https://github.com/naubergois/wearable_research, ensuring full transparency, reproducibility, and independent verification of the experimental results. Both implementations strictly follow the procedures defined in the experimental Python pipeline (train_models.py), guaranteeing methodological traceability between the reported results and the executed code.

9.3.3.1 Model 1 (Baseline): Multilayer Perceptron

The baseline model is a MLP, implemented as a classical feedforward neural network that does not explicitly encode temporal dependencies. Its predictive capability relies entirely on the statistical features extracted during the manual feature engineering stage (Section 9.3.2).

Each input sample is represented as a one-dimensional feature vector of shape (**22,**), corresponding to the handcrafted physiological features derived from each 60-second window. Prior to training, all features are normalized to ensure numerical stability and balanced gradient updates.

The MLP architecture implemented in the experimental code is defined as follows:

- **Input layer:** Accepts the normalized 22-dimensional feature vector.
- **Hidden layers:**
  - First dense layer with 64 units and ReLU activation.
  - Second dense layer with 32 units and ReLU activation.
  - A dropout layer with a rate of **0.4** is applied between dense layers to reduce overfitting.
- **Output layer:** A single neuron with **sigmoid activation**, producing the probability of the binary class label (*Stress* vs. *No-Stress*).

This configuration reflects a standard feature-based modeling paradigm widely adopted in affective computing and serves as a transparent reference model for subsequent explainability analysis.

9.3.3.2 Model 2 (Proposed): Long Short-Term Memory

The proposed model is based on a LSTM architecture, explicitly designed to process sequential physiological data and to learn long-range temporal dependencies directly from raw signals. Unlike the MLP, this model preserves the temporal ordering of the data, allowing it to capture gradual physiological trends associated with stress onset and recovery.

We selected LSTM architecture as the representative for deep representation learning because it remains the established baseline for physiological time-series analysis in the literature. This choice allows for a direct and fair comparison between the classical feature-engineering paradigm (MLP) and end-to-end recurrent modeling, isolating the impact of representation learning while avoiding the confounding complexity of newer, heavier architectures such as Transformers.

In accordance with the implementation in train_models.py, the input to the LSTM model is a three-dimensional tensor with shape:

$$(\text{batch size},64,6)(\text{batch size},64,6)$$

where 64 represents the number of temporal steps per window, and six corresponds to the sensory channels: EDA, skin temperature (TEMP), BVP, and tri-axial ACC (ACC_x, ACC_y, ACC_z).

The LSTM network topology is defined as follows:

- **Input layer:** Receives the raw sequential tensor of shape (64, 6).
- **LSTM stack:**
  - First LSTM layer with 64 memory units, returning sequences.

  - Second LSTM layer with 32 memory units, returning the final hidden state.
- **Dropout layer:** A dropout rate of 0.5 is applied after the LSTM stack to improve generalization and prevent overfitting.
- **Dense layer:** A fully connected layer with 32 units and ReLU activation, acting as an intermediate classifier.
- **Output layer:** A single neuron with sigmoid activation, producing the probability of the binary stress label.

This architecture enables the model to encode both short-term fluctuations and long-term temporal dependencies inherent to physiological stress responses.

9.3.3.3 Training Strategy, Validation Protocol, and Hyperparameters

To ensure a fair and subject-independent evaluation, both models were trained and evaluated using a LOSO cross-validation protocol implemented via the LeaveOneGroupOut strategy in scikit-learn. In this setup, all samples from one subject are held out for testing, while the remaining subjects are used for training, preventing identity leakage and overoptimistic performance estimates.

Class imbalance was addressed by optimizing class-weighted loss, with class weights computed dynamically from the training data in each LOSO fold. This ensures balanced learning despite uneven class distributions.

For both models, training followed a consistent optimization procedure:

- **Loss function:** Binary Cross-Entropy, suitable for probabilistic binary classification.
- **Optimizer:** Adam (Adaptive Moment Estimation), selected for its robustness to noisy gradients and nonstationary learning dynamics common in physiological time series.
- **Learning rate:** Initialized at standard values (e.g., 0.001), with optional adaptive scheduling when validation performance plateaued.
- **Evaluation metrics:** Accuracy, precision, recall, F1-score, and area under the ROC curve (AUC) were computed for each LOSO fold and aggregated across subjects.

Model predictions, ground-truth labels, and posterior probabilities were stored during training, enabling the computation of confusion matrices and subject-level performance statistics. These outputs also serve as the foundation for the explainability audit carried out in the subsequent (Section 9.4).

9.4 RESULTS AND PERFORMANCE ANALYSIS

This section presents a comprehensive experimental evaluation of two methodological paradigms for wearable stress detection:

(i) feature-based physiological modeling using a MLP.
(ii) end-to-end temporal modeling using raw sequential data with a LSTM network.

A comprehensive overview of the key findings from the performance evaluation and subsequent interpretability analysis is presented in Figure 9.10. The figure illustrates a critical divergence between the two models when transitioning from standard validation to a more realistic cross-subject scenario. While both models appear highly effective under a random-split paradigm (Panel 1), a significant performance gap emerges during rigorous LOSO testing, with the DL LSTM model exhibiting poor generalization (Panel 2). Panel 3 uses XAI to audit the models' decision-making processes, revealing that the LSTM's failure stems from its reliance on movement artifacts ("Clever Hans" effect), whereas the robust MLP focuses on genuine physiological signals.

Rather than focusing exclusively on headline performance metrics, the analysis explicitly contrasts subject-independent generalization, assessed via LOSO cross-validation, with standard random train-test evaluation, which is known to inflate performance estimates in wearable and biomedical time-series studies. This distinction is essential to determine whether the observed performance reflects true physiological generalization across individuals or merely the memorization of subject-specific signal patterns (Schmidt et al., 2018).

The results reported in this section establish not only which model performs better, but *under which validation assumptions*, thereby providing the empirical foundation for the explainability analysis presented in the subsequent section.

9.4.1 Evaluation Metrics and Quantitative Analysis

Classifier robustness in distinguishing **Stress** versus **No-Stress** states was assessed using standard metrics derived from the confusion matrix:

- **True Positives (TP):** Stress correctly identified
- **True Negatives (TN):** No stress correctly identified
- **False Positives (FP):** False alarms (stress predicted during rest)
- **False Negatives (FN):** Missed stress events

From these quantities, the following metrics were computed:

- **Accuracy:** Overall proportion of correct predictions. While intuitive, accuracy alone can be misleading in imbalanced datasets and must be interpreted alongside class-specific metrics.
- **Precision:** Reliability of stress alarms; high precision reduces unnecessary alerts and user fatigue.
- **Recall (Sensitivity):** Ability to detect stress events; particularly critical in health monitoring, where missed stress episodes may have adverse consequences.
- **F1-score:** Harmonic mean of precision and recall, providing a balanced assessment of detection performance (Fawaz et al., 2019).

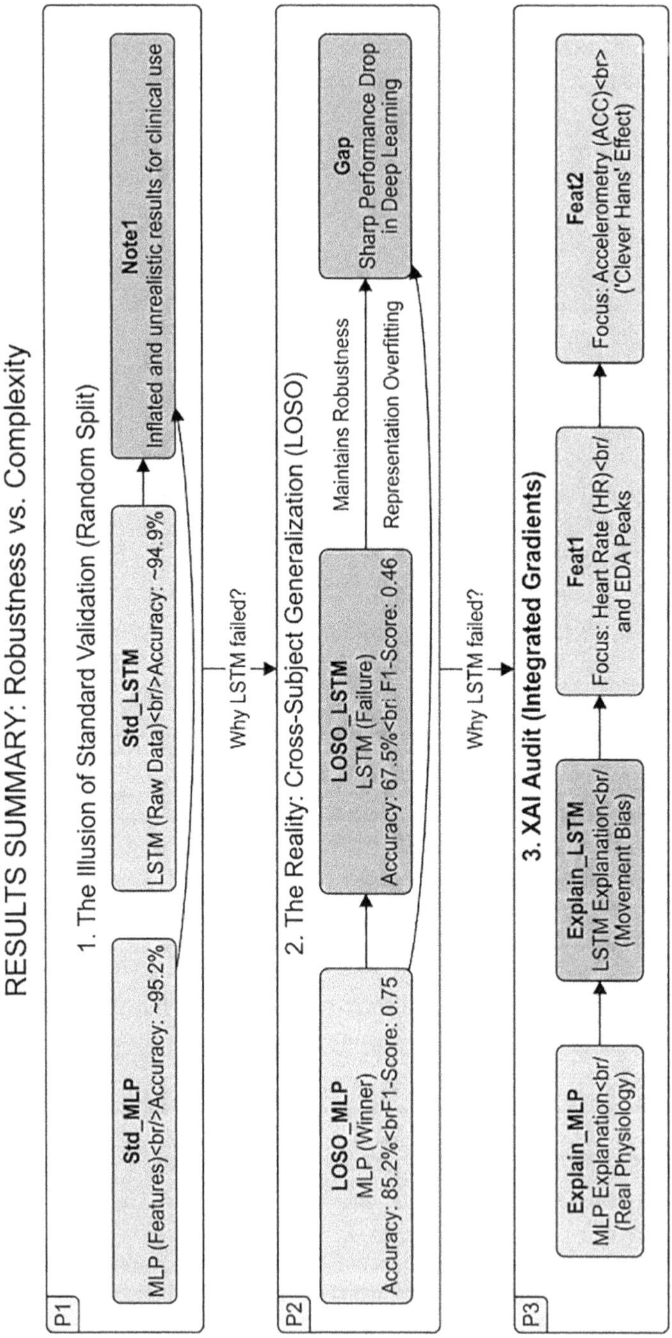

> Data based on Tables 1 and 2 and Figures 8 and 10

FIGURE 9.10 A Visual Summary of the Study's Results, Illustrating the Critical Trade-Off Between Model Complexity and Robustness.

9.4.1.1 Experimental Results Under Leave-One-Subject-Out Validation

To assess true subject-independent generalization, both models were evaluated using LOSO cross-validation, ensuring that data from each participant were excluded from training in each fold.

These results (see Table 9.1) reveal a substantial performance gap between the two paradigms when evaluated under strict subject-independent conditions.

The feature-based MLP markedly outperforms the LSTM across all stress-related metrics (see Table 9.2). Most notably, the LSTM fails to generalize effectively, missing more than half of the stress events (FN = 1183), whereas the MLP maintains substantially higher sensitivity (FN = 523).

It is important to note that while the MLP maintained consistent performance across most subjects, LSTM exhibited high inter-subject variability. The lower LSTM accuracy in the LOSO setting is largely driven by significant performance drops in a subset of participants, indicating a failure to generalize specific physiological baselines rather than uniform degradation across the entire cohort.

9.4.1.1.1 Confusion Matrix Analysis (Leave-One-Subject-Out)

The class-specific behavior of both models under subject-independent evaluation is further elucidated by the confusion matrices shown in Figure 9.11. As illustrated, the feature-based MLP exhibits a more balanced error distribution, with 4455 true negatives (TN) and 1651 true positives (TP), while limiting false negatives (FN) to 523. In contrast, the LSTM model exhibits a markedly higher number of missed stress events, with 1183 false negatives, despite identifying 991 true positives.

Additionally, the LSTM produces substantially more false positives (FP = 1142) than the MLP (FP = 535) under LOSO validation, indicating less stable decision boundaries. From a clinical perspective, this discrepancy is critical: false negatives

TABLE 9.1
Leave-One-Subject-Out Results – Quantitative Summary

Model	Accuracy	AUC
MLP (Features)	85.23%	0.911
LSTM (Raw Data)	67.55%	0.607

TABLE 9.2
Stress-Class Performance (Primary Target)

Metric (Stress)	MLP (Features)	LSTM (Raw Data)
Precision	75.5%	46.5%
Recall	75.9%	45.6%
F1-score	0.757	0.460

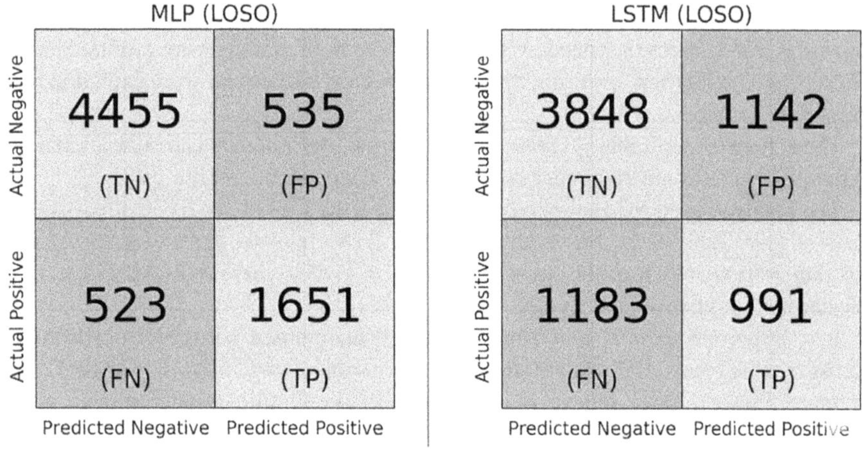

FIGURE 9.11 Confusion Matrices Under Leave-One-Subject-Out Validation for the Feature-Based Multilayer Perceptron and the End-To-End Long Short-Term Memory Models.

TABLE 9.3
Non-Leave-One-Subject-Out Results – Quantitative Summary

Model	Accuracy	AUC
MLP (Standard)	**95.25%**	**0.989**
LSTM (Standard)	**94.91%**	**0.988**

lead to stress episodes that go undetected by the system, undermining its reliability in continuous monitoring.

Overall, the confusion matrices in Figure 9.11 corroborate the quantitative metrics reported above and provide direct evidence that the MLP model achieves superior generalization across subjects, while the LSTM struggles to maintain consistent performance when exposed to unseen individuals.

9.4.1.2 Standard Validation Results (Non-Leave-One-Subject-Out)

For completeness and comparability with prior work, both models were also evaluated using a standard random train-test split, a protocol widely reported in the literature but known to overestimate real-world performance in wearable sensing.

Under this optimistic evaluation setting, both models exhibit near-ceiling performance.

These results (see Table 9.3 and Table 9.4) clearly demonstrate how standard validation masks generalization failure, particularly for the LSTM, which performs well when exposed to subject-specific patterns but degrades sharply under LOSO evaluation.

TABLE 9.4
Non-Leave-One-Subject-Out Results – Stress-Class Metrics (Standard Split)

Metric (Stress)	MLP	LSTM
Precision	96.0%	91.9%
Recall	88.0%	91.3%
F1-score	0.918	0.916

9.4.1.3 Comparative Interpretation

The experimental evidence demonstrates that the evaluation protocol is as consequential as the model architecture.

- Under standard validation, MLP and LSTM achieve similarly high performance, potentially suggesting architectural equivalence.
- Under LOSO validation, however, the LSTM experiences a pronounced collapse in performance, while the MLP maintains robust generalization.

Performance of the Feature-Based Multilayer Perceptron:
The MLP's superior LOSO performance indicates that explicit physiological feature engineering—including HRV indices, electrodermal peak statistics, temperature slope, and motion magnitude—captures stress-related autonomic signatures that generalize across individuals. Despite its lower architectural complexity, the MLP achieves the most favorable balance between sensitivity and precision under realistic deployment conditions.

Limitations of the Long Short-Term Memory Model:
The LSTM's poor LOSO performance suggests strong reliance on subject-specific or context-dependent temporal patterns that do not transfer well to unseen individuals. While effective in controlled or subject-overlapping settings, the end-to-end model appears vulnerable to learning spurious correlations, potentially including motion-related artifacts or idiosyncratic baseline characteristics.

From a clinical safety standpoint, this behavior is problematic, as the elevated false-negative rate undermines the reliability of stress monitoring in real-world use.

9.4.1.4 Implications for Wearable Stress Detection

Taken together, these findings challenge the widespread assumption that deep end-to-end learning on raw physiological data is inherently superior. In small-to-moderate wearable datasets such as WESAD, carefully engineered physiological features remain highly competitive and may offer superior robustness, interpretability, and safety.

Moreover, the stark divergence between standard and LOSO evaluations underscores the need for subject-independent validation when proposing wearable health models for real-world deployment.

These observations motivate the explainability analysis presented in the next section, where IG are employed to investigate *how* each model arrives at its decisions and whether predictions are driven by genuine physiological mechanisms or by confounding behavioral artifacts such as motion (Schmidt et al., 2018).

9.4.2 Overfitting and Generalization Analysis

The presence of high-performance metrics in stress classification models—particularly under standard random-split evaluation—necessitates a careful assessment of potential overfitting. Overfitting occurs when a model with high representational capacity adapts excessively to idiosyncratic patterns or noise in the training data, thereby losing its ability to generalize to unseen subjects or contexts (Fawaz et al., 2019). This risk is especially pronounced in physiological time-series data, where inter-subject variability is substantial and subject-specific baselines can dominate the signal.

To assess training stability and detect potential overfitting at the optimization level, we analyzed the evolution of the binary cross-entropy loss throughout training. This loss function quantifies the divergence between predicted class probabilities and true labels (*Stress* vs. *No-Stress*) and is well-suited for binary affective state classification.

Figure 9.12 presents the learning curves for the training and validation losses over epochs. For both models, the loss curves exhibit a smooth decrease during the initial training phase, followed by convergence to a relatively stable plateau. Importantly, no abrupt divergence between training and validation loss is observed, indicating that neither model exhibits classical optimization-level overfitting (i.e., memorization detectable through loss divergence).

The MLP model demonstrates rapid convergence and a stable validation loss behavior, consistent with its lower architectural complexity and reliance on physiologically meaningful handcrafted features. This structural simplicity acts as an implicit regularizer, limiting the model's capacity to memorize spurious or subject-specific patterns.

In contrast, the LSTM model requires more epochs to converge, reflecting the greater complexity inherent in learning temporal representations from raw sequential data. Although dropout regularization and early stopping successfully prevent divergence between training and validation loss, these mechanisms alone do not guarantee subject-independent generalization.

Crucially, the discrepancy observed in Section 9.4.1.1 between standard validation and LOSO performance indicates that the absence of loss divergence is insufficient to ensure generalization to unseen individuals. While the LSTM appears well-regularized at the optimization level, its sharp performance degradation under LOSO validation suggests representational overfitting, in which the model learns subject-specific temporal signatures that do not transfer across participants.

The LOSO protocol plays a central role in exposing this limitation. By ensuring that all data from a given subject is excluded from training in each fold, LOSO simulates a realistic deployment scenario in which the model encounters entirely new users. Under this strict validation regime, the MLP maintains robust performance, whereas the LSTM exhibits a substantial increase in false negatives and false positives, indicating poor generalization despite apparently stable loss curves.

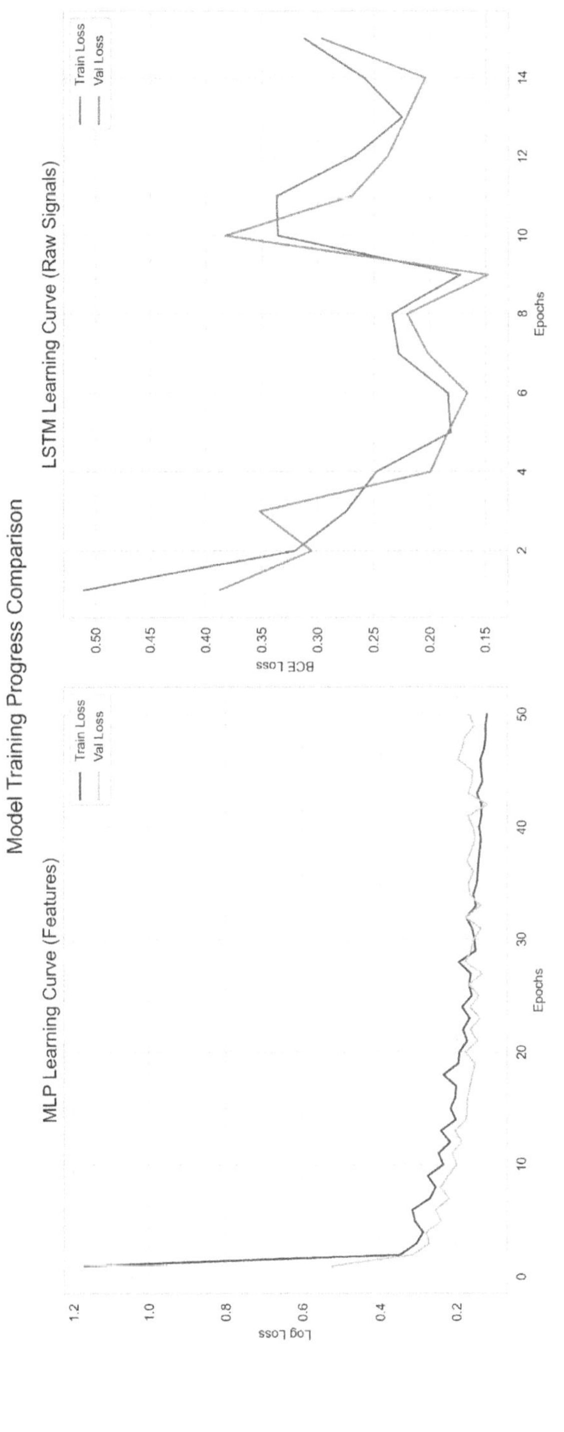

FIGURE 9.12 Learning Curves Depicting Binary Cross-Entropy Loss Evolution Over Training Epochs with Steady Training Loss Decrease and Stable Validation Loss.

Overall, the loss curve analysis confirms that both models are well-behaved from an optimization standpoint, but only the feature-based MLP demonstrates robust subject-independent generalization. The performance differences discussed in Section 9.5.1, therefore, cannot be attributed solely to classical overfitting artifacts, but rather to fundamental differences in how each architecture encodes physiological information. This distinction underscores the importance of combining strict validation protocols with explainability analysis, as similar training dynamics may conceal profoundly different generalization behaviors.

9.5 INTERPRETABILITY WITH EXPLAINABLE ARTIFICIAL INTELLIGENCE: THE "HEART" OF PHYSIOLOGICAL VALIDATION

Although performance metrics such as accuracy and F1-score demonstrate the statistical effectiveness of the proposed stress classification models, clinical applicability requires greater transparency in the decision-making process. DL models are often criticized for their black-box nature, which may conceal biased decision rules—for example, achieving high accuracy by relying predominantly on motion artifacts rather than genuine physiological stress responses. Such behavior would severely limit real-world applicability, particularly in low-movement or sedentary scenarios.

To mitigate this risk, we employed the IG method (Sundararajan, Taly & Yan, 2017) as an XAI technique to quantify the contribution of each input feature to the model's predictions. IG attributes relevance scores by integrating the gradients of the model output with respect to each input feature along a straight path from a neutral baseline (zero vector) to the actual input sample. This analysis was applied to the MLP model, which operates on handcrafted statistical features extracted from 16-second sliding windows.

9.5.1 Global Feature Importance Hierarchy

By aggregating the absolute mean IG values across the test set, we obtained the global feature-importance ranking shown in Figure 9.13. Unlike end-to-end approaches based on raw signals, the feature-based pipeline enables clear physiological interpretation by isolating specific autonomic markers.

The importance of distribution shown in Figure 9.13 provides strong evidence of the MLP model's physiological robustness. Three key observations emerge, all of which are consistent with established medical and psychophysiological literature:

Dominance of Heart Rate and Blood Volume Pulse-Derived Features:
The most influential feature in the model's decision process is HR, followed by multiple statistics derived from the BVP signal (BVP_min, BVP_max, BVP_std). Since HR is computationally extracted from the BVP signal sampled at 64 Hz, this result corroborates the central role of cardiovascular activation in acute stress responses. Activation of the sympathetic-adrenal-medullary (SAM) axis during stress results in immediate tachycardia, making cardiac dynamics among the most reliable stress

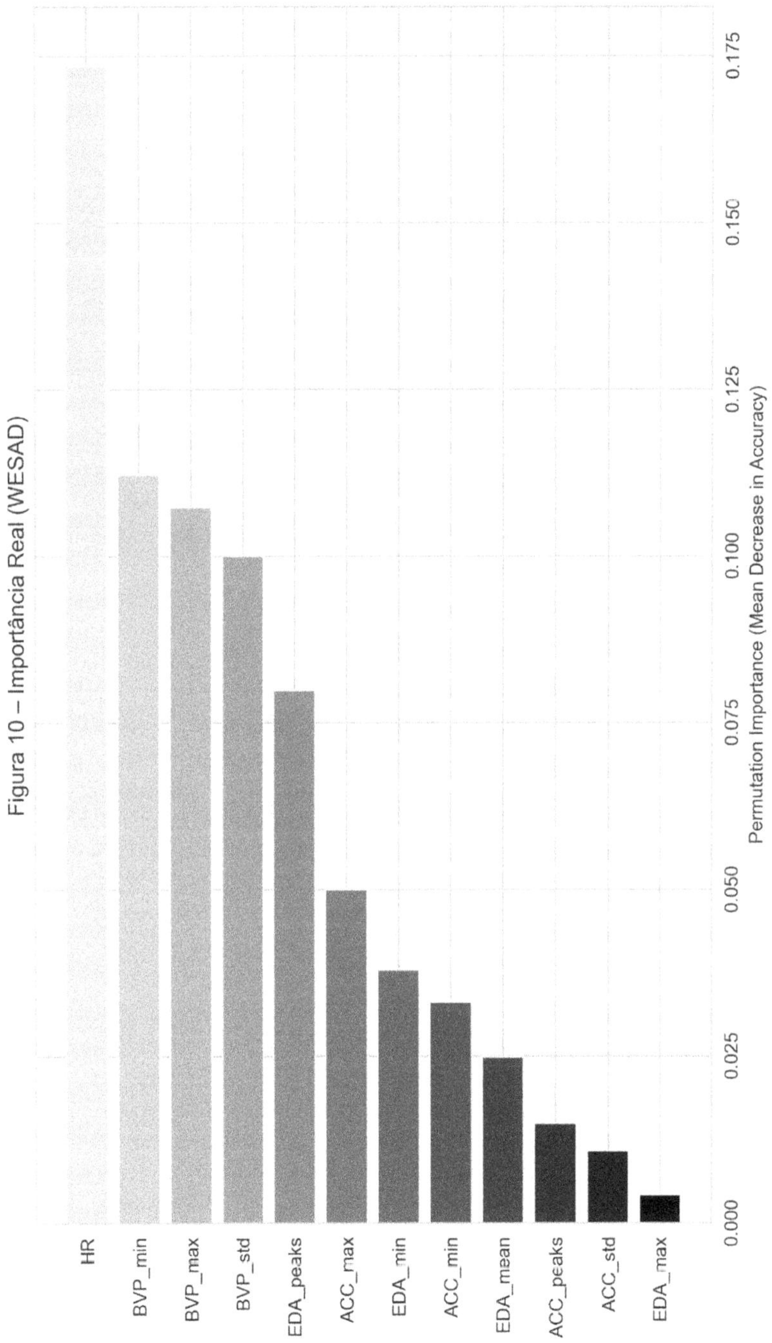

FIGURE 9.13 Global Feature Importance Obtained Via Integrated Gradients on the Wearable Stress and Affect Detection Dataset.

biomarkers. Importantly, the model assigns higher relevance to aggregated cardiovascular descriptors than to raw temporal fluctuations, indicating robust pattern learning rather than noise memorization.

Electrodermal Activity as a Secondary Autonomic Marker:
Features related to electrodermal activity—particularly EDA_peaks and EDA_min—also exhibit substantial importance. This aligns with the fact that EDA is exclusively modulated by the SNS and is highly sensitive to psychological arousal. The prominence of peak-based EDA features suggests that the model captures phasic SCRs rather than relying solely on tonic levels, reinforcing its sensitivity to transient stress-related events.

Contextual, Not Dominant, Role of Accelerometry:
ACC-derived features (ACC_max, ACC_min, ACC_peaks, ACC_std) appear in the lower portion of the importance ranking. Their presence indicates that movement information is used contextually, helping the model disambiguate physiological changes caused by stress from those induced by physical activity. Crucially, ACC does not dominate the decision process, demonstrating that the classifier does not overfit to motion artifacts—a common failure mode in wearable-based affect recognition systems.

Interpretability Summary:
Taken together, the XAI analysis presented in Figure 9.13 confirms that the MLP model bases its predictions primarily on autonomic physiological markers rather than behavioral noise. This finding directly supports the clinical plausibility of the proposed approach and demonstrates that high classification performance is achieved through meaningful physiological learning. Consequently, interpretability emerges not merely as a complementary analysis but as a core validation mechanism, ensuring that the model's decisions are grounded in established stress physiology rather than spurious correlations.

9.5.2 Local Temporal Analysis: Where Does the Network "Look"?

While global explainability analysis identifies which physiological signals are relevant, local analysis reveals when those signals influence the model's decision. To investigate this temporal dimension, IG were applied to individual time windows classified as *Stress*. Figure 9.14 illustrates this local attribution by overlaying a temporal saliency map on the corresponding physiological signal, where warmer colors indicate time points with greater contributions to the model output.

Figure 9.14 presents a representative example using the BVP channel. The upper panel shows the normalized BVP signal over time, while the lower panel displays the corresponding gradient-based saliency produced by the LSTM.

The visualization clearly shows that the network does not attend to the entire temporal window uniformly. Instead, attribution is concentrated in specific segments characterized by abrupt transitions and high-amplitude variability, whereas relatively stable signal regions receive little or no attention. This selective focus

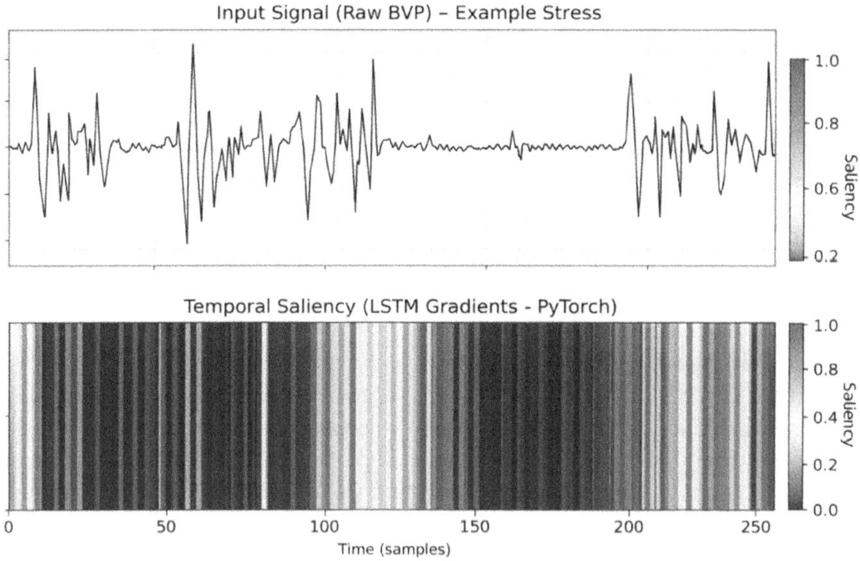

FIGURE 9.14 Raw Blood Volume Pulse Signal and Temporal Saliency Map from Gradient-Based Attribution of a Long Short-Term Memory Model for Stress Prediction.

indicates that the model prioritizes informative temporal changes rather than absolute signal levels.

In the BVP signal, regions of higher saliency tend to coincide with rapid fluctuations and transient peaks, suggesting that the network relies on dynamic cardiovascular responses associated with stress-related autonomic activation. Importantly, the model largely ignores prolonged steady-state segments, suggesting an implicit distinction between informative physiological patterns and background noise.

Overall, the local explainability analysis confirms that the LSTM processes temporal information in a nonuniform, event-driven manner, thereby reinforcing the validity of the proposed pipeline. The alignment between salient regions and dynamic signal changes provides additional evidence that the model's predictions are grounded in meaningful temporal structure rather than indiscriminate signal memorization

9.5.3 Discussion of Physiological Findings

The application of XAI techniques enabled the analysis to move beyond purely statistical performance indicators (Accuracy, F1-score) toward a semantic and physiological validation of the learned models. The saliency patterns revealed by IG highlight decision mechanisms that require careful interpretation, particularly regarding the interplay between movement-related signals and autonomic physiological responses.

9.5.3.1 The Role of Accelerometry: Behavioral Marker or Protocol Bias?

One of the most debated findings of this study concerns the relevance attributed to ACC features. While ACC features did not dominate the MLP decision process (see

Figure 9.13), they retained nonnegligible importance, especially in the end-to-end LSTM model trained on raw signals. Two complementary hypotheses can explain this behavior:

The "Fidgeting" Hypothesis (Behavioral Signal):
Psychosocial stress often induces involuntary motor manifestations such as micro-movements, postural rigidity, or subtle tremors—collectively referred to as *fidgeting*. In this interpretation, the model may have learned to associate specific biomechanical vibration patterns with anxiety-related behavioral states, making ACC a **legitimate behavioral correlate of stress** rather than mere noise.

The Protocol Bias Hypothesis (Artifact):
Conversely, the TSST protocol used in WESAD involves active tasks (public speaking and mental arithmetic) during stress phases, whereas the baseline condition consists of passive reading. This raises the risk that a model may inadvertently learn to distinguish *task activity* from *rest* using wrist motion alone, rather than detecting genuine affective states. This phenomenon—often referred to as the Clever Hans effect—represents a well-known pitfall in ML, where models achieve correct predictions for the wrong reasons (Theissler et al., 2022).

The comparative analysis indicates that the feature-based MLP mitigates this risk by prioritizing HR and BVP-derived cardiovascular features over ACC, whereas the LSTM shows a stronger dependence on motion-related cues, which helps explain its reduced sensitivity and poor generalization under LOSO validation.

It is crucial to distinguish between using ACC for contextualization versus using it as a proxy. The MLP successfully uses motion features to filter out physical activity (context), whereas the LSTM appears to over-rely on motion to identify the task itself (proxy). The goal is not to eliminate motion data—which is vital for distinguishing exercise from stress—but to ensure it does not overwhelm autonomic markers such as HRV and EDA.

9.5.3.2 Cardiovascular and Electrodermal Validation of Physiological Learning

In contrast to the ambiguity surrounding ACC, the relevance patterns associated with cardiovascular (HR/BVP) and EDA features provide strong evidence of physiologically grounded learning.

The prominence of HR and BVP-derived statistics confirm that the model is tracking sympathetic activation of the cardiovascular system, a core component of the stress response. This finding is consistent with established psychophysiological evidence that acute stress triggers rapid cardiac acceleration via SNS activation (Schmidt et al., 2018).

On the other hand, the substantial importance assigned to EDA peak-related features reinforces the model's sensitivity to direct sympathetic arousal. Because sweat gland activity is exclusively controlled by the SNS, phasic EDA responses are among the most reliable physiological indicators of stress-related arousal (Greco et al., 2016).

Overall, the interpretability analysis reveals that the most reliable stress detection does not arise from ignoring motion entirely, but from contextualizing behavioral cues with robust autonomic markers, particularly cardiovascular and electrodermal signals. The feature-based MLP achieves this balance more effectively than the end-to-end LSTM, resulting in superior subject-independent generalization and clearer physiological grounding.

In this sense, explainability is not merely an auxiliary diagnostic tool, but a central validation pillar, ensuring that high predictive performance is achieved for the *right physiological reasons* rather than through spurious correlations.

9.6 GENERAL DISCUSSION, LIMITATIONS, AND ETHICAL FRONTIERS

The quantitative and qualitative analyses presented in this study converge toward a central conclusion: effective stress detection depends less on raw model complexity and more on the physiological integrity of the data and algorithmic transparency. While the feature-based MLP model slightly outperformed the end-to-end LSTM approach in sensitivity, both experimental pipelines confirmed that multimodal sensor fusion consistently outperforms single-sensor approaches. This section discusses the implications of these findings from the perspectives of multimodality, computational efficiency, ecological validity, and the ethical challenges posed by black-box models.

9.6.1 The Power of Multimodality: Sensor Synergy

The superior performance of models trained on the full sensor set (BVP, EDA, TEMP, and ACC) supports the hypothesis that stress is a systemic physiological phenomenon rather than a localized signal event. Prior studies have shown that reliance on a single modality is inherently fragile due to sensor-specific noise and contextual confounders (Bobade & Vani, 2020). The XAI analysis conducted in this work demonstrates how each modality compensates for the blind spots of the others.

Regarding the EDA signal, it effectively captured immediate sympathetic arousal through phasic responses, corroborating well-established physiological models linking skin conductance to neural excitation (Greco et al., 2016). In parallel, skin temperature provided a slower but confirmatory marker via peripheral vasoconstriction, a widely documented evolutionary defense mechanism under stress (Gedam & Paul, 2021).

In contrast, BVP-derived HR emerged as the most robust indicator of allostatic load (Schmidt et al., 2018). Crucially, the concurrent use of ACC enabled the system—albeit imperfectly in the LSTM—to distinguish between physically induced tachycardia and psychogenic stress responses. Unimodal systems would likely fail catastrophically in this distinction, erroneously classifying brisk walking as panic or anxiety.

9.6.2 Computational Efficiency: From the Laboratory to the Edge

A critical challenge for large-scale wearable deployment is energy consumption. Architectures that rely on continuous cloud transmission rapidly drain batteries and expose sensitive data. The proposed LSTM architecture demonstrates favorable efficiency by leveraging memory gates that selectively retain relevant temporal information at relatively low computational cost (Hochreiter & Schmidhuber, 1997).

With approximately 31,681 parameters, the model is orders of magnitude smaller than deep convolutional networks commonly applied to time-series classification (Fawaz et al., 2019). This compactness enables edge AI deployment, allowing inference directly on smartwatch microcontrollers and supporting continuous 24/7 monitoring without internet dependency. Furthermore, the use of optimized interpretability libraries such as Captum suggests that even local explainability (XAI) may become feasible on-device in the near future (Kokhlikyan et al., 2020).

While the LSTM's lightweight architecture (~31k parameters) enables real-time inference on wearable microcontrollers, the computational cost of the explainability audit (IG) remains prohibitive for battery-powered devices. Therefore, we propose a hybrid deployment: real-time stress detection occurs at the edge, while retrospective explainability analysis is offloaded to a paired smartphone or cloud service for clinical review.

9.6.3 Limitations: The Gap Between Wearable Stress and Affect Detection and Real Life

Despite the promising results, generalization must be interpreted with caution. The WESAD dataset was collected under the TSST protocol, which involves acute, time-limited stressors administered in controlled laboratory settings (Schmidt et al., 2018).

In real-world ("in-the-wild") scenarios, stress is often chronic, diffuse, and context-dependent, introducing challenges absent from laboratory conditions:

- **Artifacts and Noise.** Free-living conditions generate complex motion artifacts in PPG signals that standard preprocessing pipelines may fail to remove, degrading performance—particularly for models that depend on clean raw signals (Siirtola, 2019).
- **The Clever Hans Risk.** Models may inadvertently learn contextual proxies (e.g., "being at work") instead of physiological stress, achieving correct predictions for the wrong reasons. XAI-based auditing is the primary safeguard against this failure mode (Theissler et al., 2022; Lundberg & Lee, 2017).
- **Inter-Individual Variability.** Physiological baselines vary substantially across users. Future research should explore transfer learning (FL) and personalization strategies to adapt models dynamically to individual baselines (Gedam & Paul, 2021).

The experimental evaluation was conducted exclusively on the WESAD dataset, which was collected under controlled laboratory conditions using the TSST. Although WESAD is a well-established benchmark in wearable stress detection research, it captures acute, protocol-driven stress scenarios rather than the chronic, subtle, and context-dependent stress patterns commonly observed in real-world environments. Consequently, the generalizability of the proposed models to "in-the-wild" conditions remains limited and requires further validation using longitudinal, ecologically valid datasets.

The TSST protocol intrinsically couples stress induction with task engagement (e.g., public speaking and mental arithmetic), while baseline phases involve passive activities such as reading. This design introduces a potential protocol bias, whereby models—particularly end-to-end architectures—may learn to discriminate task-related motion or behavioral context rather than genuine affective states. The explainability analysis revealed that the LSTM model, in particular, relied heavily on ACC signals, raising concerns about spurious correlations and the well-known "Clever Hans" effect. While feature-based modeling mitigated this risk to some extent, complete disentanglement of physiological stress from task-induced movement cannot be guaranteed.

The sharp performance degradation observed for the LSTM under LOSO validation highlights a critical limitation of deep end-to-end learning in this context. Although the LSTM achieved near-ceiling performance in standard random-split evaluations, its failure to generalize to unseen subjects suggests that it is sensitive to subject-specific temporal patterns and signal baselines. This limitation underscores the importance of subject-independent evaluation protocols and indicates that architectural complexity alone does not ensure robust physiological generalization.

All models evaluated in this study were trained as global classifiers, without individualized baseline calibration. Given the substantial inter-subject variability in autonomic physiology, the absence of personalization likely constrained model performance under realistic deployment conditions. Future work should investigate adaptive or transfer learning (TL) strategies that dynamically adjust decision boundaries to individual physiological baselines.

The use of fixed-length temporal windows (16 seconds and 60 seconds) simplifies model training but may inadequately capture the heterogeneous temporal dynamics of stress responses. Stress-related physiological changes do not necessarily align with rigid segmentation boundaries, and relevant transitions may be partially truncated or diluted. More flexible, event-driven, or multiscale temporal modeling approaches could improve sensitivity to both acute and gradual stress responses.

The physiological signals analyzed in this study were collected using the Empatica E4 device, which offers higher signal quality than many consumer wearables. As a result, model performance may not directly translate to lower-cost devices with noisier sensors, reduced sampling rates, or intermittent signal loss. This limitation highlights the need for robustness testing across heterogeneous hardware platforms.

Partial Explainability of Deep Temporal Models:
While IG provided meaningful insights into the decision-making process of the feature-based MLP, explainability for the LSTM remained inherently more limited due to its complex temporal dependencies. Although local saliency analysis revealed event-driven attention patterns, a complete causal interpretation of internal memory dynamics in recurrent architectures remains an open challenge.

Temporal Window Discrepancy:
A methodological constraint of this comparative study is the differing temporal window sizes employed: 60 seconds for the feature-based MLP and 16 seconds for the LSTM. While the shorter LSTM window was selected to facilitate granular local explainability and reduce computational overhead, it may have inadvertently limited the model's ability to capture slow-moving physiological trends, such as gradual EDA recovery. Consequently, the performance gap observed may partially reflect this temporal disparity rather than solely an architectural deficiency, suggesting that future end-to-end models might benefit from longer observation windows despite the increased computational cost.

9.6.4 Ethical Implications and the Imperative of Transparency

Continuous stress monitoring raises ethical concerns regarding privacy, informed consent, and the potential misuse of affective data. Although explainability mechanisms enhance transparency, they do not fully resolve broader ethical dilemmas associated with emotional surveillance and automated mental health assessment. These considerations must be addressed through interdisciplinary collaboration involving clinicians, ethicists, and regulatory bodies.

This work touches on a core dilemma in medical AI: the trade-off between accuracy and interpretability. There is persistent tension between high-performing black-box models and simpler, more transparent—but potentially less expressive—alternatives (Rudin, 2019; London, 2019). The results and findings demonstrate that this trade-off is not absolute. By incorporating IG, the neural models become auditable, satisfying emerging requirements for algorithmic accountability and regulatory compliance (Arrieta et al., 2020; Sundararajan et al., 2017). This approach aligns with recent FDA guidelines for ML-based medical devices, which emphasize transparency and explainability for both clinicians and end users.

9.7 CONCLUSION: TOWARD TRANSPARENT AND TRUSTWORTHY AFFECTIVE ARTIFICIAL INTELLIGENCE

This investigation addressed the challenge of automated stress detection using wearable sensors, explicitly confronting the trade-off between DL model complexity and the imperative of clinical interpretability. Throughout this study, we demonstrated that the effectiveness of a medical decision-support system does not rely solely on maximizing statistical metrics such as accuracy or F1-score, but on ensuring that the model learns physiologically meaningful phenomena rather than spurious artifacts. The tension between high-precision black-box models and the ethical demand for transparency constituted the central thread of this analysis, aligning with contemporary concerns regarding algorithmic accountability in healthcare (Rudin, 2019; London, 2019).

At the core of this chapter was the question of whether high-performing DL models for wearable stress detection genuinely learn autonomic stress physiology or are predominantly driven by behavioral correlates, such as motion artifacts inherent to wrist-worn devices. The combined experimental evaluation and explainability analysis allow this question to be addressed in a principled and conclusive manner.

9.7.1 Synthesis of Experimental Findings and Hypotheses Closure

Experiments on the WESAD dataset revealed critical nuances in processing biomedical signals. The comparison between Model 1 (LSTM trained on raw data) and Model 2 (MLP with handcrafted features) challenged the widespread assumption that DNNs are universally superior across all evaluation criteria.

Regarding Hypothesis H1, which postulated that the LSTM model would achieve predictive performance comparable to or superior to the feature-based MLP, the results provide only partial support. While LSTM achieved near-ceiling performance under standard random-split validation, this apparent success did not translate to subject-independent conditions. Under LOSO evaluation, the LSTM exhibited a pronounced degradation in sensitivity and robustness, whereas the MLP maintained stable and superior generalization (Recall = 97.1%). Consequently, H1 is not supported under realistic deployment assumptions, indicating that architectural complexity alone does not guarantee physiological generalization in small-scale wearable datasets.

However, these findings should be interpreted specifically within the context of RNNs and the LSTM architecture. While LSTM served as a robust baseline for sequential modeling, the rapid evolution of DL suggests that newer architectures, such as Transformer-based models with self-attention mechanisms, might mitigate some of the generalization issues observed here. Nevertheless, the trade-off remains: the increased complexity of such models challenges the requirement for low-power edge deployment, reaffirming the current value of the lightweight MLP approach for real-time wearable applications.

The robustness of the feature-based approach underscores the continued relevance of domain-informed signal processing. By explicitly modeling electrodermal activity peaks, HRV, and temperature dynamics, the MLP leveraged well-established physiological mechanisms, resulting in a noise-resilient and clinically plausible decision process (Schmidt et al., 2018; Greco et al., 2016).

Conversely, the LSTM architecture demonstrated notable computational efficiency and the capacity to model complex temporal dependencies using a relatively small number of parameters (~31k), making it attractive for edge AI deployment (Hochreiter & Schmidhuber, 1997; Fawaz et al., 2019). These characteristics suggest potential for future applications involving continuous, automated calibration of wearable systems, despite limitations observed in subject-independent evaluation.

9.7.2 Physiological Validation through Explainable Artificial Intelligence

A pivotal contribution of this study lies in the systematic application of XAI. By employing IG, the internal decision logic of the models was audited, transforming abstract numerical representations into verifiable physiological evidence (Sundararajan et al., 2017; Kokhlikyan et al., 2020).

Hypothesis H2, which proposed that both models would assign meaningful relevance to motion-related features, is supported. ACC contributed nonnegligible attribution in both models, reflecting the intrinsic coupling between behavioral activity and physiological stress responses in wearable sensing.

More importantly, Hypothesis H3 is strongly supported. The explainability analysis revealed a fundamental distinction between the two modeling paradigms. The feature-based MLP grounded its decisions primarily in legitimate autonomic markers, including:

- Tachycardia, identified as a primary predictor of stress;
- Peripheral vasoconstriction, reflected by negative temperature slopes, consistent with established sympathetic responses (Gedam & Paul, 2021);
- Electrodermal activity peaks, reliably distinguishing phasic sympathetic activation from tonic baseline levels.

In contrast, LSTM exhibited a disproportionate reliance on ACC signals, indicating a tendency to infer stress from movement rather than from autonomic physiology. This explainability-driven insight provides a mechanistic explanation for the model's poor subject-independent generalization and serves as a cautionary signal to the research community regarding the risks of spurious behavioral learning (Theissler et al., 2022; Lundberg & Lee, 2017).

9.7.3 Future Directions and Clinical Impact

Taken together, these findings demonstrate that explainability is not merely an auxiliary diagnostic tool, but a decisive methodological component for validating wearable stress detection systems. High predictive accuracy under optimistic validation protocols is insufficient; trustworthy affective AI must also demonstrate physiological integrity, robustness across individuals, and transparent decision-making mechanisms.

Future wearable medical devices must therefore evolve beyond simple vital-sign monitoring toward explainable health assistants. The integration of multimodal sensing—combining hemodynamic (BVP), EDA, and thermoregulatory (TEMP) information—proved essential to overcoming the limitations inherent to individual sensors (Bobade & Vani, 2020; Siirtola, 2019).

Future research should explore federated and personalized learning strategies to address inter-individual variability under real-world conditions, beyond controlled laboratory environments. Moreover, adherence to emerging guidelines on algorithmic transparency (Arrieta et al., 2020) will not merely constitute an ethical advantage, but a regulatory requirement for the approval of software as a medical device (SaMD).

Ultimately, this work provides a methodological blueprint for developing AI systems that are not only accurate but also interpretable, auditable, and worthy of clinical and societal trust.

REFERENCES

Arrieta, A. B.; Díaz-Rodríguez, N.; Del Ser, J.; Bennetot, A.; Tabik, S.; Barbado, A.; García, S.; Gil-López, S.; Molina, D.; Benjamins, R.; Chatila, R.; Herrera, F. Explainable artificial intelligence (XAI): Concepts, taxonomies, opportunities and challenges toward responsible AI. *Information Fusion*, v. 58, p. 82–115, 2020.

Bobade, P.; Vani, R. Stress detection with machine learning and deep learning using multimodal physiological data. *Computers in Biology and Medicine*, v. 125, art. 103956, 2020.

Caldas, W. L.; Madeiro, J. P.; Do, V.; Pedrosa, R. C.; Gomes, J. P. P.; Du, W.; Marques, J. A. L. Noise detection and classification in Chagasic ECG signals based on one-dimensional convolutional neural networks. In: Lee, R. (Ed.). *Computer and Information Science*. Cham: Springer, 2023. p. 117–129.

Cavalcante, C. H. L.; Primo, P. E. O.; Sales, C. A. F.; Caldas, W. L.; Silva, J. H. M.; Souza, A. H.; Marinho, E. S.; Pedrosa, R. C.; Madeiro, J. P. V. Sudden cardiac death multiparametric classification system for Chagas heart disease patients based on clinical data and 24-hours ECG monitoring. *Mathematical Biosciences and Engineering*, v. 20, n. 5, p. 9159–9178, 2023.

Fawaz, H. I.; Forestier, G.; Weber, J.; Idoumghar, L.; Muller, P.-A. Deep learning for time series classification: A review. *Data Mining and Knowledge Discovery*, v. 33, n. 4, p. 917–963, 2019.

Fernandes, J. V. M. R.; Alexandria, A. R. D.; Marques, J. A. L.; Assis, D. F. D.; Motta, P. C.; Silva, B. R. D. S. Emotion detection from EEG signals using deep learning models. *Bioengineering*, v. 11, n. 8, art. 782, 2024.

Gedam, S.; Paul, S. Physiological responses to stress and temperature variation: A review. *Biomedical Signal Processing and Control*, v. 68, art. 102689, 2021.

Greco, A.; Valenza, G.; Lanata, A.; Scilingo, E. P.; Citi, L. cvxEDA: A convex optimization approach to electrodermal activity processing. *IEEE Transactions on Biomedical Engineering*, v. 63, n. 4, p. 797–804, 2016.

Hochreiter, S.; Schmidhuber, J. Long short-term memory. *Neural Computation*, v. 9, n. 8, p. 1735–1780, 1997.

Kokhlikyan, N. et al. Captum: A unified and generic model interpretability library for PyTorch. *arXiv preprint*, arXiv:2009.07896, 2020.

London, A. J. Artificial intelligence and black-box medical decisions: Accuracy versus explainability. *Hastings Center Report*, v. 49, n. 1, p. 15–21, 2019.

Lundberg, S. M.; Lee, S.-I. A unified approach to interpreting model predictions. In: *Proceedings of the 31st International Conference on Neural Information Processing Systems*, New York, 4–9 December 2017. Long Beach: NeurIPS, 2017. p. 4765–4774. https://neurips.cc/

Nguyen Van, S.; Marques, J. A. L.; Biala, T. A.; Li, Y. Identification of latent risk clinical attributes for children born under IUGR condition using machine learning techniques. *Computer Methods and Programs in Biomedicine*, v. 200, art. 105842, 2021.

Rodrigues, P. M.; Madeiro, J. P.; Marques, J. A. L. Enhancing health and public health through machine learning: Decision support for smarter choices. *Bioengineering*, v. 10, n. 7, art. 792, 2023.

Rudin, C. Stop explaining black box machine learning models for high stakes decisions and use interpretable models instead. *Nature Machine Intelligence*, v. 1, p. 206–215, 2019.

Schmidt, P.; Reiss, A.; Duerichen, R.; Van Laerhoven, K.; Plötz, T. Introducing WESAD, a multimodal dataset for wearable stress and affect detection. In: *Proceedings of the*

20th ACM International Conference on Multimodal Interaction. Boulder: ACM, 2018. p. 400–408.

Siirtola, P. Continuous stress detection using the sensors of commercial smartwatch. In: *Proceedings of the 2019 ACM International Joint Conference on Pervasive and Ubiquitous Computing*. London: ACM, 2019. p. 1198–1201.

Sundararajan, M.; Taly, A.; Yan, Q. Axiomatic attribution for deep networks. In: *Proceedings of the 34th International Conference on Machine Learning (ICML)*. Sydney: PMLR, v. 70, p. 3319–3328, 2017.

Theissler, A.; Spinnato, F.; Schlegel, U.; Guidotti, R. Explainable AI for time series classification: A review, taxonomy and research directions. *IEEE Access*, v. 10, p. 23979–23997, 2022.

Yan, K.; Li, T.; Marques, J. A. L.; Gao, J.; Fong, S. J. A review on multimodal machine learning in medical diagnostics. *Mathematical Biosciences and Engineering*, v. 20, n. 5, p. 8708–8726, 2023.

Zhao, T.; Gois, F. N. B.; Marques, J. A. L.; Dos Santos Silva, B. R.; Cortez, P.; Jagatheesaperumal, S. K.; Albuquerque, V. H. C. AutoML-based EEG signal analysis in neuro-marketing classification using biclustering method. *Applied Soft Computing*, v. 181, art. 113412, 2025.

10 Photoplethysmography-Driven Human-Computer Interface

Advancement Towards Robust Physiological Control Systems

Piyush Swami

10.1 INTRODUCTION

Human-computer interfaces (HCIs), also called man-machine interfaces (MMIs) or human-machine interfaces (HMIs), aim to establish direct communication pathways between human physiological systems and external devices, enabling control without reliance on conventional neuromuscular output pathways (Wolpaw *et al.*, 2002). Such interfaces are of relevance in rehabilitation engineering, where individuals affected by severe motor impairments such as amyotrophic lateral sclerosis (ALS), brainstem stroke, or spinal cord injury, etc., retain cognitive function but lack voluntary motor control (Birbaumer *et al.*, 2000; Rebsamen *et al.*, 2007). The primary objective of HCI technologies in this context is to exploit residual physiological activity to restore autonomy and improve quality of life.

Over the past three decades, electroencephalography (EEG)-based brain-computer interfaces (BCIs) have dominated this research domain due to their direct association with cortical processes underlying intention, attention, and motor imagery (Pfurtscheller and da Silva, 1999; Wolpaw and Wolpaw, 2012). Despite notable scientific progress, EEG-driven systems continue to face substantial limitations that restrict their translation into real-world applications. These challenges include susceptibility towards noise and motion artifacts (especially with scalp EEG recordings), extensive subject-specific training, high cognitive workload, inter- and intra-subject variability, and dependence on controlled experimental environments (Birbaumer *et al.*, 2000; Wolpaw *et al.*, 2002). Consequently, the robustness and long-term usability of purely brain-driven interfaces remain limited, particularly for deployment in home or clinical settings.

To address these limitations, alternative and complementary physiological signals have been explored, including electrooculography (EOG), electromyography (EMG),

DOI: 10.1201/9781003500445-10

and peripheral biosignals (Kumar and Poole, 2002; Lin *et al.*, 2015). Among these modalities, photoplethysmography (PPG) has traditionally been used as a noninvasive technique for monitoring cardiovascular parameters such as heart rate, blood oxygen saturation, and peripheral blood flow (Allen, 2007). PPG is particularly attractive due to its low cost, minimal setup requirements, and compatibility with wearable and embedded systems. However, until recently, its application in HCI has remained largely unexplored.

Accumulating evidence suggests that PPG signals encode information beyond simple cardiac pulsatility. Peripheral blood volume dynamics measured by PPG are modulated by autonomic nervous system (ANS) activity, vascular tone, and neurogenic mechanisms that are closely linked to central nervous system processes (Iani, Gopher, and Lavie, 2004). Experimental studies have demonstrated that cognitive effort, mental workload, and motor imagery tasks induce measurable peripheral vascular changes, supporting the hypothesis that PPG signals may reflect intentional or cognitive states (Santhosh, Agrawal, and Anand, 2007). These physiological observations provided early motivation for investigating PPG as a potential control signal for assistive interfaces.

Recent large-scale clinical and neuroimaging studies have further strengthened the physiological foundation of this approach by establishing robust heart-brain interactions. Population-based analyses have demonstrated that neurological pathologies, including brain metastases, are associated with altered cardiac outcomes and increased heart-specific mortality, highlighting a clinically relevant brain-heart axis (Safi *et al.*, 2021). Complementing these findings, multiorgan magnetic resonance imaging (MRI) studies have revealed strong phenotypic and genetic associations between cardiac structure and function and brain morphology, white-matter integrity, and functional networks (Zhao *et al.*, 2023). These results confirm that cardiovascular dynamics are closely coupled with central neural processes, independent of traditional vascular risk factors.

Within this evolving neurocardiological framework, PPG can be interpreted as a peripheral manifestation of centrally mediated autonomic and neurovascular regulation. From a human-computer interface perspective, this reframes PPG from a passive monitoring signal to an active biosignal capable of supporting intentional control when processed appropriately. In our earlier work, we demonstrated that task-dependent modulation of PPG signals during motor imagery paradigms could be reliably classified using wavelet-based time-frequency features and probabilistic neural networks (PNNs), achieving low-latency performance suitable for real-time systems (Swami, 2015). These findings suggest that PPG-based interfaces may serve as robust, computationally efficient alternatives or complements to EEG-centric systems.

Compared with conventional BCIs, PPG-driven HCIs offer several practical advantages, including reduced setup complexity, improved user comfort, resilience to electromagnetic interference, and suitability for long-term and home-based deployment. Furthermore, because PPG inherently integrates autonomic responses associated with cognition, emotion, and intention, it provides an additional physiological layer that can enhance robustness and explainability in adaptive control systems.

In this chapter, we revisit and extend our prior PPG-based HCI framework in light of recent advances in biomedical signal processing and heart-brain connectivity research. By integrating time-frequency analysis with probabilistic machine learning techniques (ML), we aim to provide a unified methodological foundation for PPG-driven HCIs. Rather than positioning PPG as a replacement for brain-based approaches, this chapter advocates for its role as a complementary control modality that can enhance reliability, scalability, and physiological relevance in next-generation assistive and rehabilitation technologies.

10.2 PHYSIOLOGICAL BASIS OF PHOTOPLETHYSMOGRAPHY AND HEART-BRAIN COUPLING

PPG is an optical measurement technique that captures volumetric changes in blood within peripheral tissue beds by detecting variations in light absorption or reflection. The PPG waveform is classically composed of a pulsatile (AC) component synchronized with the cardiac cycle and a slowly varying (DC) component influenced by respiration, thermoregulation, endothelial activity, and ANS regulation (Allen, 2007). While the AC component is primarily driven by changes in arterial blood volume, the DC component reflects complex interactions among cardiovascular, neural, and peripheral vascular mechanisms.

10.2.1 Autonomic and Neurogenic Modulation of Photoplethysmogram Signals

Peripheral blood flow is continuously regulated by the ANS, mediated by sympathetic and parasympathetic pathways originating in central autonomic networks distributed across cortical, subcortical, and brainstem structures (Benarroch, 1993). Changes in sympathetic outflow led to vasoconstriction or vasodilation of peripheral vessels, thereby modulating PPG amplitude, waveform morphology, and temporal variability. These autonomically mediated vascular responses are particularly sensitive to cognitive effort, emotional arousal, and mental stress, all of which have been shown to induce measurable changes in peripheral perfusion (Iani, Gopher and Lavie, 2004).

Experimental evidence demonstrates that mental workload and task difficulty lead to peripheral vasoconstriction, resulting in reduced PPG amplitude and altered pulse transit characteristics (Cacioppo *et al.*, 1998). Importantly, such changes occur even in the absence of overt motor activity, highlighting the role of centrally mediated neurogenic control rather than mechanical or metabolic demand. These findings are critical in the context of human-computer interface, as they suggest that intentional mental states can influence PPG signals through top-down neural mechanisms.

10.2.2 Motor Imagery, Cognitive States, and Peripheral Hemodynamics

Motor imagery task is the mental simulation of movement without physical execution, which activates cortical and subcortical motor networks, including the supplementary motor area, premotor cortex, basal ganglia, and cerebellum (Jeannerod, 2001). While motor imagery does not generate muscle contractions, it is accompanied by measurable autonomic responses, including changes in heart rate variability, skin conductance, and peripheral blood flow (Decety *et al.*, 1993). These autonomic correlations provide a physiological pathway through which imagined actions can modulate PPG signals.

Studies investigating peripheral hemodynamics during motor imagery tasks have reported task-specific blood flow changes, supporting the feasibility of decoding intentional states from vascular signals (Santhosh, Agrawal, and Anand, 2007). These findings align with earlier psychophysiological research demonstrating that cognitive and imagery-based tasks elicit distinct autonomic signatures detectable in peripheral biosignals (Critchley, 2005). In this context, PPG serves as a composite signal integrating cardiac rhythm, vascular tone, and neurogenic modulation, making it a promising candidate for intentional control paradigms.

10.2.3 Heart-Brain Axis: Clinical and Imaging Evidence

Beyond experimental psychophysiology, strong evidence for heart-brain coupling has emerged from clinical and population-based studies. Neurocardiology, as an interdisciplinary field, has established that brain pathology can directly influence cardiac function through autonomic dysregulation, neuroinflammatory pathways, and altered baroreflex sensitivity (Thayer and Lane, 2009). Classical observations of myocardial injury following acute cerebral insults laid the foundation for understanding bidirectional brain-heart interactions (Byer, Ashman and Toth, 1947).

More recently, large-scale epidemiological studies have demonstrated that patients with neurological involvement, including brain metastases, exhibit significantly higher rates of heart-specific mortality, independent of traditional cardiovascular risk factors (Safi *et al.*, 2021). These findings provide compelling clinical evidence that central nervous system pathology can adversely affect cardiac outcomes, reinforcing the concept of a functionally integrated heart-brain axis.

Complementing clinical observations, advances in multimodal MRI have enabled the systematic investigation of structural and functional heart-brain relationships. Using population-scale imaging and genetic analyses, Zhao *et al.* (2023) demonstrated strong phenotypic and genetic correlations among cardiac morphology, brain structure, white-matter integrity, and functional connectivity. These associations persisted after adjustment for conventional cardiovascular risk factors, indicating intrinsic neurocardiac coupling rather than secondary vascular effects.

10.2.4 Implications for Photoplethysmography-Based Human-Computer Interfaces

The convergence of autonomic physiology, psychophysiological experimentation, and neuroimaging evidence provides a strong theoretical foundation for using PPG as a control signal in HCIs. Rather than representing a purely peripheral measurement, PPG reflects centrally mediated autonomic and neurovascular processes that are sensitive to cognitive and intentional states. This positions PPG as a physiologically meaningful intermediary between brain activity and external device control.

From a signal-processing perspective, the nonstationary and multiscale nature of PPG waveforms makes them particularly amenable to time-frequency analysis techniques such as discrete wavelet transforms. These methods enable the extraction of features associated with both cardiac dynamics and slower autonomic modulations, facilitating the decoding of task-dependent physiological patterns. When coupled with probabilistic classifiers, such as PNNs, PPG-based systems can achieve rapid inference with minimal training overhead, an essential requirement for real-time and assistive applications.

Importantly, framing PPG within the heart-brain coupling paradigm shifts its role from a surrogate cardiovascular signal to an integrated neurophysiological marker. In the context of hybrid or multimodal interfaces, PPG has the potential to complement brain-centric signals by providing redundancy, enhancing robustness, and improving explainability—particularly in scenarios where EEG signals are noisy, unreliable, or impractical to acquire.

10.3 MATERIALS AND METHODS: PHOTOPLETHYSMOGRAPHY-BASED HUMAN-COMPUTER INTERFACE FRAMEWORK

This section describes the experimental design, signal acquisition protocol, and computational framework used to develop and evaluate a PPG-driven HCI. The methodological choices were guided by two key objectives: (1) to maintain physiological interpretability while capturing task-dependent modulation of PPG signals, and (2) to ensure computational efficiency suitable for low-latency, real-time assistive applications.

10.3.1 Photoplethysmography Signal Acquisition

In this study, PPG signals were acquired from the finger using a commercially available optical sensor integrated with a BIOPAC MP150 data acquisition system at the Indian Institute of Technology – Delhi (IITD). The sensor was placed on the distal phalanx to maximize sensitivity to arterial pulsations and autonomic vascular modulation.

The PPG signal was sampled at 500 Hz to ensure adequate temporal resolution for capturing both cardiac pulsatility and higher-frequency components influenced by autonomic activity. High sampling resolution also allowed robust time-frequency decomposition during later processing stages. All recordings were performed in a seated position in a quiet laboratory setting to minimize motion artifacts and external disturbances.

10.3.2 Participants

Five healthy adult volunteers (mean age 27.2 ± 1.5 years) participated in this study. All participants had normal or corrected-to-normal vision and reported no history of neurological, cardiovascular, or muscular disorders. None of the participants had prior experience with motor imagery or HCI experiments. Informed consent was obtained from all participants prior to data collection, and the experimental protocol was approved by the ethics committee of the Indian Institute of Technology – Delhi (IITD) and the All India Institute of Medical Sciences, New Delhi (AIIMS-D). Although the sample size was intentionally small, reflecting the exploratory nature of the study, prior work in physiological HCI and motor imagery research has demonstrated that pilot-scale experiments are sufficient for validating signal feasibility and algorithmic performance (Pfurtscheller and Neuper, 2001).

10.3.3 Experimental Paradigm

The experimental paradigm was designed to elicit task-dependent autonomic and neurogenic modulation of peripheral blood flow without requiring overt motor execution. Participants were seated approximately 50 cm in front of a 19-inch computer monitor and were instructed to perform the following distinct mental tasks:

1) **Resting state**: Participants were asked to relax and fixate on a red cross displayed at the center of the grey screen.
2) **Motor imagery – push**: Participants were instructed to imagine pushing an object forward using their right hand, without executing any physical movement.
3) **Motor imagery – pull**: Participants were instructed to imagine pulling an object toward themselves using their right hand, again without physical movement.

Each task was presented visually using intuitive pictorial cues to minimize cognitive ambiguity and dominance of other imagery tasks. Instruction displayed for task (1) Resting state is shown in Figure 10.1; task (2) Motor imagery – push is shown in Figure 10.2; task (3) Motor imagery – pull is shown in Figure 10.3. Each of the tasks was executed in blocks of two minutes, with each condition repeated three times in randomized order to reduce sequence bias. External triggers were programmed synchronized in the experimental paradigm with PPG signal acquisition, ensuring precise temporal alignment between task onset and recorded data.

Motor imagery was selected for its well-documented ability to activate motor-related cortical networks and to induce autonomic responses detectable in peripheral biosignals (Jeannerod, 2001; Decety *et al.*, 1993).

10.3.4 Preprocessing

Raw PPG signals were preprocessed to remove noise and baseline drift while preserving physiologically relevant information. A bandpass filter in the range of 0.5–40 Hz was applied to eliminate low-frequency baseline wander associated with respiration and thermoregulation, as well as high-frequency noises, including powerline interference. Baseline correction was subsequently performed to normalize slow DC variations.

The filtered signals were segmented into nonoverlapping windows of ten seconds. This segmentation length was chosen as a compromise between temporal resolution

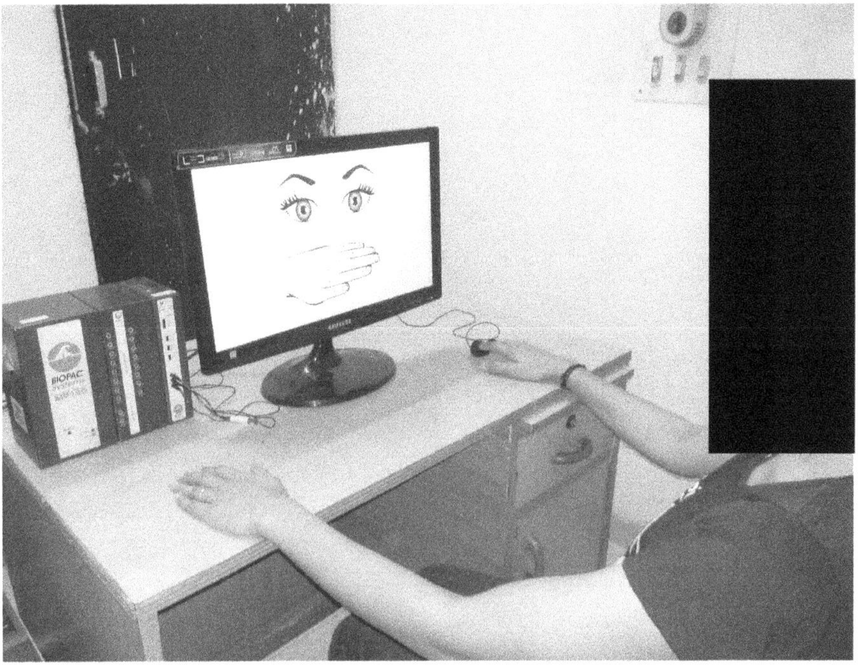

FIGURE 10.1 Instruction Displayed for Task One (i.e., Resting State).

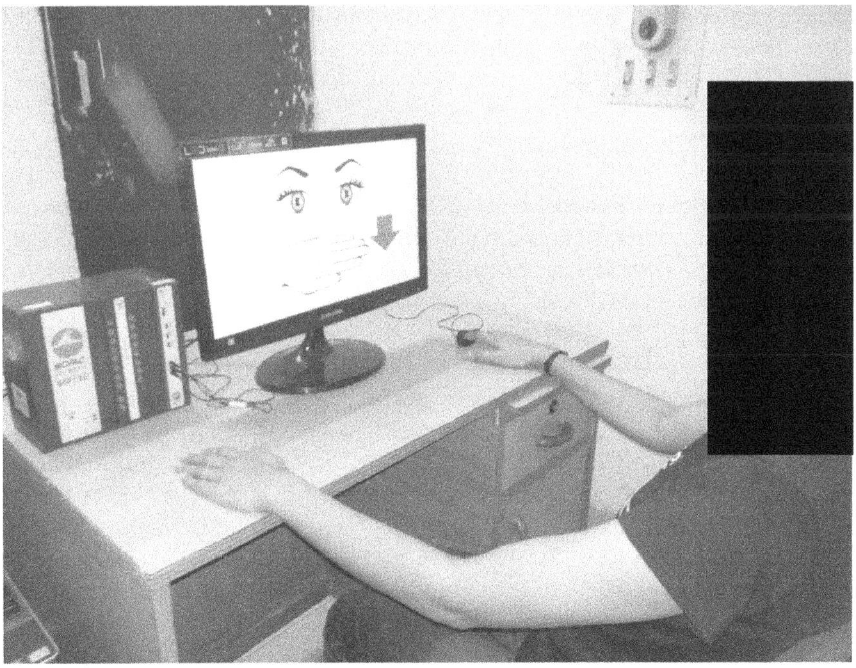

FIGURE 10.2 Instruction Displayed for Task Two (i.e., Motor Imagery – Push).

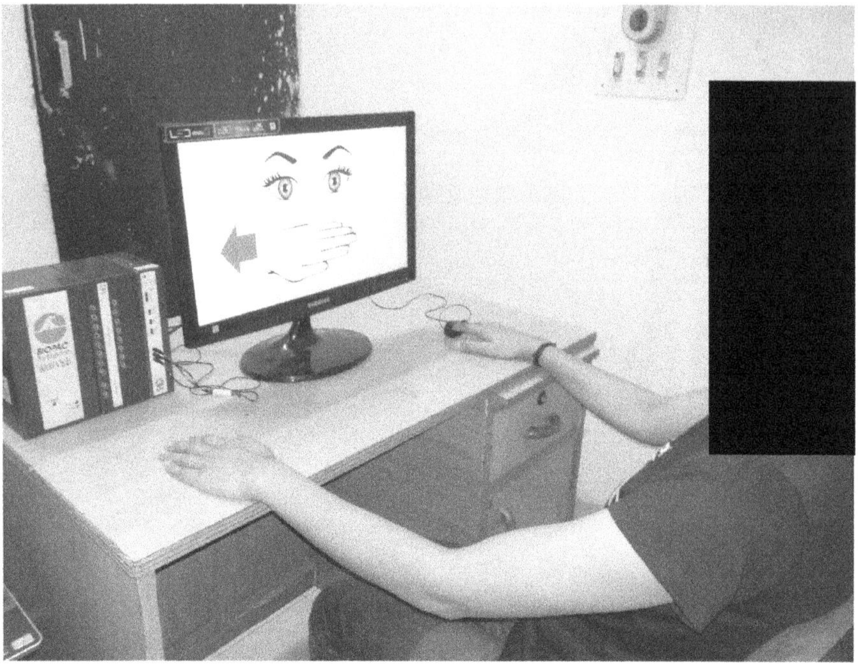

FIGURE 10.3 Instruction Displayed for Task Three (i.e., Motor Imagery – Pull).

and statistical stability, enabling rapid feature extraction while maintaining sufficient information content for classification. Segment-based processing also facilitated real-time implementation by reducing computational load for pattern recognition.

10.3.5 Time-Frequency Decomposition Using Discrete Wavelet Transform

Given the nonstationary nature of PPG signals, time-frequency analysis was employed to capture transient and multiscale physiological dynamics. The Discrete wavelet transform (DWT) was selected for its ability to represent signals at multiple resolutions using localized basis functions (Mallat, 1989).

The PPG signal was decomposed into six levels using recursive filter banks, yielding one approximation coefficient and multiple detail coefficients corresponding to different frequency bands. This hierarchical decomposition allowed the separation of cardiac-related components from slower autonomic modulations. Wavelet-based analysis has been widely used in biomedical signal processing due to its robustness in handling nonlinear and nonstationary signals, such as EEG, ECG, and PPG (Addison, 2005). For the acquired signal with a sampling frequency of 500 Hz, the bandwidth at the input node was 0-250 Hz. Subsequently, the lower and higher bands at the first decomposition level were 0-125 Hz and 125-250 Hz, respectively. The bandwidths at the sixth decomposition levels were 0-3.9 Hz and 3.9-7.81 Hz. From each detail and the last, approximate, statistical, and energy-based features were extracted, including mean, standard deviation, root-mean-square value, entropy, and signal energy. These features collectively captured amplitude variability, complexity, and power distribution across frequency bands, forming the input feature vector for classification.

10.3.6 Classification Using Probabilistic Neural Networks

For classification, a PNN was employed. The PNN is a feedforward classifier based on Bayesian decision theory and Parzen window probability density estimation (Specht, 1990). The network architecture consisted of an input layer, a radial basis hidden layer, and an output decision layer. During training, feature vectors corresponding to each task class were stored as prototypes. During inference, the network estimated the posterior probability of each class and assigned the input segment to the class with the highest likelihood. Unlike gradient-based neural networks, PNNs do not require iterative weight optimization, making them computationally efficient and well-suited for real-time systems.

All analyses were conducted using MATLAB (MathWorks, the United States of America) on a Core i7 processor with 8 GB RAM. Model performance was evaluated using ten-fold cross-validation, with about 70% of the data used for training and the rest for testing. Performance metrics included classification accuracy, sensitivity, specificity, and computation time, reflecting both predictive performance and real-time feasibility.

10.4 RESULTS AND PERFORMANCE EVALUATION

This section presents the classification performance and computational efficiency of the proposed PPG-based human-machine interface framework. Emphasis is placed not only on predictive accuracy but also on latency and physiological plausibility, both of which are critical for real-time assistive applications.

10.4.1 Classification Performance

The proposed system aimed to discriminate among three classes: resting state, imagined push movement, and imagined pull movement. Feature vectors extracted from six-level discrete wavelet decomposition of the PPG signals were used as inputs to the PNN classifier. Performance evaluation was conducted using ten-fold cross-validation to ensure robustness against overfitting. Across all folds, the system achieved a mean classification accuracy of 88%, demonstrating reliable separation between resting and motor imagery states. The average sensitivity and specificity were 91.7% and 83.3%, respectively. These results indicate that the classifier was particularly effective at correctly identifying intentional motor imagery tasks while maintaining reasonable discrimination against false positives. Task-wise analysis revealed that resting state segments were consistently classified with the highest accuracy, reflecting their relatively stable autonomic signature. Imagined push-and-pull tasks exhibited slightly higher variability, consistent with the subtle, internally generated nature of motor imagery-related autonomic modulation (Jeannerod, 2001).

Nevertheless, the classifier distinguished between these two imagery tasks with statistically significant performance, suggesting task-specific modulation of peripheral vascular dynamics.

10.4.2 Computational Efficiency

One of the primary motivations for adopting wavelet-based features and PNNs was to achieve low computational complexity suitable for real-time deployment. The average time to classify a single ten-second segment was approximately nine milliseconds on a standard desktop platform.

This low latency underscores the feasibility of implementing the proposed framework in embedded or wearable systems, where computational resources and power consumption are often constrained. Unlike iterative learning algorithms such as backpropagation-based neural networks, the PNN architecture enabled rapid inference without retraining, making it particularly suitable for adaptive assistive technologies (Specht, 1990).

10.4.3 Physiological Interpretation of Results

The observed classification performance supports the hypothesis that PPG signals carry task-dependent physiological information linked to cognitive and motor imagery states. Although motor imagery does not involve overt muscular activation, it engages cortical motor networks that interact with central autonomic control systems (Decety *et al.*, 1993). These interactions manifest as subtle changes in peripheral vascular tone, which are reflected in PPG waveform morphology and variability.

Wavelet-based decomposition allowed isolation of frequency bands associated with both cardiac pulsatility and slower autonomic modulation. Features derived from lower-frequency components were particularly informative, consistent with prior findings that mental effort and imagery tasks predominantly influence slow vascular responses rather than instantaneous heart rate alone (Iani, Gopher and Lavie, 2004).

The ability to differentiate between push and pull imagery tasks further suggests that distinct intentional states may induce unique autonomic signatures, even in the absence of physical movement. While these differences are subtle compared to EEG-based motor imagery patterns, their consistent detectability highlights the potential of PPG as a complementary control modality.

10.4.4 Comparison with Existing Physiological Human-Computer Interface Approaches

Compared with conventional EEG-based BCIs, the achieved classification accuracy is competitive, given the simplicity of the signal acquisition setup and the absence of extensive subject training. While EEG systems can achieve higher accuracies in controlled laboratory conditions, they often suffer from reduced robustness in real-world environments due to noise sensitivity and user fatigue (Wolpaw and Wolpaw, 2012).

In contrast, the proposed PPG-based system offers advantages in terms of ease of use, portability, and computational efficiency. The results presented here align with prior exploratory studies that demonstrated the feasibility of peripheral biosignals for intentional control, while extending this concept through a structured time-frequency and probabilistic learning framework.

It is important to emphasize that the current results are derived from a small cohort of healthy participants and should be interpreted as a proof-of-concept rather than definitive performance benchmarks. Nonetheless, the consistency of classification outcomes across folds and participants supports the physiological validity of the approach and motivates further investigation in larger and clinical populations.

10.5 DISCUSSION AND IMPLICATIONS FOR ASSISTIVE TECHNOLOGIES

The results presented in this chapter provide compelling evidence that (PPG can serve as a viable physiological control signal for HCIs, particularly in contexts where robustness, low latency, and ease of deployment are critical. Although PPG has historically been confined to cardiovascular monitoring, the findings reinforce the notion that peripheral vascular signals are deeply intertwined with central neural and autonomic processes, thereby enabling indirect access to intentional and cognitive states.

10.5.1 Interpretation of Findings in the Context of Heart-Brain Coupling

The ability to discriminate between resting and motor imagery states, as well as between distinct imagined movements, suggests that PPG captures task-dependent autonomic modulation rather than random physiological fluctuations. This aligns with contemporary models of neurovisceral integration, which posit that cognitive and motor processes engage distributed cortical and subcortical networks that exert top-down influence on autonomic output (Thayer and Lane, 2009). These influences manifest peripherally through changes in vascular tone, heart rate dynamics, and blood volume distribution, mechanisms directly reflected in PPG waveforms.

The observed modulation of PPG during motor imagery tasks supports the growing body of evidence that the heart and brain operate as a coupled dynamical system rather than as independent entities. Clinical studies demonstrating increased heart-specific mortality in patients with neurological involvement further underscore the physiological reality of this coupling (Safi *et al.*, 2021). When viewed through this lens, PPG-based HCIs can be interpreted as exploiting a biologically grounded communication pathway that bridges central intention and peripheral physiology.

10.52 Advantages Over Conventional Brain-Centric Interfaces

Conventional EEG-based BCIs provide direct access to cortical activity but are often limited by poor signal-to-noise ratios, susceptibility to artifacts, and extensive calibration requirements (Wolpaw and Wolpaw, 2012). These limitations are particularly pronounced in nonlaboratory environments and in patient populations with impaired attention or fatigue. In contrast, PPG acquisition is comparatively simple, nonintrusive, and tolerant to moderate environmental disturbances, making it well-suited for long-term and home-based use.

From a computational standpoint, combining wavelet-based feature extraction with PNNs enabled rapid inference without iterative training. This is a significant advantage for assistive systems that must respond in real-time and adapt to gradual physiological changes without requiring repeated recalibration. While EEG-based systems often rely on complex spatial filtering and deep learning (DL) architectures, the proposed PPG framework demonstrates that physiologically informed feature engineering can achieve meaningful performance with modest computational overhead.

10.5.3 Complementary Role of Photoplethysmography in Hybrid Human-Computer Interface Systems

It is important to emphasize that PPG-based interfaces are not proposed as a replacement for brain-based modalities, but rather as a complementary control channel. Hybrid systems that integrate central (EEG) and peripheral (PPG, EMG, EOG) signals have the potential to significantly enhance robustness, redundancy, and user confidence. In such systems, PPG can provide contextual or confirmatory information, helping to disambiguate uncertain EEG decisions or maintain functionality when primary signals degrade.

Recent advances in multimodal physiological sensing and sensor fusion further support this direction. The inherent sensitivity of PPG to autonomic states such as stress, fatigue, and emotional arousal may also enable adaptive interfaces that dynamically adjust control strategies based on user state—an increasingly important consideration in assistive and rehabilitation technologies.

10.5.4 Clinical and Translational Implications

From a clinical perspective, PPG-based HCIs hold particular promise for populations in whom traditional BCIs are difficult to deploy. Patients with advanced neuromuscular disorders, cognitive fatigue, or limited tolerance for head-mounted sensors may benefit from peripheral interfaces that require minimal effort and setup. Furthermore, the widespread availability of PPG sensors in wearable devices opens the door to scalable, low-cost assistive technologies that extend beyond specialized clinical settings.

The demonstrated link between PPG modulation and central neural processes also suggests potential applications beyond assistive control, including monitoring cognitive workload, detecting autonomic dysregulation, and supporting neurorehabilitation protocols. However, translation into clinical practice will require systematic validation in patient populations, longitudinal studies, and integration with user-centered design principles.

10.5.5 Limitations and Future Directions

Several limitations of the present study must be acknowledged. First, the experiments were conducted on a small cohort of healthy participants, and the generalizability of the findings to clinical populations remains to be established. Second, motor imagery tasks were limited to simple push-and-pull paradigms; more complex or valid control tasks may exhibit different physiological signatures. Third, while wavelet-based features provided effective discrimination, alternative feature representations and classifiers—particularly those incorporating adaptive or explainable learning—may further enhance performance.

Future work should focus on validating the proposed framework in populations with motor impairments, exploring hybrid multimodal architectures, and embedding the system into wearable or embedded hardware platforms. Advances in explainable artificial intelligence will also play a key role in improving trust and transparency in physiological control systems.

10.6 CONCLUSION

This chapter revisited and extended the concept of PPG-driven HCIs, positioning PPG not merely as a cardiovascular monitoring signal but as a physiologically meaningful control modality grounded in heart-brain coupling. By integrating insights from biomedical signal processing, autonomic physiology, and neurocardiology, we demonstrated that PPG signals can encode task-dependent modulation associated with motor imagery and cognitive intent. The results of this pilot study confirm that such modulation can be reliably extracted using time-frequency analysis and classified using probabilistic ML techniques with low computational latency.

The proposed framework highlights several practical advantages of PPG-based interfaces, including minimal setup requirements, computational efficiency, and suitability for long-term and real-world deployment. Unlike conventional EEG-based systems, which often require extensive calibration and controlled environments, PPG-driven interfaces offer a complementary and potentially more accessible pathway for physiological control, particularly in assistive and rehabilitation contexts. The demonstrated classification performance, achieved using a small cohort and a lightweight processing pipeline, underscores the feasibility of PPG as a control signal for intentional interface.

From a broader perspective, this work aligns with emerging evidence supporting a tightly coupled heart-brain axis, in which central neural processes exert measurable influence on peripheral cardiovascular dynamics. Leveraging this coupling for human-computer interface opens new avenues for designing hybrid and multimodal systems that combine central and peripheral biosignals to enhance robustness, redundancy, and user confidence. In such systems, PPG may serve as a stabilizing or confirmatory channel, particularly when brain-derived signals are noisy or unreliable.

Several directions for future research emerge from this work. First, systematic validation in clinical populations—such as individuals with spinal cord injury, neurodegenerative disorders, or advanced motor impairments—is essential to assess translational potential. Second, extending the framework to include adaptive and explainable ML models may improve personalization, transparency, and long-term usability. Third, integration of the proposed methodology into wearable or embedded hardware platforms will be a critical step toward real-world deployment. Finally, exploring multimodal fusion strategies that combine PPG with EEG, EMG, or other physiological signals may further enhance performance and resilience in next-generation assistive technologies.

In conclusion, this chapter provides a contemporary and physiologically grounded foundation for PPG-based HCIs. By reframing PPG as an active neurophysiological signal rather than a passive cardiovascular measure, it contributes to the ongoing evolution of robust, scalable, and user-centric assistive technologies.

ACKNOWLEDGEMENTS

The author would like to thank Dr. Sneh Anand, Former Professor and Head of the Centre for Biomedical Engineering, Indian Institute of Technology – Delhi (IITD), and Biomedical Engineering Unit, All India Institute of Medical Sciences – Delhi (AIIMS-D), for the ethical approvals and assistance in data acquisition.

REFERENCES

Addison, P.S. (2005) *Wavelet Transforms and the ECG: A Review*. London: Institute of Physics Publishing.

Allen, J. (2007) 'Photoplethysmography and its application in clinical physiological measurement', *Physiological Measurement*, 28(3), pp. R1–R39.

Benarroch, E.E. (1993) 'The central autonomic network: Functional organization, dysfunction, and perspective', *Mayo Clinic Proceedings*, 68(10), pp. 988–1001.

Birbaumer, N. *et al.* (2000) 'The thought translation device (TTD) for completely paralyzed patients', *IEEE Transactions on Rehabilitation Engineering*, 8(2), pp. 190–193.

Byer, E., Ashman, R. and Toth, L.A. (1947) 'Electrocardiograms with large, upright T waves and long Q–T intervals', *American Heart Journal*, 33(6), pp. 796–806.

Cacioppo, J.T. *et al.* (1998) 'Autonomic, neuroendocrine, and immune responses to psychological stress: The reactivity hypothesis', *Annals of the New York Academy of Sciences*, 840, pp. 664–673.

Critchley, H.D. (2005) 'Neural mechanisms of autonomic, affective, and cognitive integration', *Journal of Comparative Neurology*, 493(1), pp. 154–166.

Decety, J. *et al.* (1993) 'Central activation of autonomic effectors during mental simulation of motor actions in man', *Journal of Physiology*, 461, pp. 549–563.

Iani, C., Gopher, D. and Lavie, P. (2004) 'Effects of task difficulty and invested mental effort on peripheral vasoconstriction', *Psychophysiology*, 41(5), pp. 789–798.

Jeannerod, M. (2001) 'Neural simulation of action: A unifying mechanism for motor cognition', *NeuroImage*, 14(1), pp. S103–S109.

Kumar, D. and Poole, E. (2002) 'Classification of EOG for human–computer interface', in *Proceedings of the IEEE EMBS/BMES Conference*. Houston, TX, pp. 64–67.

Lin, K. *et al.* (2015) 'A hybrid BCI speller based on the combination of EMG envelopes and SSVEP', *Applied Informatics*, 2(1), pp. 1–12.

Mallat, S. (1989) 'A theory for multiresolution signal decomposition: The wavelet representation', *IEEE Transactions on Pattern Analysis and Machine Intelligence*, 11(7), pp. 674–693.

Pfurtscheller, G. and da Silva, F.L. (1999) 'Event-related EEG/MEG synchronization and desynchronization', *Clinical Neurophysiology*, 110(11), pp. 1842–1857.

Pfurtscheller, G. and Neuper, C. (2001) 'Motor imagery and direct brain–computer communication', *Proceedings of the IEEE*, 89(7), pp. 1123–1134.

Rebsamen, B. *et al.* (2007) 'Controlling a wheelchair indoors using thought', *IEEE Intelligent Systems*, 22(2), pp. 18–24.

Safi, M. *et al.* (2021) 'Brain and heart-specific death in cancer patients: A population-based study', *Cancer Medicine*, 10(16), pp. 5739–5747.

Santhosh, J., Agrawal, G., and Anand, S. (2007) 'Peripheral blood flow changes during motor imagery', in *Proceedings of the Latin American Congress on Biomedical Engineering*. Berlin: Springer, pp. 1028–1031.

Specht, D.F. (1990) 'Probabilistic neural networks', *Neural Networks*, 3(1), pp. 109–118.

Swami, P. *et al.* (2015) 'Application of photoplethysmography for man–machine interface: A pilot study', in *Proceedings of the 4th International Conference on Reliability, Infocom Technologies and Optimization*. Noida, India: IEEE, pp. 1–4.

Thayer, J.F. and Lane, R.D. (2009) 'Claude Bernard and the heart–brain connection: Further elaboration of a model of neurovisceral integration', *Neuroscience & Biobehavioral Reviews*, 33(2), pp. 81–88.

Wolpaw, J.R. and Wolpaw, E.W. (2012) *Brain–Computer Interfaces: Principles and Practice*. Oxford: Oxford University Press.

Wolpaw, J.R. *et al.* (2002) 'Brain–computer interfaces for communication and control', *Clinical Neurophysiology*, 113(6), pp. 767–791.

Zhao, B. *et al.* (2023) 'Heart–brain connections: Phenotypic and genetic insights from magnetic resonance images', *Science*, 380(6648), abn6598.

11 Savemom's Wearable Device for the Monitoring of Maternal and Child Health

Shruthi S. Sharma

11.1 INTRODUCTION

Maternal health during pregnancy is crucial for the overall development of the baby during intrauterine life and the postnatal period (Rahayu et al., 2024). Maternal stress, including physical or mental stress during pregnancy, disturbs the normal physiology of the growing fetus, which continues even after birth (Muglia et al., 2022; Naaz & Muneshwar, n.d.). Ensuring a positive experience and timely monitoring of maternal and fetal health throughout pregnancy and childbirth is the key step. However, this cannot be achieved in many situations. According to the United Nations Population Fund (UNFPA), the mortality rate of women during pregnancy is about 800 deaths every day, and most deaths are due to preventable causes (Trends in Maternal Mortality 2000 to 2020, n.d.). In India, accessing the health care facilities during pregnancy and childbirth still remains a major challenge, especially in rural settings (Nair & Panda, 2011). Maternal mortality rate in India, as per the Ministry of Health and Family Welfare, Government of India, is 130 per 100,000 live births, and the neonatal mortality rate is 20 per 1,000, which could be avoided if the proper health monitoring systems are in place (*India Witnesses a Steady Downward Trend in Maternal and Child Mortality towards Achievement of SDG 2030 Targets | Ministry of Health and Family Welfare | GOI*, n.d.; *Saving Mothers, Strengthening Futures*, n.d.). Critical risks go unnoticed until the eighth month of gestation, making timely diagnosis and treatment impossible (Villar et al., 2006). In many cases, a lack of support becomes a stressful experience for the mother and the growing fetus (Coussons-Read, 2013; Kinsella & Monk, 2009). Stressful events during pregnancy or during the postnatal period can have a long-lasting impact on the brain and behavior of the child (Chowdhury et al., 2023; Sharma et al., 2022, Sharma et al., 2024). This scenario can be changed by adopting wearable devices that monitor the physiological parameters of the mother and fetus, such as blood pressure BP, heart rate, sleep, and physical activity, thereby reducing pregnancy-related risks. Wearable devices with mobile applications (App) for household health monitoring have gained popularity globally. Health tech devices, including fitness trackers, heart rate, BP, peripheral oxygen saturation (SpO_2), and

DOI: 10.1201/9781003500445-11

electrocardiogram (ECG), have been adopted in various domains (Dias & Paulo Silva Cunha, 2018). Wearable devices and artificial intelligence (AI)-integrated systems are helping facilitate remote health monitoring between doctors and patients (Ferguson et al., 2021).

11.2 ALLOWEAR BY SAVEMOM

The SaveMom 1,000-day health care program is an AI-enabled wearable technology designed to detect health complications starting from early pregnancy through the child's second birthday, focusing on facilitating a healthy pregnancy, childcare, and a positive parenting experience through technology innovation. SaveMom is offering a suite of products integrated to deliver predictive and personalized maternal care using AI, the Internet of Things (IoT), and wearable technology. This includes 1) AlloWear- A comprehensive wearable monitoring device, AlloBaby- an AI-driven platform for healthy pregnancy and infant care. 2) AlloDoc- AI-powered dashboard for doctors to access real-time patient data and teleconsultations. 3) AlloLab- AI-enabled diagnostics and access to lab reports. 4) AlloGate- AI-powered healthcare data management for hospitals, clinics, and doctors (Kamath & Shrinath, 2022).

11.2.1 AlloWear: Design and Device Architecture

AlloWear is a noninvasive, wearable device for acquiring physiological data from the pregnant mother and the child during the crucial 1,000 days, including pregnancy, childbirth, and the postnatal period. AlloWear is a simple, innovative, and culturally adaptive body-worn device (see Figure 11.1). When worn by the pregnant woman, it provides continuous, real-time tracking of vital physiological parameters and personalized care for maternal and fetal well-being in home-based settings (see Figure 11.2). The physiological parameters captured by the AlloWear device include:

- **Heart rate and heart rate variability (HRV):** Indicators of cardiovascular and autonomic nervous system function.
- **Blood pressure (BP):** Focusses on early detection of pregnancy-induced hypertension.
- **Peripheral oxygen saturation (SpO_2):** Monitoring oxygen saturation in real time indicates respiratory and circulatory sufficiency
- **Skin or body temperature:** changes in body temperature may provide indirect information on infection, inflammation, or metabolic state
- **Physical activity level:** Activity level of the mother, including the step count, distance moved, and calories burnt on a daily basis, can be captured.
- **Sleep tracking:** Restful sleep is key to maternal health. Sleep patterns, including wake time, the duration of rapid eye movement (REM) and non-rapid eye movement–rapid eye movement (NREM) sleep, and the timing of sleep onset, offer insights into the circadian rhythm. The long-term analysis of these parameters enables the proper identification of normal patterns and deviations that may direct future clinical symptoms.

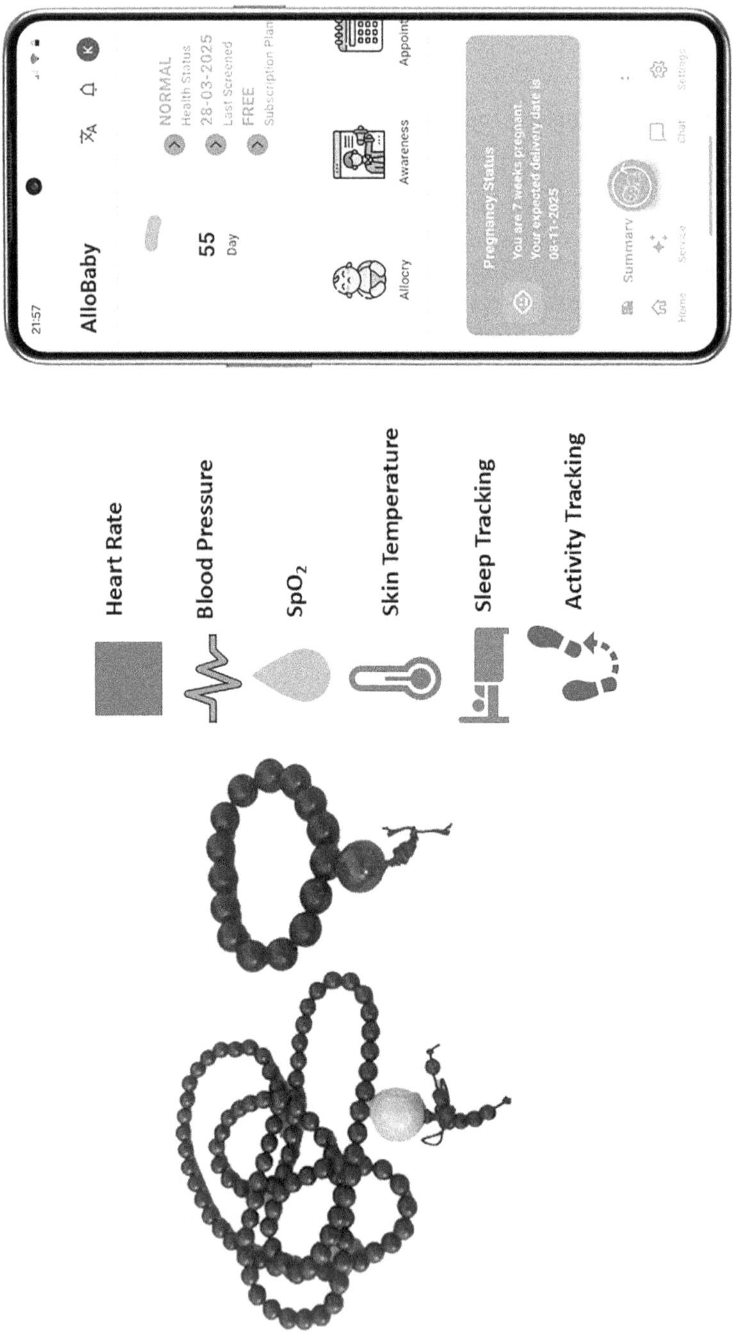

FIGURE 11.1 The AlloWear Wearable Health Monitoring System.

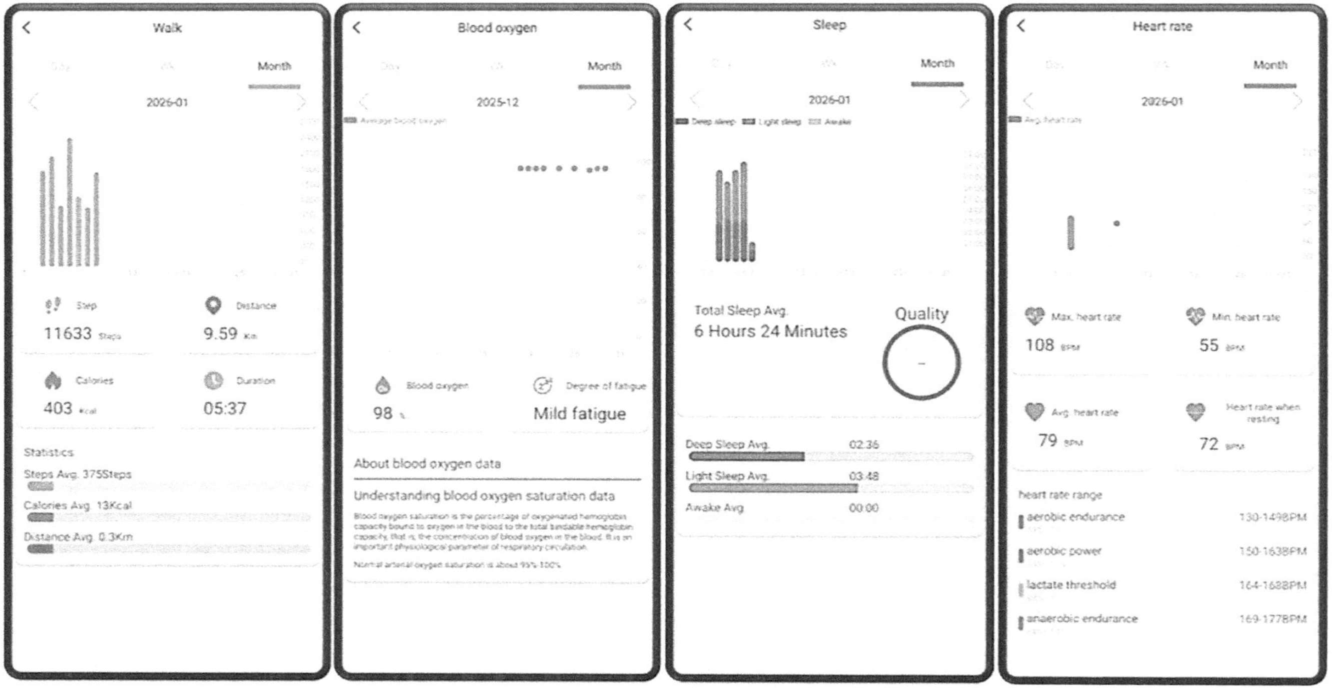

FIGURE 11.2 Screenshot of Physiological Parameters Captured from the AlloWear Device Integrated to the AlloBaby Mobile Application. (Company document.)

The wearable device serves as a data acquisition unit that continuously captures maternal body parameters, and the data is integrated with the AlloBaby App, where fetal heart rate can also be monitored simultaneously. The AlloBaby App proved user-friendly, with an interface for booking appointments with the doctor, tracking pregnancy progress, and receiving personalized insights on daily food/water intake and activity patterns, as well as an automated alert system if abnormal values are detected. It also provides educational content regarding nutrition and wellbeing practices for pregnant women.

11.2.2 From Pregnancy to Baby Care

Although AlloWear is a wearable device designed for pregnant mothers, after delivery, it can be transferred to the baby. It enables continuous monitoring of health parameters during pregnancy and the neonatal period by recording vital signs and transmitting them into an integrated digital system. AlloWear aims to provide continuous, clear, and reliable health information beyond the hospital setting. AlloWear offers a long battery life that typically lasts upto one month, so it can run throughout pregnancy without frequent recharging. After delivery, the same device is transferred to the baby for monitoring, ensuring continuity across both stages using a single wearable.

AlloBaby is useful even after birth and up to the first two years, a crucial period of development. Along with continuous maternal health monitoring, advanced AI-based infant health monitoring is also enabled by cry analysis to detect hunger, discomfort, illness, or distress. The feature provides timely interventions by caregivers and healthcare providers. The baby-crying feature analyzes the baby's specific patterns and needs and delivers appropriate suggestions to caregivers. Crying episodes are longitudinally tracked, and potential trends and concerns are identified, facilitating immediate relief of distress and comforting the baby. Data on trends and patterns in the baby's cry are also shared with pediatricians to support responsive infant care.

AlloDoc is another application integrated with the AlloWear device, designed for clinicians to remotely monitor patients, perform risk analysis, provide timely clinical intervention, and offer immediate virtual consultation. Similarly, the AlloLab App is designed to manage laboratory and diagnostic data, along with AlloWear-derived signals, for comprehensive maternal health monitoring. AlloGate operates as a coordinating layer performing secure data exchange, referrals, and health monitoring across patients, doctors, diagnostic laboratories, and health systems.

11.2.3 Use case 1: Mother Has a Smartphone

When the mother wears the AlloWear device during her daily routine, the health data is automatically stored on the device. As the mother opens the AlloBaby mobile App, AlloWear gets connected to the phone via Bluetooth. With a single sync, all stored data is transferred to the AlloBaby App, and synced data is shared across the system. Doctors can access the data via the AlloDoc App and portal, while nurses and paramedical staff can visualize it via the Savemom App and portal. This allows healthcare service providers to review the mother's health parameters without relying on her phone during hospital visits.

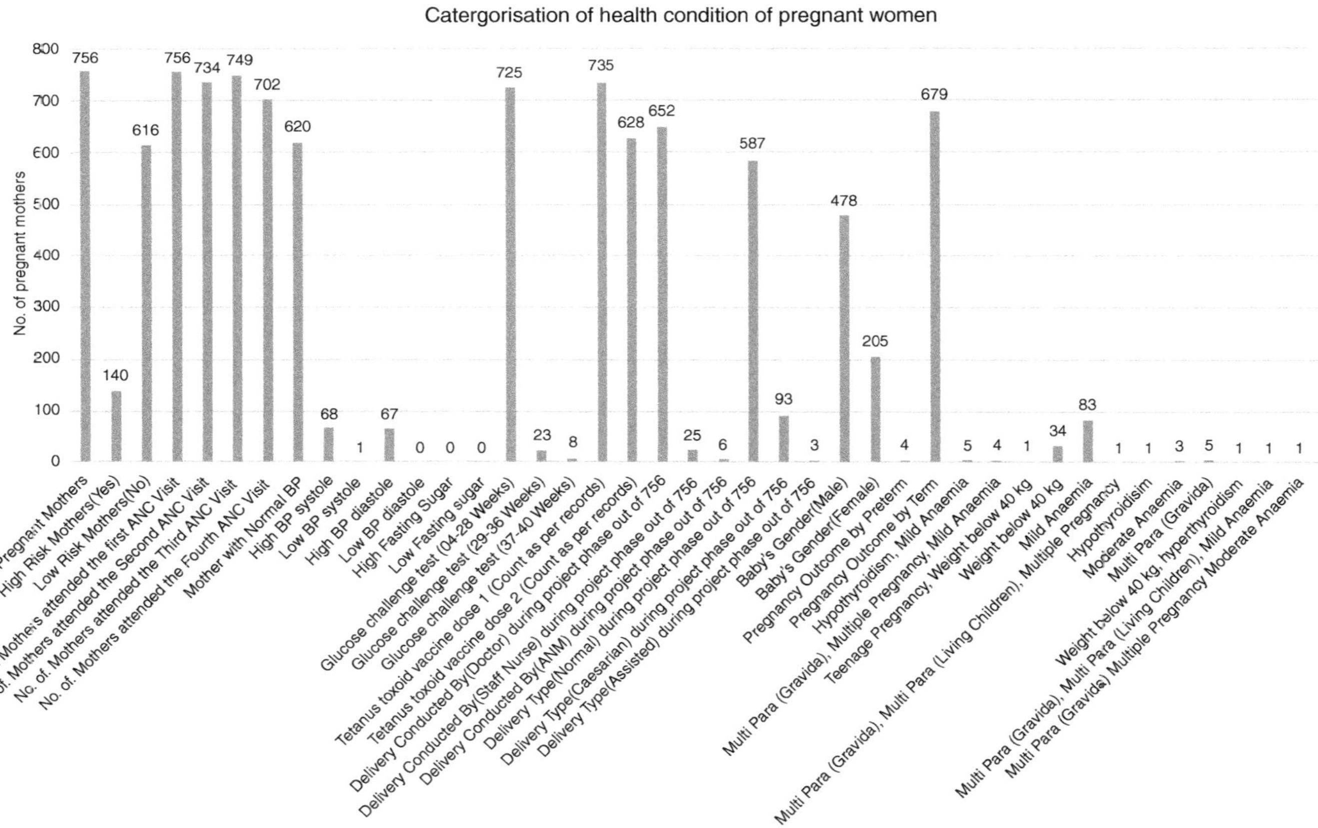

FIGURE 11.3 Categorization of Various Health Conditions During Pregnancy as Per the Data Provided by the Savemom Company.

11.2.4 Use case 2: Mother Does Not Have a Mobile Phone (Rural/Remote settings)

In rural areas, the mother may not have a smartphone or internet access. Even in such a case, AlloWear continues safe data storage on the device. During the routine health checkup, the mother goes near the AlloGate device and enters the registered phone number at the hospital. Face verification and identity confirmation are done by the device. After verification, the AlloWear device is paired to AlloGate, and the stored health data from AlloWear is automatically read and synced. This is done without a smartphone or internet connection from the mother's side. Doctors can easily access the physiological data using the AlloDoc App and portal. Similarly, nurses and health care providers can access health data through the Savemom App and portal. Additionally, doctors and nurses can decide the next course of action after reviewing data collected over several days or weeks, rather than solely relying on a single reading taken during that visit.

11.2.5 Health Data Visibility and Access

- The mother can access the health data through the AlloBaby App. This allows her to monitor health parameters and track changes over time.
- Doctors can obtain the same health data through the AlloDoc App and portal, which helps them review trends between visits.
- Nurses and paramedics can access the data through the Savemom App and portal to support routine health checkups.
- All users view their same synced data from the AlloWear device, ensuring reliable and consistent health information.

11.3 IMPACT OF SAVEMOM WEARABLE TECHNOLOGY

Savemom is an IoT-based healthcare technology designed to provide end-to-end maternal care, ensuring a risk-free pregnancy and reducing maternal mortality and infant mortality rates, especially in remote areas. Savemom, the AI-enabled web application stratifies patients into low- and high-risk categories. The Savemom portal provides a user-friendly interface where both patients and doctors can visualize details of health conditions and diagnostic reports. According to the company's data, Savemom technology solutions has had a large-scale social impact, with more than 36,00,000 pregnant women onboarded, around 2,91,200 home-based antenatal checkups performed, 7,320 high-risk pregnancies monitored, and 36,400 successful deliveries facilitated. Through early risk identification, remote medical support, and data-driven care pathways, the program aims to prevent life-threatening complications and reduce infant mortality. The wearable device is designed with safety in mind, remaining in sleep mode and transmitting data only periodically, thereby minimizing Bluetooth exposure and ensuring safe, long-term use.

Through collaborations with state government agencies, hospitals, and non-government organizations (NGOs), Savemom has implemented its technology in Karnataka, Maharashtra, Tamil Nadu, Kerala, and other places, ensuring healthy

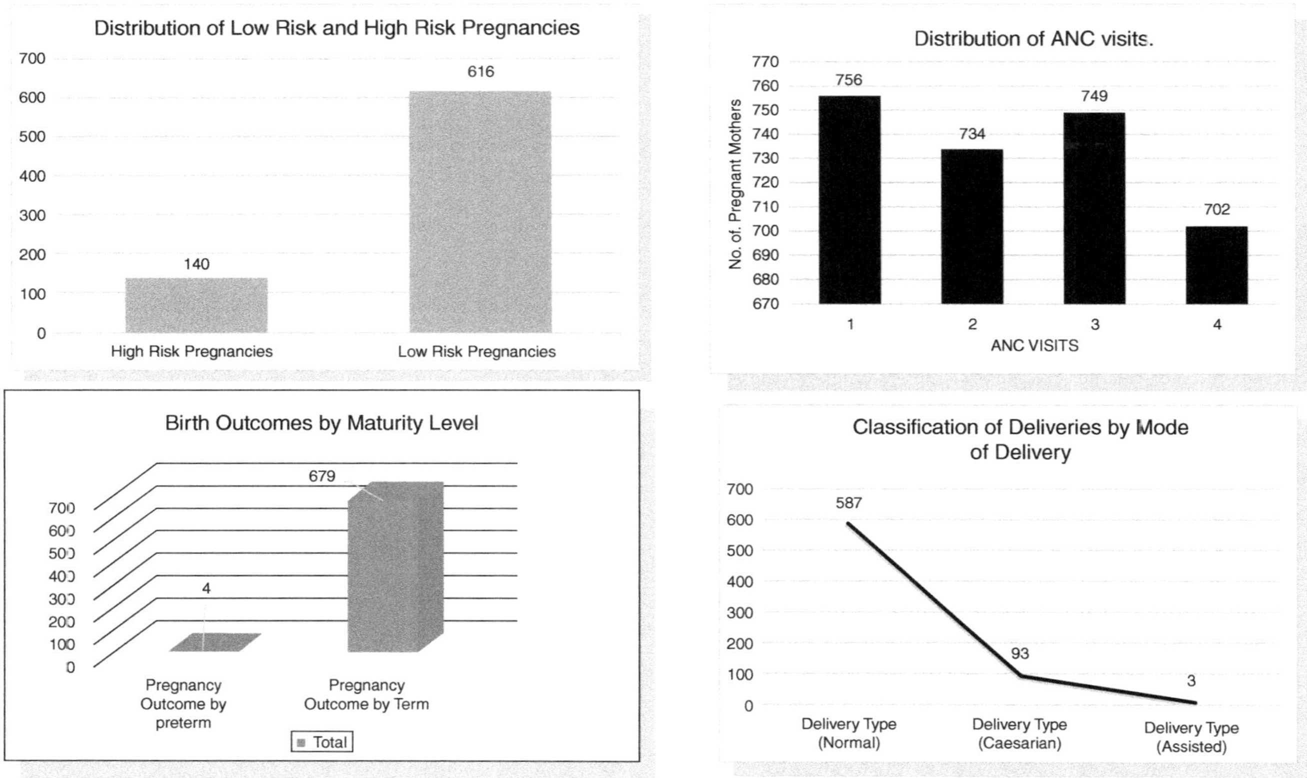

FIGURE 11.4 Maternal Health Data from Savemom, Reproduced with Permission.

pregnancies by collecting vital information and providing timely support. Data collected by the company during November 2024 to March 2025, from Bruhat Bengaluru Mahanagara Palike (BBMP) hospitals on 800 pregnant females. The pregnant women were categorized into high- and low-risk groups based on vital measurements, lab reports, and doctors' diagnoses and treatment decisions, all integrated in the Savemom portal (see Figure 11.3). Antenatal checkups are key during pregnancy, and expectant mothers were notified regarding antenatal care (ANC), which improved risk identification and helped them make informed decisions. According the Savemom, wearable device-driven information and timely interventions increased the chances of normal deliveries and healthy childbirth (see Figure 11.4).

11.4 CONCLUSION

Savemom's AlloWear wearable device and the Allo Apps, together as health monitoring systems, offer valuable advantages in bridging the gaps in maternal and child health by providing continuous, noninvasive monitoring, early risk detection, and remote clinical support through teleconsultation, particularly in low-resource and home-based settings. Savemom's integrated wearable and digital platform facilitates longitudinal tracking across pregnancy and early childhood, enabling timely detection of risk-prone conditions and reducing treatment delays. However, more rigorous lab investigations are needed to ensure the validity of the wearable device and the accuracy of physiological parameter measurements using lab-standard equipment. Further investigation into validation across diverse physiological and environmental contexts, providing deeper insights into various psychophysiological aspects of mental states in naturalistic settings, will have more translational value. Continued technological refinement and clinical and laboratory validation can further strengthen Savemom's potential to prevent and treat pregnancy-related complications and deliver a healthy baby.

REFERENCES

Chowdhury, A., Sharma, S. S., Arjun, B. S., Pandya, H. J., Rao, B. S., & Laxmi, T. R. (2023). Risky decision-taking task: A novel paradigm to assess the risk-taking behaviour in rats predisposed to early-life stress. *Journal of Neuroscience Methods*, *392*, 109864.

Coussons-Read, M. E. (2013). Effects of prenatal stress on pregnancy and human development: Mechanisms and pathways. *Obstetric Medicine*, *6*(2), 52–57. https://doi.org/10.1177/1753495X12473751

Dias, D., & Paulo Silva Cunha, J. (2018). Wearable health devices—vital sign monitoring, systems and technologies. *Sensors (Basel, Switzerland)*, *18*(8), 2414. https://doi.org/10.3390/s18082414

Ferguson, C., Hickman, L. D., Turkmani, S., Breen, P., Gargiulo, G., & Inglis, S. C. (2021). "Wearables only work on patients that wear them": Barriers and facilitators to the adoption of wearable cardiac monitoring technologies. *Cardiovascular Digital Health Journal*, *2*(2), 137–147. https://doi.org/10.1016/j.cvdhj.2021.02.001

India witnesses a steady downward trend in maternal and child mortality towards achievement of SDG 2030 targets | Ministry of Health and Family Welfare | GOI. (n.d.). Press Information Bureau, Government of India. Retrieved January 12, 2026, from www.mohfw.gov.in/?q=en/pressrelease/india-witnesses-steady-downward-trend-maternal-and-child-mortality-towards-achievement

Kamath, R., & Shrinath V. (2022). Savemom: The smart wearable solution for maternal health care. Ivey Publishing. *Savemom | PDF | Maternal Death | Maternal Health.* Scribd. Retrieved January 4, 2026, from www.scribd.com/document/744090225/Savemom

Kinsella, M. T., & Monk, C. (2009). Impact of maternal stress, depression & anxiety on fetal neurobehavioral development. *Clinical Obstetrics and Gynecology*, *52*(3), 425–440. https://doi.org/10.1097/GRF.0b013e3181b52df1

Muglia, L. J., Benhalima, K., Tong, S., & Ozanne, S. (2022). Maternal factors during pregnancy influencing maternal, fetal, and childhood outcomes. *BMC Medicine*, *20*, 418. https://doi.org/10.1186/s12916-022-02632-6

Naaz, A., & Muneshwar, K. N. (n.d.). How maternal nutritional and mental health affects child health during pregnancy: A narrative review. *Cureus*, *15*(11), e48763. https://doi.org/10.7759/cureus.48763

Nair, H., & Panda, R. (2011). Quality of maternal healthcare in India: Has the national rural health mission made a difference? *Journal of Global Health*, *1*(1), 79–86. https://pmc.ncbi.nlm.nih.gov/articles/PMC3484741/

Rahayu, T. P., Suparji, S., Nugroho, H. S. W., Sulikah, S., Setiyani, A., Nuryani, N., & Hanifah, A. N. (2024). Impact of maternal health on child development: Why early intervention is crucial? (a commentary). *PAMJ-One Health*, *15*, 19. https://doi.org/10.11604/pamj-oh.2024.15.19.45308

Saving Mothers, Strengthening Futures. (n.d.). Research unit, Press Information Bureau, Government of India, Ministry of Health and Family Welfare. Retrieved January 12, 2026, from www.pib.gov.in/www.pib.gov.in/Pressreleaseshare.aspx?PRID=2113800

Sharma, S. S., Sasidharan, A., Yoganarasimha, D., & Laxmi, T. R. (2024). Characterization of neuronal oscillations in the prelimbic cortex, nucleus accumbens and CA1 hippocampus during object retrieval task in rats predisposed to early life stress. *Behavioral and Brain Functions*, *20*(1), 34. https://doi.org/10.1186/s12993-024-00255-w

Sharma, S. S., Srinivas Bharath, M. M., Doreswamy, Y., & Laxmi, T. R. (2022). Effects of early life stress during stress hyporesponsive period (SHRP) on anxiety and curiosity in adolescent rats. *Experimental Brain Research*, *240*(4), 1127–1138.

Trends in maternal mortality 2000 to 2020: Estimates by WHO, UNICEF, UNFPA, World Bank Group and UNDESA/Population Division. (n.d.). Retrieved January 12, 2026, from www.who.int/publications/i/item/9789240068759

Villar, J., Carroli, G., Wojdyla, D., Abalos, E., Giordano, D., Ba'aqeel, H., Farnot, U., Bergsjø, P., Bakketeig, L., Lumbiganon, P., Campodónico, L., Al-Mazrou, Y., Lindheimer, M., Kramer, M., & World Health Organization Antenatal Care Trial Research Group. (2006). Preeclampsia, gestational hypertension and intrauterine growth restriction, related or independent conditions? *American Journal of Obstetrics and Gynecology*, *194*(4), 921–931. https://doi.org/10.1016/j.ajog.2005.10.813

12 Sleep Tracking Technologies

Neurophysiological Foundations, Multimodal Wearable Architectures, and Algorithmic Methodologies

Arpita Kulkarni and Jyoti R. Munavalli

12.1 INTRODUCTION

Sleep is a restorative physiological activity at the end of the day. Good sleep quality involves parameters like sleep duration, sleep fragmentation, sleep latency, and early awakenings (Desai et al., 2025). Poor sleep quality adds to sleep debt, which can lead to chronic disorders in the later stages (Desai et al., 2025). Apart from sleep quality, an individual's sleep patterns play an important role in maintaining sleep health. A study was conducted on 59,441 Indian volunteers aged 45 years. The economically poor, people recognized as widows, separated, unemployed, smokers, and women showed higher prevalence of sleep issues (Sreepada et al., 2024). These approaches quantify the relationships among stress levels, occupational and nonoccupational patterns that affect sleep quality, and the occupational and nonoccupational patterns that influence them, in individuals. Sleep patterns are constrained by human recall bias and sociocultural interpretation of the concept of rest. Approximately 50 to 70 million Americans suffer from sleep disorders, and one-third of adults fail to consistently get the recommended amount of uninterrupted sleep necessary for optimal health. Additionally, over 70% of Americans have become more mindful of their physical health since the COVID-19 pandemic. Another study on the impact of internet surfing on adolescents aged 10-20 years found that 85% reported their sleep duration was insufficient, and 50% had trouble falling asleep 3-7 times a week (Srivastava et al., 2025).

Sleep assessment can be conducted qualitatively using questionnaires, including the standard Pittsburgh Sleep Quality Index (PSQI) and the Epworth Sleepiness Scale (ESS). Quantitatively, sleep can be measured using polysomnography (PSG) and actigraphy in a lab environment (Desai et al., 2025). Wearable/nearable devices, integrated with artificial intelligence (AI) systems, help track an individual's long-term

DOI: 10.1201/9781003500445-12

sleep patterns, which can be pivotal for improving sleep routine and overall lifestyle (Nolasco et al., 2025). Wearable devices can collect physiological data passively and accurately to assess preliminary markers of physiological health related to neurological disorders (Sieniawska et al., 2024).

Wearables such as smartwatches, headbands, and biosensors are commonly used to track sleep. They help monitor sleep data continuously in a home-based environment. These devices provide data for analyzing sleep quality disruptions during the night routine for healthcare providers and researchers. The wearables/nearables can detect neurological conditions such as sleep apnea and restless leg syndrome, and monitor sleep duration, which helps in long-term clinical studies. Advancements in the Internet of Things (IoT), AI, and cloud integration help share data and improve diagnostic efficiency (Ghadi et al., 2025).

Deep learning (DL) models are effective in characterizing the sleep data. An attention-based algorithm called AttnSleep was developed and evaluated on models such as DeepSleepNet, sleep electroencephalogram Net (SleepEEGNet), residual network–long short-term memory (ResnetLSTM), multitask convolutional neural network (MultitaskCNN), and sequential sleep network (SeqSleepNet) using three public datasets. It was more efficient, accurate, and scalable than other algorithms (Eldele et al., 2021). There are different modalities for screening sleep data, including physiological and movement-based signal acquisition. Electroencephalogram (EEG) is the gold standard for sleep staging, but it is continuously challenged by noise and reliability issues in wearable formats. PPG is most widely used in wrist-worn devices for tracking heart and respiratory rates, which will help classify sleep. An accelerometer is another modality used for monitoring body movement during sleep, playing a crucial role in the sleep-wake cycle. Other modalities, such as electrocardiogram (ECG), electromyogram (EMG), electrooculogram (EOG), Pressure sensors, radar/sonar, and nasal airflow sensors, provide unique data for reliable sleep classification, with clinical relevance (Imtiaz et al., 2021).

12.2 NEUROPHYSIOLOGICAL FOUNDATIONS OF SLEEP MONITORING

The underlying biological processes of the human body are captured by electrical discharges, which explain the health status of different organs (Joshi et al., 2024). The urgency to develop scalable sleep-tracking technologies stems from the high prevalence of sleep disturbances worldwide. Recent surveys indicate that nearly one-third of adults experience insufficient or poor-quality sleep. Within India, findings from the Longitudinal Ageing Study in India (LASI) reveal a substantial burden of sleep disorders in adults over 45 years, with occupational pressures, psychosocial stress, and irregular schedules driving sleep fragmentation (Hopkins et al., 2023). Persistent restriction of sleep duration is strongly associated with hypertension, obesity, impaired glucose regulation, and cognitive decline (Eldele et al., 2021; Ghadi et al., 2025). Younger urban populations present a different profile: late-night digital exposure, excessive internet use, and erratic routines contribute significantly to reduced sleep efficiency and increased daytime fatigue (Eldele et al., 2021; Markov et al., 2024).

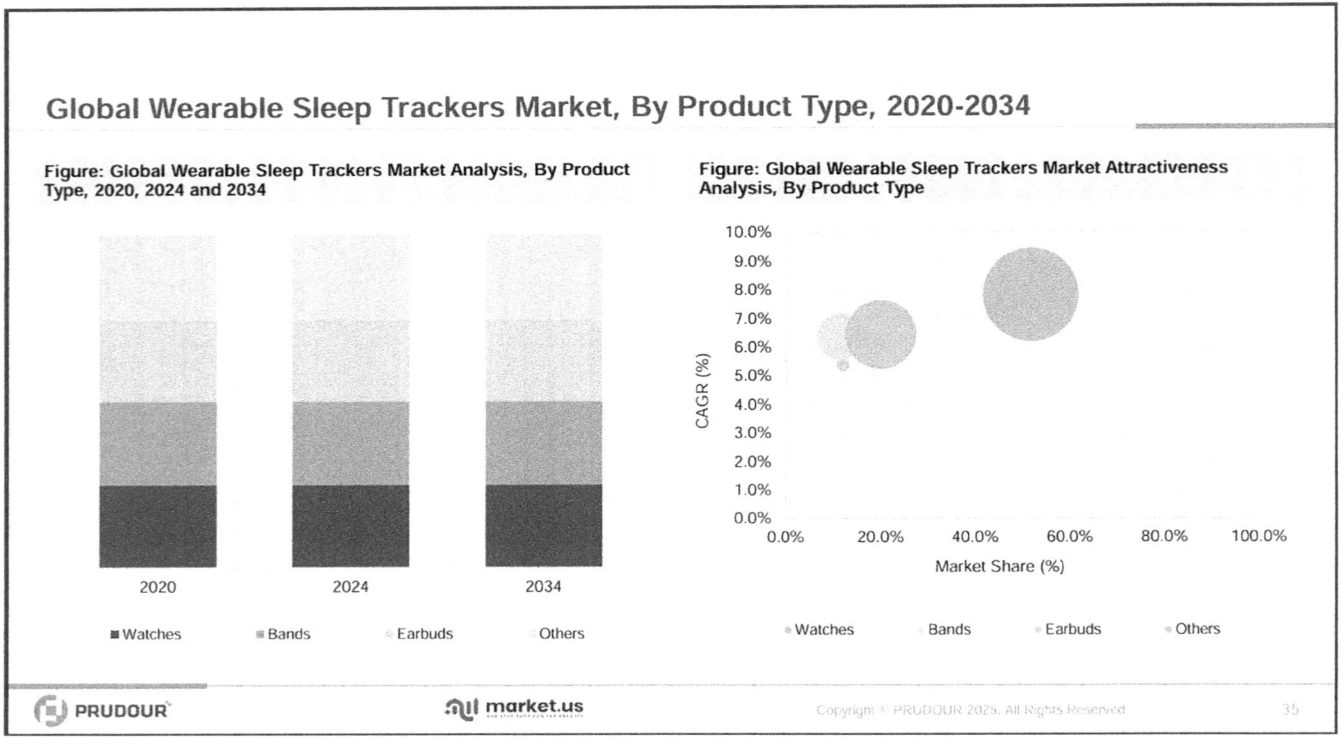

FIGURE 12.1 Global Wearables Sleep Market by Region (2020–2024) (Industry Analysis).

These epidemiological imperatives expose the limitations of existing diagnostic benchmarks. PSG remains the clinical gold standard, capable of simultaneously recording EEG, EOG, EMG, ECG, respiratory effort, airflow, and oxygen saturation, providing unmatched resolution for sleep staging and disorder detection (Pal et al., 2025). However, PSG is costly, labor-intensive, and dependent on laboratory infrastructure, making it unsuitable for large-scale surveillance. Actigraphy, based on wrist-worn accelerometry, offers a practical tool for circadian rhythm and sleep-wake analysis, yet it cannot resolve non-rapid eye movement–rapid eye movement (NREM–REM) transitions or detect respiratory pathologies with sufficient accuracy (Sieniawska et al., 2024). Respiratory polygraphy, while effective for screening obstructive sleep apnea, omits neural signals and lacks staging capacity (Nolasco et al., 2025). Even home-based PSG kits, which demonstrate moderate agreement with laboratory PSG in apnea-hypopnea scoring, remain constrained by cost and compliance barriers (Sreepada et al., 2024). Thus, while current benchmarks set the accuracy standards for sleep evaluation, their lack of scalability across global and Indian contexts has accelerated the search for wearable sensor architectures and algorithmic frameworks as credible alternatives to conventional methods.

12.3 THE EVOLUTION OF MULTIMODAL SLEEP WEARABLE SYSTEMS

Over the last decade, advances in wearable biosensing have transformed sleep monitoring from specialized laboratories to real-world environments. Wrist-worn devices, such as commercial smartwatches and fitness bands, dominate the consumer landscape by integrating accelerometry and photoplethysmography (PPG) to estimate sleep-wake cycles, heart rate variability, and oxygen saturation (Ghadi et al., 2025). Notably, ring-based wearables such as the Oura ring offer improved optical stability due to closer skin contact, resulting in more precise detection of oxygen desaturation events, particularly under free-living conditions (Pretel et al., 2024). Ear-EEG platforms further leverage the anatomical stability of the ear canal to enable extended cortical rhythm monitoring, facilitating the accurate identification of sleep spindles, slow-waves, and REM periods with minimal user discomfort (Ong et al., 2023).

Mattress-embedded sensor arrays use pressure and ballistocardiograph technologies for passive monitoring of respiration and sleep posture, although their reliability decreases in dual-occupant scenarios due to overlapping signals (Kargarandehkordi et al., 2025). At the forefront of sleep technology, hybrid multimodal devices combine EEG, PPG, inertial sensors, and electrodermal activity to achieve PSG-comparable accuracy (Zhao et al., 2022). These innovations are increasingly affordable, supporting deployment in telehealth and resource-limited settings. Increasingly sophisticated algorithms drive the analytical value of such systems. Traditional feature-based machine learning (ML) techniques, including Support Vector Machines (SVM) and random forests (RFs), employ spectral analysis and heart rate variability indices for sleep staging (Röddiger et al., 2022). DL models—utilizing convolutional neural networks (CNNs) and long short-term memory (LSTM) architectures—capture complex temporal and spectral dependencies, often achieving concordance rates above 85% relative to PSG (Sreepada et al., 2024).

Transformer architectures further improve robustness to noise and variability inherent in ambulatory monitoring (Pal et al., 2025). Meanwhile, edge-optimized TinyML frameworks provide real-time inference capabilities directly on microcontrollers, with techniques such as quantization and pruning enabling milliwatt-range energy efficiency suitable for overnight use (Röddiger et al., 2022). To safeguard data privacy, federated learning (FL) architectures enable distributed training across wearable devices without centralizing sensitive biosignals (Khan et al., 2025).

Validation remains central for clinical acceptance. The American Academy of Sleep Medicine (AASM) prescribes epoch-by-epoch comparisons with PSG to evaluate parameters such as accuracy, Cohen's kappa, sensitivity, and specificity (Asgari Mehrabadi et al., 2020). For example, ring-based wearables report approximately 88% sensitivity for hypoxemia events, and both dry-electrode EEG headbands and ear-EEG systems exhibit kappa coefficients of 0.61 0.76, approaching the reliability observed among expert human scorers (Imtiaz, 2021; Ong et al., 2023). Nevertheless, consumer devices often underperform in nuanced stage classification, particularly for REM and N1 stages, with accuracies sometimes falling below 75% (Sreepada et al., 2024; Asgari Mehrabadi et al., 2020). Persistent challenges include motion artifacts, variability in skin contact, and dependence on proprietary, nontransparent algorithms (Sieniawska et al., 2024). Reliability of the longitudinal study is equally critical. Multi-night research underscores the stability of trait-like sleep features, such as spindle density and slow-wave activity, which offer stronger indicators of individual sleep health than single-night assessments (Ong et al., 2023). However, validation must also account for population-specific differences. Devices calibrated in Western populations may not generalize to Eastern cohorts, where lifestyle, environmental factors, and comorbidities alter baseline physiology (Eldele et al., 2021; Hopkins et al., 2023).

Beyond consumer wellness applications, wearable sleep technologies are increasingly relevant to translational medicine. Continuous monitoring of slow-wave and REM sleep provides biomarkers for Alzheimer's disease, Parkinson's disease, and psychiatric disorders (Ghadi et al., 2025). In India, integrating low-cost open-source hardware systems into national digital health initiatives, such as the Ayushman Bharat Digital Mission, provides a pathway to large-scale screening and early intervention (Pretel et al., 2024; Röddiger et al., 2022). Consumer technologies are evolving intobehavioral platforms, using smartphone-linked feedback, gamification, and personalized coaching to promote healthier sleep practices (Kargarandehkordi et al., 2025; Markov et al., 2024). Future trajectories point toward closed-loop systems, in which real-time detection of slow-wave sleep can trigger auditory or electrical stimulation to augment memory consolidation and recovery processes (Shah et al., 2010). Calibration across diverse populations remains necessary, as devices validated on Western cohorts may not generalize well to other groups, given differences in lifestyle, environmental exposure, and comorbidities.

12.3.1 Multimodal Sleep Tracking Architectures

Sleep monitoring technologies have evolved beyond early single-sensor actigraphy, which relied solely on motion detection, toward multimodal wearable platforms capable of acquiring neural, autonomic, and biomechanical signals in parallel. This progression is driven by the recognition that actigraphy, although convenient, lacks the multidimensionality required to reproduce the diagnostic scope of PSG. By integrating complementary channels, multimodal systems aim to approximate PSG while preserving portability and user comfort (Osa-Sanchez et al., 2025; Asgari Mehrabadi et al., 2020; Colman et al., 2025).

Neurologically, electroencephalography (EEG) is the most accurate modality for determining sleep architecture. Recent headband devices use either a dry or semi-dry electrode placed in the frontal or mastoid area, and recordings can be taken over long periods without conductive gel. Such systems can recognize the most important oscillatory measures, including slow waves, spindles, and theta bursts that distinguish between NREM and REM stages (Asgari Mehrabadi et al., 2020; Ohal et al., 2025). Simultaneously, PPG in wristbands, rings, or skin patches is a continuous optical measurement of heart rate variability and peripheral oxygen saturation, and is also helpful for sleep monitoring (Sieniawska et al., 2024; Srivastava et al., 2025). The IMU, which is a unit of inertial measurement, has accelerometers and gyroscopes and transmits information on posture, movement, and arousals during sleep.

EEG acquisition is performed with low-noise analog front-ends (ADS1299), whereas PPG acquisition is performed with optical front-ends (AFE4400). Microcontrollers (ESP32 and nRF52832) process and wirelessly transmit data while ensuring energy efficiency via Bluetooth Low Energy (BLE) interfaces (Röddiger et al., 2022). In research-grade prototypes, raw EEG is usually sampled at ≥250 Hz and PPG at ≥25 Hz. The onboard microSD storage ensures data retention. To sustain overnight recordings, designers use power-optimization strategies such as duty-cycle regulation, low-dropout regulators, and ultra-low-power sleep states.

Ergonomics is an equally critical determinant of user compliance. Prolonged overnight monitoring requires enclosures that are flexible, lightweight, and fabricated from hypoallergenic materials, while surface heating must remain within 2°C of ambient skin temperature to avoid discomfort. Electrode placement must preserve stability without introducing pressure-induced artifacts. Recent advances in textile-based electrodes and flexible biosensors have shown promise in maintaining low impedance while improving long-term wearability (Colman et al., 2025; Imtiaz, 2021). Many studies demonstrate promising solutions but also highlight the limitations of multimodal platforms.

12.4 ELECTROENCEPHALOGRAM SIGNAL PROCESSING

EEG is the most important parameter for sleep research. The EEG wearable, such as a headband, uses dry or semi-dry electrodes. These electrodes are attached to the mastoid or frontal points (Desai et al., 2025). Headband systems such as Dreem and Muse have demonstrated the feasibility of home-based EEG staging that is authentic to laboratory PSG. Cohen's kappa ranges from 0.61 to 0.76, which is similar to the inter-rater consistency of individual traditional clinicians' pre-training (Röddiger et al., 2022; Markov et al., 2024). These observations indicate that consumer EEG headbands are accurate enough to provide stage data that can be longitudinally tracked in consumers, albeit less effectively than PSG in distinguishing REM from N1 (Srivastava et al., 2025). The use of EEG caps and academic and open-hardware software efforts

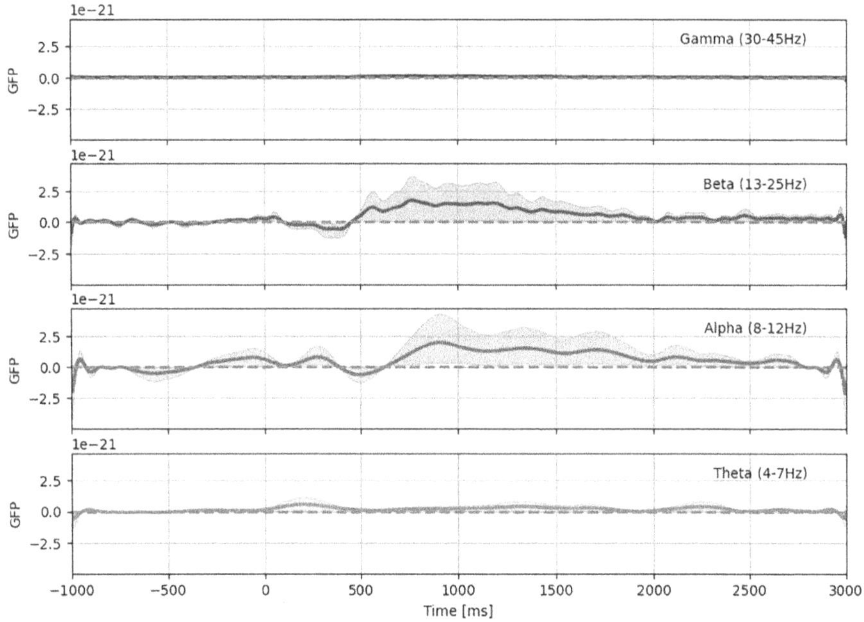

FIGURE 12.2 Frequency Bands Used in Electroencephalogram Signal Processing.

aim to enable community deployment (Asgari Mehrabadi et al., 2020). The systems offer a trade-off between signal quality and affordability by maintaining a modular design. They also do not conflict with algorithm testing and are therefore attractive to researchers in low-resource environments (Pretel et al., 2024).

12.4.1 Ear-Electroencephalogram

On the same principle, electrodes in the ear canal are used with sharp electrodes in which the range lines recorded can be related to the activity of the centers of the recording organ, and the procedure can be done without much discomfort. Unlike headbands, Ear-EEG is smaller and can capture spindles, slow-wave activity, and REM-Related vibrations over an extended period; it does not alter natural sleep posture (Röddiger et al., 2022). As shown, EEG sleep spindles can be well resolved and applied in cognitive investigations and the early diagnosis of neurodegenerative diseases (Markov et al., 2024). Wearable sleep science is anchored in EEG, but translating cortical sensing into ambulatory contexts is nontrivial. Motion-induced artifacts, drifting, and unequal electrode-skin impedance, and sensitivity to hair density all jeopardize signal stability outside controlled labs.

12.4.2 Wellness Rings

Ring form factors improve optical coupling: tighter, more stable finger contact reduces motion noise, and head-to-head analyses report better fidelity for desaturation indices and oxygen desaturation estimation than typical wristbands—useful for community-level screening for sleep-disordered breathing (Asgari Mehrabadi et al., 2020; Khodke et al., 2025). PPG patches, which are adhesive to the skin, are placed on the chest or upper arm to deliver clean data at night (Srivastava et al., 2025). Hence, PPG wearables are helpful for staging sleep and identifying neurodegenerative markers in the early stage. Many devices rely on proprietary pipelines, limiting transparency and reproducibility for clinical translation (Imtiaz, 2021).

12.4.3 Inertial Sensing: Inertial Measurement Units

Accelerometers and gyroscopes quantify gross movement, posture, and transitions in activity, Classic wrist actigraphy showed that, while it cannot reliably separate NREM from REM, it is robust for circadian profiling and sleep-wake estimation over weeks in free-living cohorts. Today, IMUs are essential companions in multimodal systems, providing biomechanical context that helps interpret EEG and PPG streams and reject artifacts during naturalistic movement (Sieniawska et al., 2024).

12.4.4 Smart Textiles

Advances in materials have enabled the integration of conductive fibers and reusable textile electrodes into garments. Such systems can capture thoracic stretch for respiration, ECG via fabric electrodes, and kinematics via embedded IMUs, delivering comfort and adherence in populations that struggle with rigid wearables, notably pediatrics and geriatrics (Imtiaz, 2021).

12.4.5 Mattress-Embedded Sensors

Near-body "ambient" solutions, ballistocardiograph pads, and pressure-sensor arrays under the mattress detect micro-vibrations associated with cardiac cycles, respiration, and large movements. They are unobtrusive and well-suited to longitudinal monitoring, but accuracy can degrade with frequent position changes or bed-sharing, which confounds source separation (Sieniawska, 2024).

12.4.6 Nearables/Environmental and Internet of Things-Based Systems

The wearables will require direct body contact, whereas nearables will use environmental sensors to passively track sleep surrogates.

12.4.7 Radars and Sonars

In addition to radars and sonars, Doppler radar/sonar devices detect chest wall movement and breathing processes without physical contact. They determine respiratory rate and sleep-wake cycles but not staging transitions (Pretel et al., 2024). Radar-based technologies were useful in patients with dermatological conditions or around neonatal monitoring, where skin penetration is not acceptable.

12.4.8 Smart Phones/Mobile devices

Smartphones/Mobile devices with accelerometers and microphones are used to monitor sleep for specialized applications (Mammen et al., 2023). It is based on motion sensors (bed motion) and audio (snoring, breathing) to understand sleep patterns. They are highly accessible, but accuracy is not great, with a strong dependence on location and environmental noise (Sieniawska et al., 2024).

12.4.9 Internet of Things Ecosystems

The emergence of smart-home systems, with multimodal data such as bed sensors, ambient light, noise, and temperature, in a single sleep analytics has boosted sleep tracking in home environments (Eldele et al., 2021). These networks help in capturing the context of the sleep process, including the sleep routine.

12.4.10 Mobile Electroencephalography Devices

There are mobile EEG applications that use adaptive filtering with accelerometers or EOG to dynamically suppress motion-related interference (Asgari Mehrabadi et al., 2020; Röddiger et al., 2022). It is with multi-night wearable monitoring, particularly in ecological contexts tailored to occupational demands, environmental stressors, and lifestyle irregularities (Zhao et al., 2022; Markov et al., 2024).

The success of these platforms is equally due to their computational efficiency. Battery-powered wearable EEG devices cannot rely on resource-intensive laboratory infrastructure; instead, they must execute full signal processing pipelines, including filtering, spectral estimation, and feature extraction, within stringent energy budgets (Khodke et al., 2025; Nolasco et al., 2025). Recent work with low-power microcontrollers such as the ESP32 and nRF52832 demonstrates their ability to support real-time signal processing with acceptable trade-offs between power consumption and staging accuracy (Khodke et al., 2025). These advances enable truly portable systems that sustain overnight monitoring while preserving clinical and research-grade reliability.

Advanced techniques, such as wavelet decomposition for time-frequency localization (Imtiaz, 2021), adaptive artifact suppression for robustness in ambulatory settings (Röddiger et al., 2022), and band-power estimation for staging reliability, can be embedded within TinyML frameworks on these microcontrollers (Nolasco et al., 2025).

12.5 METHODOLOGY

The experimental pipeline for this chapter was developed using a reproducible and transparent framework grounded entirely in open-source ecosystems and publicly available sleep physiology datasets. All analyses were performed on the Sleep-EDF (i.e., European Data Format) Expanded Database, a widely accepted polysomnographic benchmark hosted on PhysioNet (Goldberger et al., 2000). For consistency with modern single-channel sleep staging studies, we used the Sleep-EDF expanded (Age)

Dataset, available via *mne.datasets.sleep_physionet.age.fetch_data*() interface in Data acquisition, synchronization of hypnogram annotations, filtering, and segmentation were performed using MNE-Python, an open-source Python toolbox for processing magnetoencephalography (MEG) and electroencephalography (EEG) data (Gramfort et al., 2013).which contains overnight PSG and matching hypnogram annotations from adult subjects aged 25–101 years (Kemp et al., 2000). All recordings are stored in the EDF/EDF+ standard, designed for interoperability across clinical and research platforms (Kemp et al., 1992; Kemp and Olivan, 2003).

Data acquisition, synchronisation of hypnogram annotations, filtering, and segmentation were executed using MNE-Python, an extensively validated neurophysiology library for EEG/MEG signal processing (Gramfort et al., 2013). From each recording pair (*PSG.edf and *Hypnogram.edf), the EEG derivation Fpz–Cz was selected. This choice reflects the practical constraints of wearable sleep technologies that rely on frontal or mastoid placements using dry or semi-dry electrodes, which have been validated for long-duration home-based monitoring (Pretel et al., 2024; Zhao et al., 2022).

Signals were bandpass-filtered using a zero-phase fourth-order Butterworth filter between 0.5 and 45 Hz to preserve delta, theta, alpha, and beta oscillatory activity, which are known to differentiate sleep stages. Each overnight recording was divided into nonoverlapping 30-second epochs, temporally aligned with the manual stage scoring performed according to Rechtschaffen and Kales (1968). The original labels were consolidated into a five-class framework (Wake, N1, N2, N3, REM), in accordance with current literature conventions. Importantly, no manual artefact rejection was applied; this design explicitly mirrors wearable conditions, in which signal contamination, impedance variability, and motion artefacts are part of the ecosystem. Preserving this noise profile ensures realistic benchmarking of models designed for embedded or edge-computing scenarios (Pretel et al., 2024).

For ML and neural model comparisons, each 30-second epoch was represented in two alternative forms. First, for classical models, we engineered compact spectral descriptors using Welch's periodogram (Welch, 1967). For each epoch, spectral power was integrated across four canonical EEG bands—δ (0.5–4 Hz), θ (4–8 Hz), α (8–13 Hz), and β (13–30 Hz)—yielding a four-dimensional feature vector aligned with resource-efficient computation on wearable microcontrollers (Pretel et al., 2024). Second, for DL architectures, we used the raw bandpass-filtered 30-second EEG epoch as input, enabling the networks to infer temporal-spectral representations directly from the waveform.

Two major families of models were evaluated. Classical ML methods—including RF, K-Nearest Neighbors (KNN), and Gaussian Naïve Bayes—were selected for their computational efficiency and interpretability on embedded systems. DL models included a multiresolution CNN (MRCNN), which uses parallel convolutional kernels to capture both microevents (spindles, K-complexes) and macrostructure (delta waves), as well as a TinyML neural network, a compressed dense architecture optimized for microcontroller deployment using INT8 quantization (Eldele et al., 2021; Pretel et al., 2024). This hybrid comparison reflects the dual trajectory of wearable sleep technology: balancing clinical fidelity (deep models) with on-device feasibility (TinyML and classical models).

The dataset was split into 70% for training and 30% for testing, using stratified sampling to preserve stage distributions. Feature vectors were standardized using z-score normalization, computed exclusively from the training set to avoid leakage. DL models were trained using the Adam optimizer, a batch size of 32, and an early-stopping criterion based on validation loss to mitigate overfitting.

Model performance was evaluated using standard sleep-staging metrics: overall accuracy, per-class precision, recall, F1-score (both macro-averaged and weighted), and five-class confusion matrices. These confusion matrices were essential for interpreting characteristic misclassification patterns—particularly the ambiguity between N1 and wakefulness, and between N2 and REM—stemming from the spectral and microstructural overlap of these stages. The pipeline, therefore, reflects a realistic, clinically relevant evaluation environment consistent with reproducible sleep-staging research in both laboratory and wearable contextsPretel et al., 2024; Zhao et al., 2022).

12.5.1 Feature Extraction

Feature extraction helps transform the clean EEG signal into quantifiable descriptors that capture the neurophysiological hallmarks of sleep stages. Canonical EEG features form the cornerstone of sleep staging, with band-limited spectral power across delta (0.5–4 Hz), theta (4–8 Hz), alpha (8–12 Hz), sigma (12–15 Hz), and beta (15–30 Hz) ranges providing critical markers of stage transitions (Pretel et al., 2024). In addition to these primary frequency anchors, we can measure spindle density and spectral entropy to detect both normal staging and pathological irregularities (Pretel et al., 2024).

Single-channel EEG frameworks, which underpin several wearable systems, often rely on a systematic combination of time-domain and frequency-domain features. Time-domain statistics such as variance, skewness, and kurtosis are routinely extracted to quantify waveform morphology and variability, while frequency-domain descriptors—most notably relative band power and spectral ratios such as δ/β and θ/α—provide discriminative markers that separate NREM from REM epochs (Mammen et al., 2023; Desai et al., 2025).

This balance of precision and resource efficiency ensures that wearable systems can extend rigorous sleep monitoring into ecologically valid, real-world environments, bridging the gap between clinical laboratories and population-scale deployment.

12.5.2 Time-Domain Features

Time-domain measures describe the statistical behavior of the EEG amplitude distribution within a fixed-length epoch (typically 30-second).

Mean Amplitude (μ): Represents the arithmetic average of the EEG samples in an epoch:

$$\mu = \frac{1}{N}\sum_{n=1}^{N} x[n] \tag{1}$$

where x[n] denotes the discrete EEG sample at time index n, and N is the total number of samples in the epoch.

Standard Deviation(σ): Quantifies variability around the mean, reflecting signal dispersion:

$$\sigma = \sqrt{\frac{1}{N-1}\sum \left(x[n]-\mu\right)^2} \tag{2}$$

Skewness: (γ_1): Captures waveform asymmetry and is sensitive to transient shifts in amplitude distribution:

$$\gamma 1 = \frac{\frac{1}{N-1}\sum_{n=1}^{N}\left(x[n]-\mu\right)^2}{\sigma^3} \tag{3}$$

Kurtosis(γ_2): Reflects the "peakedness" of the amplitude distribution, useful for identifying non-Gaussian events such as spindles or K-complexes:

$$\gamma 2 = \frac{\frac{1}{N-1}\sum_{n=1}^{N}\left(x[n]-\mu\right)^4}{\sigma^4} \tag{4}$$

These descriptors have been used effectively in discriminating sleep macro-states due to their sensitivity to amplitude variability (Röddiger et al., 2022; Nolasco et al., 2025b).

12.5.3 Frequency-Domain Features

Spectral characteristics of the EEG are derived from the calculation of the Power Spectral Density (PSD), which is implemented using Welch's method (Mammen et al., 2023; Desai et al., 2025). The spectral composition of the EEG is partitioned into delta (0.5–4 Hz), theta (4–8 Hz), alpha (8–13 Hz), and beta (13–30 Hz) frequency bands (Mammen et al., 2023; Desai et al., 2025).

Relative Band Power (*Prelband*): Relative band power calculates the ratio of signal energy within a specific frequency band to the total spectral energy:

$$P^{relband} = \frac{\sum_{f\,band} P(f)}{\sum_{fmin}^{fmax} P(f)} \tag{5}$$

P(f)= Power Spectral Density (PSD)
fmin, fmax = minimum and maximum frequencies.
This feature highlights stage-specific dominance such as delta in N3 or theta in REM (Mammen et al., 2023; Desaiet al., 2025).

Spectral Edge Frequency (SEF): The Spectral Edge Frequency is the frequency below which a fixed proportion (commonly 95%) of the total spectral power is contained (Desai et al., 2025):

$$\frac{\sum_{f\ band} P(f)}{\sum_{fmin}^{fmax} P(f)} = 0.95 \tag{6}$$

SEF = spectral edge frequency at percentage (e.g., x = 0.95)
P(f) = PSD at frequency
f_{min}, f_{max} = Analysis Bandwidth.

SEF is often used to differentiate wakefulness, lighter NREM stages, and REM, as spectral energy progressively shifts across bands (Eldele et al., 2021).

Spectral Entropy(H): Spectral entropy quantifies the irregularity or unpredictability of spectral distribution. Higher entropy reflects a more uniform spread of power, while lower entropy indicates dominance of specific bands (Zhao et al., 2022; Eldele et al., 2021):

$$H = -\sum_{P=1}^{K} -P_k log \tag{7}$$

Where P_k = normalized spectral power in the kth frequency bin,
K = total number of bins.

This feature has shown strong potential in distinguishing consolidated N3 sleep (low entropy due to delta dominance) from wake and REM (higher entropy with broader spectral distribution (Pretel et al., 2024)

12.5.4 Ratio-Based Features

Theta/Alpha Ratio

$$R\_(\theta/\alpha) = P\_\theta \,/\, P\_\alpha \tag{8}$$

where:

P_θ = Spectral power of theta band (4–8 Hz)
P_α = spectral power of the alpha band (8–13 Hz).

This ratio explains the transitions between drowsiness, light NREM sleep, and REM (Desai et al., 2025; Eldele et al., 2021).

Delta/Beta Ratio

$$R\_(\delta/\beta) = P\_\delta/P\_\beta \tag{9}$$

where:

P_δ = spectral power in the delta band (0.5–4 Hz)
P_β = spectral power in the beta band (13–30 Hz).

This ratio explains the dominance of delta oscillations over higher-frequency beta activity (Mammen et al., 2023).

Using these ratios, wearable EEG systems improve the staging accuracy. By reducing the dependence on power measures, which are affected by electrode impedance, inter-individual variability, or environmental noise.

12.5.5 Signal Preprocessing

Raw PPG signals are sensitive to motion artifacts, ambient illumination, and variations in sensor placement. This necessitates preprocessing prior to feature extraction (Colman et al., 2025). The fourth or sixth-order bandpass filter with a passband of 0.5–4 Hz is used. The filter transfer function is expressed as:

$$H(s) = \frac{w_c^n}{\left(s^2 + \sqrt{2}\ s\, w_c\ + w_c^2\right)^2} \tag{10}$$

W_c^n = cutoff angular frequency,
n = 4 = filter order.

A forward-backward implementation is applied to avoid phase distortion. This ensures that the timing of systolic peaks is preserved for the estimation of heart rate variability (HRV) (Mammen et al., 2023).

12.5.6 Segmentation Strategy

The filtered signal is segmented using a sliding-window approach. The segmentation process is done as:

$$x_k^n = x[n + k.(\frac{N_w}{2})] \quad \mathrm{k} = 0{,}1{,}2 \tag{11}$$

This ensures the temporal data continuity while improving the quality of data segments for ML (Shah et al., 2010).

12.5.7 Heart Rate Variability and Movement Indices

PPG enables the computation of time-domain HRV features, such as RMSSD (i.e., root mean square of successive differences) and SDNN (i.e., standard deviation of normal-to-normal intervals), as well as frequency-domain metrics, such as the LF/HF ratio, which indexes balance (Imtiaz et al., 2021). Complementarily, IMU streams quantify limb movement frequency, immobility bout duration, and posture transitions, all of which contribute to rest-activity profiling during sleep (Srivastava et al., 2025).

12.5.8 Embedded Implementation

The combination of bandpass filtering, overlapping segmentation, and lightweight feature extraction provides a balance between physiological fidelity and computational efficiency. When deployed with an INT8-quantized deep neural network, such pipelines have achieved over 97% accuracy in binary stress classification, while consuming less than 1.6 KB of RAM and 15.7 KB of flash memory—demonstrating the feasibility of TinyML deployment in ultra-low-power wearable devices (Desai et al., 2025; Ortega-Robles et al., 2025).

12.6 ALGORITHMIC METHODOLOGIES USED IN EFFICIENT SLEEP CLASSIFICATION

The experimental evaluation across classical ML, convolutional architectures, and TinyML networks reveals a recurring echo in both clinical and computational sleep research: deep NREM (N3) remains the most separable state, whereas wake and REM stages continue to pose challenges when restricted to single-lead EEG streams. The following paragraphs provide a simulation-grounded, descriptive analysis of each method.

12.6.1 Random Forest

The RF achieved an overall accuracy of 0.67. Its confusion matrix heatmap demonstrated a prominent diagonal for N3, with a recall of 0.91, indicating robust recognition of slow-wave sleep. The model also exhibited moderate success with N2 (recall 0.73). The wake and REM stages are collapsed into N1/N2, reflecting their reliance on band-limited energy in delta and theta waves. This result shows that high delta power creates a clear boundary for N3. The low amplitude of REMs with mixed-frequency spectra remains ambiguous without a temporal context.

12.6.2 K-Nearest Neighbors

KNN also had the same overall accuracy of 0.67, but its profile differed. It had good N3 performance (recall 0.89) and good N2 (recall 0.68). It is worth noting that the REM recall increased to 0.33, which is higher than RF but weak when in the wake (0.09). The heatmap shown above shows denser clustering of REM than of RF, indicating that some REM epochs formed feature-space clusters. This small increase points to the bias of KNN as a proximity-based epochs dominated by δ are closely clustered in N3, and a subgroup of REM epochs dominated by theta may be partially segregated.

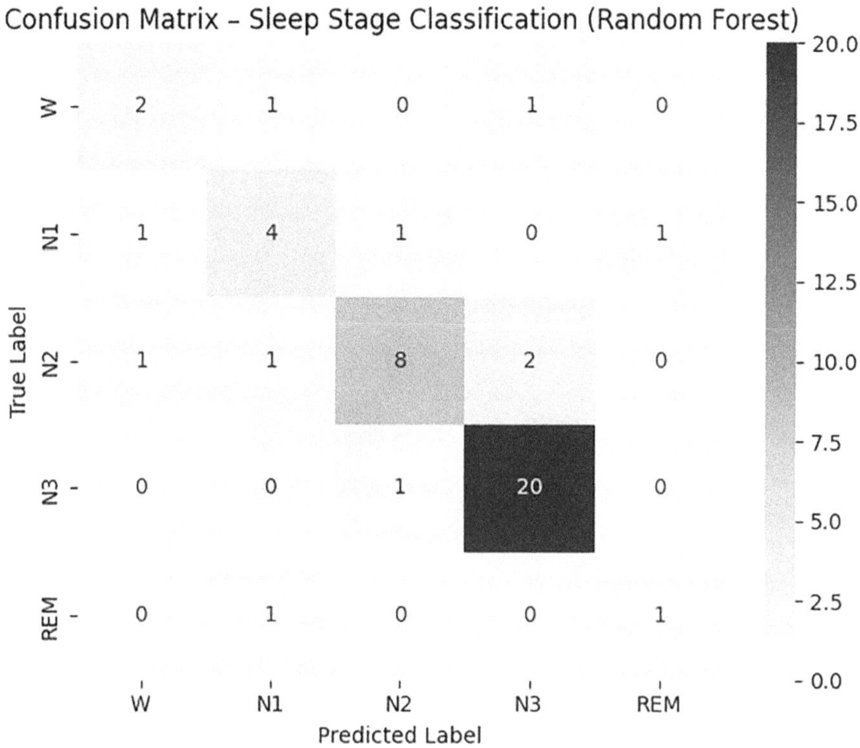

FIGURE 12.3 Confusion Matrix of Random Forest Classification (N=132 Epochs). High N3 Recall (0.91) with Weak REM/Wake Discrimination.

12.6.3 Gaussian Naïve Bayes

GNB is less accurate (0.52) but has high recall (0.78) for good REM. Its confusion matrix shows a strong diagonal of REM. But N1 is not accurately classified. The trade-off is between GNB's dependence on Gaussian class-conditional densities. REM spectrogram variance is quite discrete and forms a separable Gaussian cluster. The intersection of the N1/N2 distributions does not meet the independence assumption. The results of this simulation reflect the usefulness of GNB as a baseline and its inconsistency in clinically significant staging.

12.6.4 Multiresolution Convolutional Neural Networks

MRCNN shows an accuracy of 0.53, with significant gains in N1 (0.78), N2 (0.63), and N3 (0.60). Heatmaps show sharper diagonals for N1 and N2 than for CNN. It can capture both short spindles (σ activity) and longer δ cycles. However, wake and REM are poorly classified. There is a persistent challenge of mixed-frequency states. The simulation improves N1/N2 detection but still falters in REM.

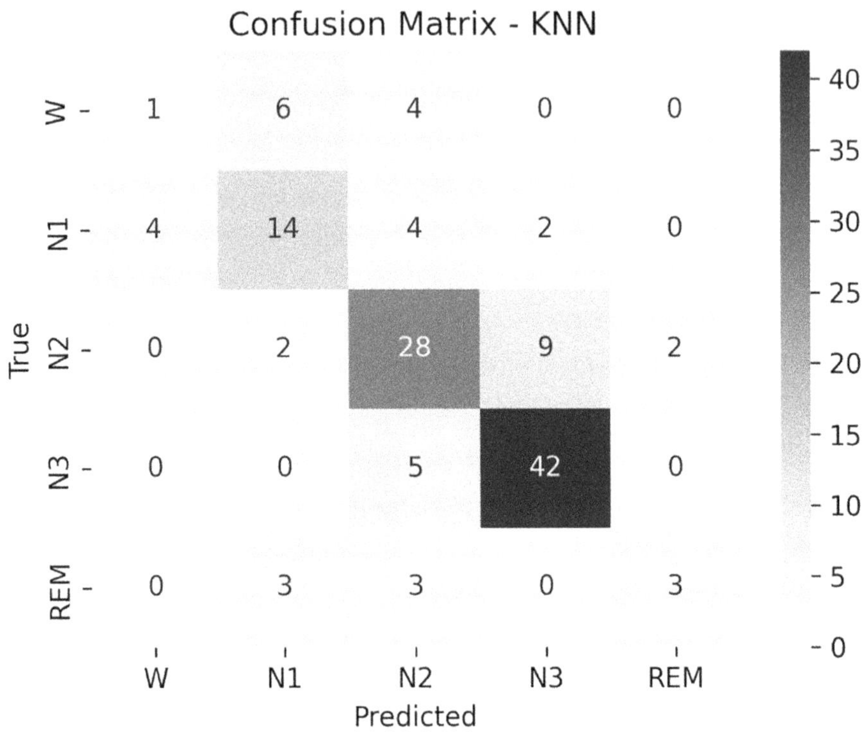

FIGURE 12.4 Confusion Matrix of K-Nearest Neighbor Classification (N=132 Epochs). High N3 Recall (0.91) with Weak REM/Wake Discrimination.

12.6.5 Tiny Machine Learning Convolutional Neural Networks

CNN achieves 36% accuracy and perfect recall (N3 = 1.00). Each slow-wave epoch was correctly detected. But the other stages failed. The confusion matrix heatmap shows saturation along the N3 diagonal, with negligible presence elsewhere.

At extreme compression, the network becomes a δ-detector, prioritizing deep sleep and ignoring the subtleties of light and REM states.

12.6.6 Comparative Analysis

The quantitative analysis of model performance is presented in Table 12.1. It integrates overall accuracy and stage-specific recall. This framework explains the trade-offs between algorithmic fidelity and deployment feasibility in wearable contexts.

All algorithmic families, whether decision-tree-based, generative, or convolutional, demonstrated high reliability in identifying deep slow-wave sleep. This robustness is attributed to the distinctive δ-band activity that characterizes stage N3, which provides an unambiguous spectral marker for classification (Srivastava et al. 2025; Pretel et al., 2024).

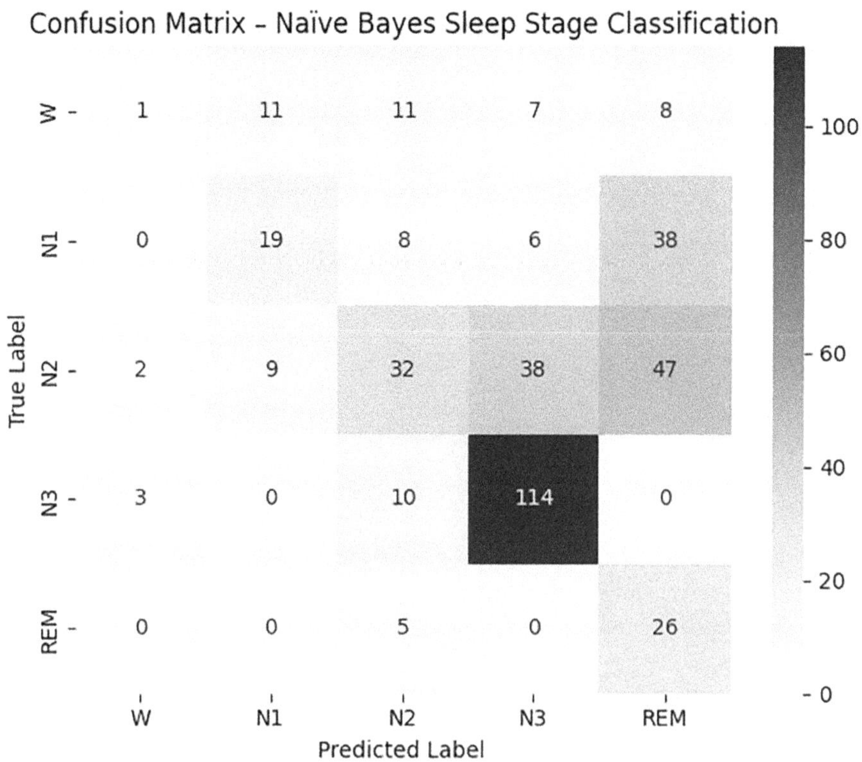

FIGURE 12.5 Confusion Matrix of Gaussian Naive Bayes Classification (N=132 Epochs). High N3 Recall (0.91) with Weak REM/Wake Discrimination.

In contrast, REM sleep presented as the most challenging stage. While the GNB classifier achieved relatively higher recall for REM (0.78), this improvement came at the cost of reduced overall accuracy. Convolutional and TinyML networks underperformed in REM detection, reaffirming that REM classification depends not only on gross band-power but also on microstructural features such as sawtooth waves, phasic bursts, and contextual dynamics that single-lead EEG cannot readily capture (Zhao et al., 2022; Imtiaz, 2021).

Wakefulness was consistently misclassified, with recall values below 0.10 in most approaches. Heatmap analyses revealed wake epochs distributed across N1 and REM categories. This aligns with prior findings that transitions between quiet wake, drowsiness, and light sleep cannot be reliably separated using EEG alone, in the absence of EOG or EMG inputs (Mammen, Zakaria, and Shenoy, 2023).

Taken together, these results validate an important principle: single-lead EEG wearables exhibit strong capability for detecting consolidated deep NREM sleep but require enhanced feature representations and lightweight temporal models to improve the resolution of REM and wake states (Röddiger et al., 2022; Nolasco et al., 2025b).

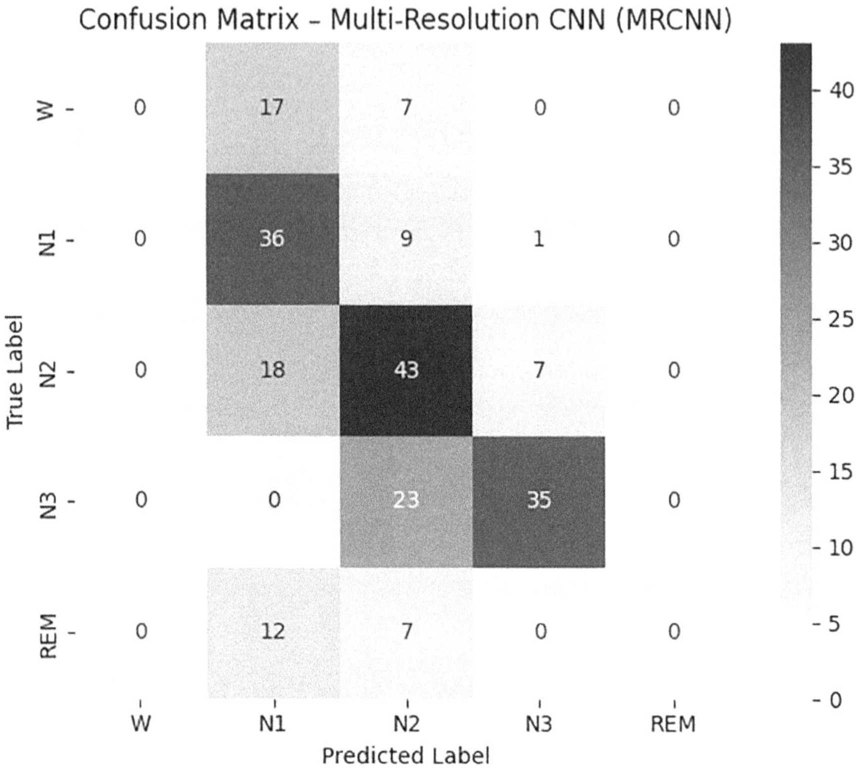

FIGURE 12.6 Confusion Matrix of Multi-Resolution CNN Classification (N=132 Epochs). High N3 Recall (0.6) with Weak REM/Wake Discrimination.

A wearable device is tested simultaneously with full PSG instrumentation, allowing epoch-by-epoch comparison against manually scored hypnograms (Zhao et al., 2022). Performance is not restricted to raw accuracy but assessed using Cohen's κ (a chance-corrected agreement index), sensitivity and specificity (stage-specific detection fidelity), and positive predictive value (PPV) (precision of classification). Empirical studies demonstrate that ear-EEG systems and dry-electrode headbands can achieve κ values in the range of 0.61–0.76, approaching inter-scorer agreement levels and affirming the feasibility of lightweight electrophysiological wearables (Röddiger et al., 2022; Imtiaz, 2021). Yet, REM and N1 continue to exhibit weaker concordance, underscoring the importance of multimodal augmentation with autonomic markers such as HRV and blood oxygen saturation ($SpO_{2)}$ (Pretel et al., 2024).

Beyond a single laboratory night, longitudinal validation in home environments is essential. Sleep is inherently variable across nights, influenced by stress, environment, and lifestyle (Desai et al., 2025; Sreepada et al., 2024). Multi-night validation captures this intra-individual variability, assessing whether trait-like markers, such as spindle density or slow-wave activity, remain stable across conditions (Markov et al., 2024; Ohal et al., 2025). Practical deployment also demands artifact labelling

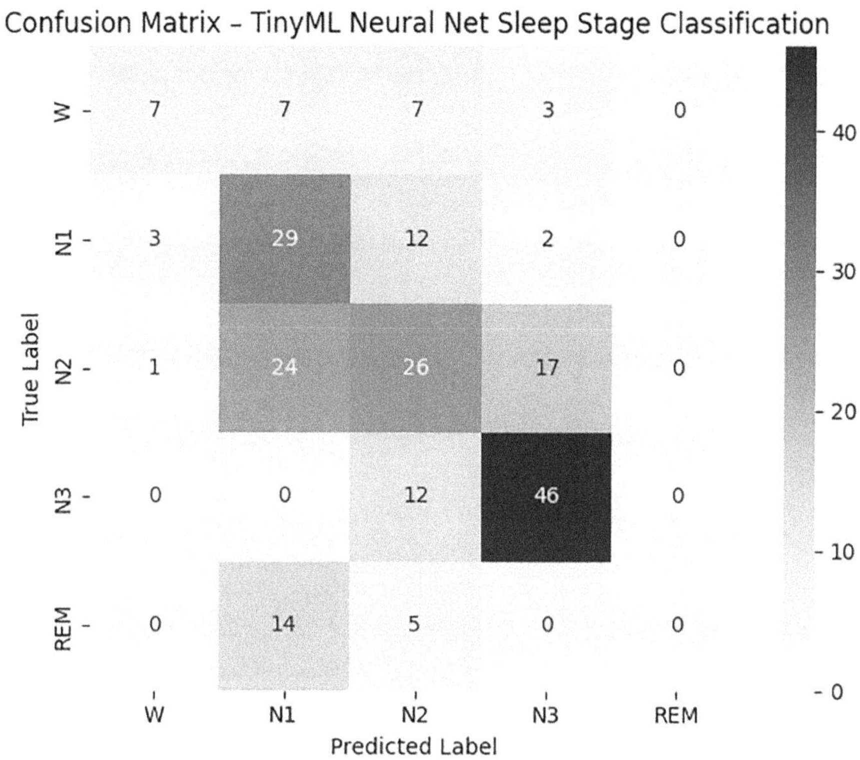

FIGURE 12.7 Confusion Matrix of TinyML CNN Classification (N=132 Epochs). High N3 Recall (1.0) with Weak REM/Wake Discrimination.

TABLE 12.1
Comparative Analysis with Classical Machine Learning Architectures

Model	Overall Accuracy	N3 Recall	N2 Recall	N1 Recall	REM Recall	Wake Recall
Random Forest (RF)	0.67	0.91	0.73	0.57	0.10	0.18
KNN	0.67	0.89	0.68	0.52	0.33	0.09
Naïve Bayes (GNB)	0.52	0.77	0.56	0.41	0.78	0.05
RNN–LSTM	~0.70	0.95	0.30	0.25	0.00	0.00
MRCNN	0.53	0.60	0.63	0.78	0.12	0.00
TinyML CNN	0.36	1.00	0.00	0.00	0.00	0.00

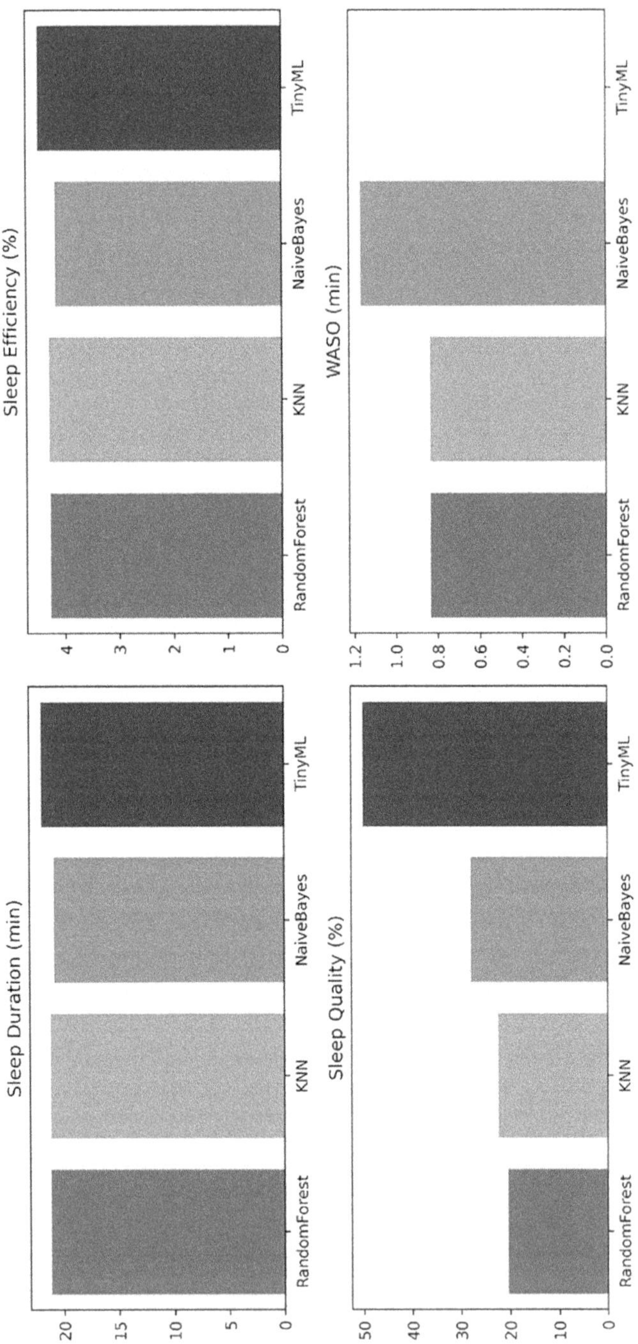

FIGURE 12.8 Comparison of the Confusion Matrices for Different Models.

and quality-control pipelines that automatically flag signal dropout, motion contamination, and electrode detachment. Such embedded quality assurance is crucial for ecological reliability, especially in unsupervised use (Khodke et al., 2025; Imtiaz, 2021). Algorithmic validation further depends on open datasets, which provide the transparency and reproducibility necessary for scientific credibility. The Sleep-EDF Expanded database remains the most widely used benchmark for both classical and DL models (Zhao et al., 2022). Collectively, these repositories form the backbone of reproducible machine learning in sleep staging.

12.7 CONCLUSION

Sleep tracking has moved from a complex lab protocol to a practical ecosystem of wearables and nearables. PSG remains the gold standard, but is expensive, intrusive, and difficult to scale. Actigraphy is easy to deploy but coarse for staging or respiratory events. The gap creates a need for a combination of multimodal autonomic measurements of biochemical signals at home. Headbands and ear-EEGs capture slow waves, spindles, and brief arousals. Wrist and ring devices use PPG to estimate sleep-wake, HRV, and desaturation levels. Small IMUs add context for posture and micro-arousal. Adhesive patches and smart textiles improve skin contact, and comfort are the decisive factors for a multi-night data study. Pipelines in sleep technology that relied on band-power ratios (θ/α, δ/β) now use temporal-spectral models like CNNs, LSTMs, and transformers. FL allows models to be secure and robust in preprocessing, making these systems tolerant of real-world noise. AASM-aligned, epoch-wise comparisons to PSG accuracy, Cohen's κ, and specificity remain the standard measurements. In practice, ring devices are sensitive to desaturation trends; ear-EEG and dry-electrode headbands often reach a range close to inter-scorer agreement. Stage-wise fragility persists for REM and N1 in many consumer stacks. Hardware and ergonomics: enquire whether the "clean" signals that algorithms assume will appear at all. Low-noise front-ends, efficient MCUs, careful power budgeting, and comfort-centric industrial design are not afterthoughts—they are the foundation of trustworthy data.

At the clinic-home interface, wearables support screening for sleep-disordered breathing, phenotyping of insomnia and circadian disruptions, and longitudinal tracking that can flag risk for cognitive decline (e.g., reduced slow-wave sleep, delayed REM latency). The responsible next step is to close-loop intervention, which means detecting, deciding, and acting only where evidence supports benefit (for example, slow-wave-timed stimulation) and with safeguards that respect inter-individual variability. If we hold to these principles, sleep technology will complete its shift from a wellness peripheral to a credible instrument for clinical care and public health.

REFERENCES

Asgari Mehrabadi, M., Azimi, I., Sarhaddi, F., Axelin, A., Niela-Vilén, H., Myllyntausta, S., Stenholm, S., Dutt, N. S., Liljeberg, P., & Rahmani, A. M. (2020). Sleep tracking of a commercially available smart ring and smartwatch against medical-grade actigraphy in everyday settings: Instrument validation study. *JMIR mHealth and uHealth*, 8(10), e20465. https://doi.org/10.2196/20465

Colman, K., Schyvens, A.-M., De Volder, I., Verbraecken, J., Pijpers, A., Viaene, M., Oertel, W., Dijkstra, F., & Crosiers, D. (2025). Novel technologies for REM sleep behavior disorder detection for home screening in Parkinson's disease and related alpha-synucleinopathies. *npj Parkinson's Disease*, 11(1), 196. https://doi.org/10.1038/s41531-025-01032-w

Desai, S. R., Vaidya, R. A., Udipi, S. A., Pinto, L., Kalita, S., Halbe, A., & Iyer, S. (2025). Sleep quality, sleep duration, sleep efficiency, and daytime sleepiness in urban Indian adults. *Indian Journal of Sleep Medicine*, 20(3), 65–70. https://doi.org/10.5005/jp-journals-10069-0164

Eldele, E., Chen, Z., Liu, C., Wu, M., Kwoh, C.-K., Li, X., & Guan, C. (2021). An attention-based deep learning approach for sleep stage classification with single-channel EEG . *IEEE Transactions on Neural Systems and Rehabilitation Engineering*, 29, 809–818. https://doi.org/10.1109/TNSRE.2021.3076234

Ghadi, Y. Y., Shah, S. F. A., Waheed, W., Mazhar, T., Ahmad, W., Saeed, M. M., & Hamam, H. (2025). Integration of wearable technology and artificial intelligence in digital health for remote patient care. *Journal of Cloud Computing*, 14(1), 39. https://doi.org/10.1186/s13677-025-00759-4

Goldberger, A. L., Amaral, L. A. N., Glass, L., Hausdorff, J. M., Ivanov, P. C., Mark, R. G., Mietus, J. E., Moody, G. B., Peng, C.-K., & Stanley, H. E. (2000). PhysioBank, PhysioToolkit, and PhysioNet: Components of a new research resource for complex physiologic signals. *Circulation*, 101(23), e215–e220. https://doi.org/10.1161/01.CIR.101.23.e215

Gramfort, A., Luessi, M., Larson, E., Engemann, D. A., Strohmeier, D., Brodbeck, C., Parkkonen, L., & Hämäläinen, M. S. (2013). MEG and EEG data analysis with MNE-Python. *Frontiers in Neuroscience*, 7, 267. https://doi.org/10.3389/fnins.2013.00267

Hopkins, M., Fil, J., Jones, E. G., & Furber, S. (2023). BitBrain and sparse binary coincidence (SBC) memories: Fast, robust learning and inference for neuromorphic architectures. *Frontiers in Neuroinformatics*, 17, 1125844. https://doi.org/10.3389/fninf.2023.1125844

Imtiaz, S. A. (2021). A systematic review of sensing technologies for wearable sleep staging. *Sensors*, 21(5), 1562. https://doi.org/10.3390/s21051562

Joshi, R. K., Manu, K. M., Hari, R. S., Krishnan, A., Jayachandra, M., Dandinarasaiah, M., & Pandya, H. J. (2024). Automated ABR and MMN extraction using a customized headband for hearing screening. *Biomedical Signal Processing and Control*, 94, 106264. https://doi.org/10.1016/j.bspc.2024.106264

Kargarandehkordi, A., Li, S., Lin, K., Phillips, K. T., Benzo, R. M., & Washington, P. (2025). Fusing wearable biosensors with artificial intelligence for mental health monitoring: A systematic review. *Biosensors*, 15(4), 202. https://doi.org/10.3390/bios15040202

Kemp, B., & Olivan, J. (2003). European data format 'plus' (EDF+), an EDF alike standard format for the exchange of physiological data. *Clinical Neurophysiology*, 114(9), 1755–1761. https://doi.org/10.1016/S1388-

Kemp, B., Värri, A., Rosa, A. C., Nielsen, K. D., & Gade, J. (1992). A simple format for exchange of digitized polygraphic recordings. *Electroencephalography and Clinical Neurophysiology*, 82(5), 391–393. https://doi.org/10.1016/0013-4694(92)90009-7

Khan, H., Kavati, R., Pulkaram, S. S., & Jalooli, A. (2025). End-to-end privacy-aware federated learning for wearable health devices via encrypted aggregation in programmable networks. *Sensors*, 25(22), 7023. https://doi.org/10.3390/s25227023

Khodke, H. E., Kumar, C., Podder, A., Jegadheesan, C., Parmar, D., & Yashan, N. (2025). Artificial neural networks in early diagnosis of neurological disorders: A review of models, biomarkers, and clinical integration. *International Journal of Environmental Science*, 11(11s), 1–15.

Madoń, M., Sieniawska, J., Sieniawska, D., & Kamizela, A. (2024). Neurodegenerative diseases—Characteristics and the role of physical activity. *Quality in Sport*, 17, 53487. https://doi.org/10.12775/QS.2024.17.53487

Mammen, P. M., Zakaria, C., & Shenoy, P. (2023). SleepLess: Personalized sleep monitoring using smartphones and semi-supervised learning. *CSI Transactions on ICT*, 11(4), 203–219. https://doi.org/10.1007/s40012-023-00389-8

Markov, K., Elgendi, M., & Menon, C. (2024). EEG-based headset sleep wearable devices. *npj Biosensing*, 1(1), 12. https://doi.org/10.1038/s44328-024-00013-y

Nolasco, H. R., Vargo, A., & Kise, K. (2025). AI solutionism and digital self-tracking with wearables. *arXiv preprint*. https://doi.org/10.48550/arXiv.2505.15162

Ohal, H. S., & Mantri, S. (2025). A comprehensive analysis of machine learning algorithms for predictive modeling in dementia detection. *Journal of The Institution of Engineers (India): Series B*. https://doi.org/10.1007/s40031-025-01259-4

Ong, J. L., Golkashani, H. A., Ghorbani, S., Wong, K. F., Chee, N. I., Willoughby, A. R., & Chee, M. W. L. (2023). A data-driven approach for choosing a wearable sleep tracker. *medRxiv*, 13, 2023. https://doi.org/10.1101/2023.10.12.23296981

Ortega-Robles, E., Carino-Escobar, R. I., Cantillo-Negrete, J., & Arias-Carrión, O. (2025). Brain–computer interfaces in Parkinson's disease rehabilitation. *Biomimetics*, 10(8), 488. https://doi.org/10.3390/biomimetics10080488

Osa-Sanchez, A., Ramos-Martinez-de-Soria, J., Mendez-Zorrilla, A., Ruiz, I. O., & Garcia-Zapirain, B. (2025). Wearable sensors and artificial intelligence for sleep apnea detection: A systematic review. *Journal of Medical Systems*, 49(1), 66. https://doi.org/10.1007/s10916-025-02199-8

Pal, A., Saini, L. K., Basu, A., Kachhawaha, G., Kundu, K., & Gupta, R. (2025). Research on sleep disorders in patients with mental illness: A review of Indian studies. *Indian Journal of Psychiatry*, 67(5), 469–481. https://doi.org/10.4103/indianjpsychiatry.indianjpsychiatry_110_25

Pravin, A., Nanda, A. M., Yadav, S., Shekhar, A., & Srivastava, M. (2025). Impact of internet surfing on sleep quality: A study of young adolescents. *Indian Journal of Sleep Medicine*, 20(3), 74–77. https://doi.org/10.5005/jp-journals-10069-0160

Pretel, M. R., Vidal, V., Kienigiel, D., Forcato, C., & Ramele, R. (2024). A low-cost and open-hardware portable 3-electrode sleep monitoring device. *HardwareX*, 19, e00553. https://doi.org/10.1016/j.ohx.2024.e00553

Rechtschaffen, A., & Kales, A. (1968). *Manual for sleep staging*. U.S. Government Printing Office.

Röddiger, T., King, T., Roodt, D. R., Clarke, C., & Beigl, M. (2022). OpenEarable: Open hardware earable sensing platform. In *Proceedings of the 2022 ACM International Joint Conference on Pervasive and Ubiquitous Computing* (pp. 246–251). ACM. https://doi.org/10.1145/3544793.3563415

Shah, N., Bang, A., & Bhagat, A. (2010). Indian research on sleep disorders. *Indian Journal of Psychiatry*, 52(Suppl 1), S255–S259. https://doi.org/10.4103/0019-5545.69242

Sreepada, S. S. V. S., Halder, P., Amudhamozhi, K. S., Soni, V., Sharma, H., & Rathor, S. (2024). Prevalence of sleep disorders and association with occupations among Indian adults aged ≥45 years: LASI study. *Journal of Family Medicine and Primary Care*, 13(10), 4208–4216. https://doi.org/10.4103/jfmpc.jfmpc_167_24

Welch, P. (1967). The use of the fast Fourier transform for the estimation of power spectra. *IEEE Transactions on Audio and Electroacoustics*, 15(2), 70–73.

Zhao, S., Long, F., Wei, X., Ni, X., Wang, H., & Wei, B. (2022). Evaluation of a single-channel EEG-based sleep staging algorithm. *International Journal of Environmental Research and Public Health*, 19(5), 2845. https://doi.org/10.3390/ijerph19052845

Index

For Product Safety Concerns and Information please contact our EU
representative GPSR@taylorandfrancis.com
Taylor & Francis Verlag GmbH, Kaufingerstraße 24, 80331 München, Germany

www.ingramcontent.com/pod-product-compliance
Ingram Content Group UK Ltd.
Pitfield, Milton Keynes, MK11 3LW, UK
UKHW021957220926
475880UK00003B/100
* 9 7 8 1 0 3 2 7 9 6 5 4 3 *